Neurologic
Rehabilitation

Neurologic Rehabilitation

A Guide to Diagnosis, Prognosis, and Treatment Planning

Edited by

Virginia M. Mills, MS, PT, CCM, Lic. NHA
President
Community Rehabilitation Care, Inc.
Newton, Massachusetts;
Neurorehabilitation Associates of New England
Wellesley, Massachusetts

John W. Cassidy, MD
Baylor College of Medicine;
Neurobehavioral Healthcare Systems
Houston, Texas

Douglas I. Katz, MD
Assistant Professor, Neurology
Boston University School of Medicine
Boston, Massachusetts;
Director
Neurorehabilitation Programs
Braintree Hospital Rehabilitation Network
Braintree, Massachusetts

b

Blackwell
Science

Blackwell Science

Editorial offices:

Commerce Place, 350 Main Street, Malden,
  Massachusetts 02148, USA
Osney Mead, Oxford OX2 0E1, England
25 John Street, London WC1N 2BL, England
23 Ainslie Place, Edinburgh EH3 6AJ, Scotland
54 University Street, Carlton, Victoria 3053,
  Australia

Other Editorial offices:

Blackwell Wissenschafts-Verlag GmbH
  Kurfürstendamm 57, 10707 Berlin, Germany
Blackwell Science KK, MG Kodenmacho Building,
  7-10 Kodenmacho Nihombashi, Chuo-ku,
  Tokyo 104, Japan

Distributors:

USA
Blackwell Science, Inc.
Commerce Place
350 Main Street
Malden, Massachusetts 02148
(Telephone orders: 800-215-1000 or 617-388-8250;
fax orders: 617-388-8270)

Canada
Copp Clark, Ltd.
200 Adelaide St. West, 3rd Floor
Toronto, Ontario
Canada, M5H 1W7
(Telephone orders: 416-597-1616 or 800-815-9417;
fax orders: 416-597-1617)

Australia
Blackwell Science Pty, Ltd.
54 University Street
Carlton, Victoria 3053
(Telephone orders: 03-9347-0300;
fax orders: 03-9349-3016)

Outside North America and Australia
Blackwell Science, Ltd.
c/o Marston Book Services, Ltd.
P.O. Box 269
Abingdon
Oxon OX14 4YN
England
(Telephone orders: 44-01235-465500;
fax orders: 44-01235-465555)

The Blackwell Science logo is a trade mark of Blackwell Science Ltd., registered at the United Kingdom Trade Marks Registry

Acquisitions: Chris Davis
Development: Karin Commeret
Production: Irene Herlihy
Manufacturing: Lisa Flanagan
Typeset by Best-set Typesetter Ltd., Hong Kong

Printed and bound by Braun-Brumfield, Inc.

© 1997 by Virginia M. Mills, John W. Cassidy, and
Douglas I. Katz
Printed in the United States of America

97 98 99 00 5 4 3 2 1

Library of Congress Cataloging-in-Publication Data

Neurologic rehabilitation: a guide to diagnosis,
  prognosis, and treatment planning / edited by
  Virginia M. Mills, John W. Cassidy, Douglas I.
  Katz.
       p.   cm.
    Includes bibliographical references and index.
    ISBN 0-86542-514-0
    1. Nervous system—Diseases—Patients—
Rehabilitation.   I. Mills, Virginia M.
II. Cassidy, John W.   III. Katz, Douglas I.
    [DNLM: 1. Nervous System Diseases—
rehabilitation.   WL 140 N4918   1997]
RC350.4.N47   1997
616.8'043—dc21
DNLM/DLC
for Library of Congress   97-24813
                                                CIP

To Michael P. Alexander, MD, our mentor and friend

Contents

Contributors

Michael P. Alexander, MD
Associate Professor of Neurology
Boston University School of Medicine;
Research Scientist
Memory Disorders Research Center
Boston VA Medical Center
Boston, Massachusetts

David Bachman, MD
Associate Professor of Neurology and Psychiatry
Division of Behavioral Neurology
Medical University of South Carolina
Charleston, South Carolina

John W. Cassidy, MD
Baylor College of Medicine;
Neurobehavioral Healthcare Systems
Houston, Texas

Mark D'Esposito, MD
Assistant Professor
Cognitive Neurology Section
Department of Neurology
University of Pennsylvania School of Medicine
Philadelphia, Pennsylvania

Ann Gillespie, MBA, CTRS
Chief Operating Officer
Community Rehabilitation Care, Inc.
Newton and Medford, Massachusetts

Kathy Joy, PT, MBA
Clinical Supervisor
Balance and Gait Disorders Program
Braintree Hospital
Braintree, Massachusetts

Douglas I. Katz, MD
Assistant Professor, Neurology
Boston University School of Medicine
Boston, Massachusetts;
Director
Neurorehabilitation Programs
Braintree Hospital Rehabilitation Network
Braintree, Massachusetts

Jeffrey S. Kixmiller, PhD
Research Psychologist
Memory Disorders Research Center, Boston VA Medical Center;
Assistant Clinical Professor in Neurology
Boston University School of Medicine
Boston, Massachusetts;
Neuropsychologist
Community Rehabilitation Care, Inc.
Newton and Medford, Massachusetts

Virginia M. Mills, MS, PT, CCM, Lic. NHA
President
Community Rehabilitation Care, Inc.
Newton and Medford, Massachusetts;
Neurorehabilitation Associates of New England
Wellesley, Massachusetts

Susan Pierson, MD, PT
Director, Neurology and Neurorehabilitation
Heather Hill Hospital Health and Care Center
Chardon, Ohio

Eileen Wusteney, MS, PT
Consultant
Private Practice
Elihu White Nursing Rehabilitation Center
Braintree, Massachusetts

Foreword

The ultimate goal of every health care professional and, indeed, the true objective of medical research is to maximize the quality of life of the individual patient. Rehabilitation should be the context where this intent is most fully achieved. In practice, unfortunately, this is not always the case.

The editors of this book, Virginia Mills, John Cassidy, and Douglas Katz, respond to this challenge in neurologic rehabilitation in several ways. First, and in my opinion, most important, they present a conceptual approach to rehabilitation that they label the "neurologic rehabilitation model." This model is a consistent, unifying theme in the various chapters of this text. Second, they have assembled contributors with extensive experience in the field. Third, the structure of the book and the chapters themselves are not overly ambitious. In the first half of the book, they limit themselves to presenting the model and its application in common neurologic disorders. The second half illustrates how the model is used to treat specific deficits, such as disorders of memory and balance. Fourth, the method of presentation makes the book easy to read and a handy reference. Tables are appropriately used to summarize the main points in a chapter, and case studies present practical examples of the approach.

While the entire work should be read to understand the model and its applications fully, certain lessons deserve highlighting. The primary one is that accurate diagnosis and understanding of a disorder's natural history provide the only hope of generating a sensible rehabilitation plan. This demands a diagnosis that precisely delineates the neuropathophysiologic basis of disability in each patient and accounts for important factors, such as age, that affect outcome. This dynamic approach must be extended to prognosis that is grounded by the natural history of the disorder under consideration. While the model is labeled a "neurologic rehabilitation model," it is a focused approach to rehabilitation that takes into consideration the total person as well as the disease process.

Neurologic rehabilitation practitioners from many disciplines will benefit from reading this book. Students using it as a text will build a foundation that can support evolving rehabilitation practices; seasoned professionals will find the approach a refreshing change of perspective. As such, even if the sole benefit of the volume is a change in rehabilitation philosophy, it will have served an important purpose for all of us.

Donald T. Stuss, PhD
Director, Rotman Research Institute
of Baycrest Centre for Geriatric Care
North York, Ontario;
Professor, Departments of Psychology and Medicine (Neurology)
University of Toronto
Toronto, Ontario
Canada

Preface

Neurorehabilitation has entered its turbulent adolescence. Under attack from within for promising more than it can deliver and from without for its perceived inefficiency and increasing cost, it is struggling to define its adult identity. Lest we despair, these conflicts must be viewed in a historical context that recognizes that these rites of passage are no different than those faced by many of its older, medical siblings. This is especially true for those that had to confront equally chronic and seemingly incurable disorders. One recent example comes to us from the mid-1950s with medicine's response to the poliomyelitis epidemic. Those who witnessed them can never forget the enormous "iron lungs" that once filled the polio pavilions of most major hospitals. These machines were the technological marvels of their time and like all "compensatory technologies," to paraphrase Lewis Thomas, they were extremely expensive to own and operate. Yet they never cured polio, never killed one virus. Rather, they kept a polio victim alive while the ravages of the disease ran its course. Over forty years ago, the then *American Journal of Physical Medicine* devoted an entire issue to the subject of poliomyelitis. In an article by Harold Dinken, he reminded clinicians that in spite of the marked advances in understanding the disease and improvements in its treatment, "the basic facts about the epidemiology and prevention of poliomyelitis are still unknown." Furthermore, he wrote, "the proper management of the poliomyelitis patient whether seen during the acute, convalescent or chronic phase of the disease required a team approach . . . insuring the total physical, psychosocial, educational, and vocational rehabilitation of the afflicted individual." Dinken concluded with the admonition that there was no shortcut to such an approach: "It is detailed and time consuming and there are no standard techniques for teaching the most important activities a patient must learn . . . Every case presents a unique problem and retraining methods have to be adapted to the special requirements of each individual."

In the 1990s, neurologic disorders raise the same specter as poliomyelitis. Their remediation has all the characteristics of those now obsolete iron lungs. Neurorehabilitation is an immense, expensive, "compensatory technology" that does not cure the underlying pathophysiology of these disorders. Similar to all treatments directed at the surface manifestations of a disorder, it attempts to help an individual compensate for the handicapping conditions created by an injury or disease process, but does not truly remediate it. Therefore, it serves as a prosthesis that is structurally sophisticated, but therapeutically primitive. Yet, it is all that can be done until there is a genuine understanding of the biomechanical perturbations that create the condition and ways found to reverse it safely. When this level of understanding is reached, the industry of neurorehabilitation will vanish and no longer pose the huge problems of logistics, cost, and ethics that it poses today. However, what do we do in the interim?

Perhaps the best that can be hoped for in this "decade of the brain" is the adoption of a neurologic rehabilitation paradigm that models Dinken's approach to polio. Such a development would recognize the inherently primitive nature of all our interventions, while advancing a more coherent model of treatment based on an increasingly sophisticated understanding of a disorder's underlying neuropathology and natural history. It would emphasize the psychosocial, educational, and vocational outcome of the afflicted individual, rather than a composite FIM score. Furthermore, this construct would integrate an awareness of an individual's premorbid attributes with his or her injury characteristics when attempting to predict outcome accurately.

To that end, *Neurologic Rehabilitation: A Guide to Diagnosis, Prognosis, and Treatment Planning* begins with an overview of this way of thinking about patients and their underlying disorders. It also provides a concise but very functional review of normal central nervous system anatomy and physiology. Chapters 2 through 6 focus on developing the model as it applies to the most common types of neuropathology seen in rehabilitative settings. Beginning with Chapter 7, the focus shifts to dealing with specific issues that clinicians confront on a daily basis with their neurologically impaired patients. Chapter 7 evolves the constructs developed earlier to their logical conclusion in assessment and treatment planning. In Chapter 8, an activities assessment algorithm is outlined that is designed to improve our understanding of why a patient fails to perform a specific activity of daily living. When we have a better understanding of how things go wrong in this process, we can develop more rational strategies to achieve the desired functional outcome. Balance problems constantly frustrate both patients and clinicians as we so often feel powerless to intervene successfully. Chapter 9 challenges this sense of therapeutic nihilism by offering a rational way to evaluate these conditions and teach the patient strategies to improve his or her situation. Post-acute traumatically brain injured patients often complain of memory deficits, and Chapter 10 addresses these issues in the context of a comprehensive, community-based outpatient program. Finally, Chapter 11 extends the neurologic model of rehabilitation to the difficult outlier patient population, which is often very behaviorally disordered as well as cognitively impaired.

All in all, we hope that the practicing clinician or student will ruminate on the model and not pass judgment too quickly. It may produce more work for busy clinicians on the front end, but its use drastically improves the effectiveness and timing of their therapeutic interventions. The case studies presented should provide a good basis to help clarify some of the more abstract concepts and demonstrate the applicability of the techniques discussed in the text. The implications of adopting this model are profound because it is obvious that it involves changing the way most rehabilitation teams think about their work and approach their patients. Nevertheless, we hope that they will move toward its implementation with this patient population.

In addition, we would like to thank Chris Davis of Blackwell Science for his invaluable help in the evolution of the text. Not only did he provide much needed encouragement when our energy was waning, but several dinners at some of Boston's most wonderful restaurants. Finally, although we hope this model will advance the practice of rehabilitation, it, too, can be supplanted by new paradigms generated by basic research. Despite the shift in focus seen in medicine during these cost-conscious times, basic research remains the hope of the future, just as it was over forty years ago. The hope is that, like the iron lung, the neurologic rehabilitation model will become another historical footnote supplanted by a newer technology as elegant as the polio vaccine.

John W. Cassidy

Reference

Dinken H. Physical medicine and rehabilitation and poliomyelitis. Am J Phys Med 1952;31:282–284.

Neurologic Rehabilitation

The Neurologic Rehabilitation Model in Clinical Practice

Douglas I. Katz, Virginia M. Mills, and John W. Cassidy

Why yet another book on rehabilitation? The answers are complicated, but ultimately converge on the aspiration to propose a distinct paradigm for the treatment of neurologically impaired individuals. To that end, this text places great emphasis on accurate diagnosis and an integral understanding of the natural history of the disorders under consideration. It also presupposes that the organ of the mind is the brain and, as such, its reach extends beyond traditional neurologic constructs to include those of neuropsychiatry, which help explicate the rehabilitative process in terms of the individual being rehabilitated. As complex as this tapestry may seem at first glance, it is woven with understandable skeins of knowledge that can be taught and that, once learned, will enhance the evaluation and treatment of those who come for help for these incurable afflictions.

This chapter begins with a brief reintroduction of basic neuroanatomy and physiology, principally because dysfunction is best understood from the vantage point of knowing what is normal. Therefore, an appreciation of how these disorders disrupt normal brain function is essential for their appropriate evaluation, proper prognostication, and judicious treatment. Then, in subsequent chapters, the pathophysiology of the common neurologic disorders (cerebral vascular disease, traumatic brain injury, anoxic encephalopathy, encephalitis, and multiple sclerosis) that beset patients who present for rehabilitation is reviewed in detail.

Despite some similar clinical manifestations, such as hemiparesis or behavioral dyscontrol, these syndromes cause diverse patterns of damage to the central nervous system (CNS) that have vastly different ramifications for prudent rehabilitation. This awareness allows a clinician to plan interventions and set realistic goals in the context of the anticipated natural history of the disease; that is, what deficits are expected from this type of CNS insult, which are amenable to treatment and which are not, what types of remediation make sense, when can improvement be expected, and, ultimately, what is the likely outcome for the patient following therapy.

Chapter 1 closes with a description of the *neurologic model of rehabilitation*. The following chapters fully elaborate this approach by reviewing the neuropathology, clinical features, natural history, and prognosis of a variety of neurologic syndromes. They include patient examples that illustrate how this model can help guide clinicians in performing their assessments and making rational choices about remediation. We believe that this text provides a much-needed synthesis of the available information about the evaluation and treatment of these disorders that, to date, has not been fully appreciated or methodically used in most rehabilitation settings.

NORMAL NEUROANATOMY AND PHYSIOLOGY

The human CNS consists of a vast array of hierarchically controlled structures that subserve behavioral regulation. Classical anatomists consider the whole modern human brain to consist of five subdivisions, based on their distinct embryologic origins (1). Hence, the brainstem, subserving vegetative functions such as the regulation of respiration, heart rate, and blood pressure, consists of the myelencephalon (*medulla*), the metencephalon (*pons and cerebellum*), and the mesencephalon (*midbrain*), and includes the reticular formation that extends the length of the three regions. The more rostral diencephalon consists of the thalamus and hypothalamus, as well as the hypophysis (*pituitary gland*) and the epiphysis (*pineal gland*). Structures in this subdivision are considered to be intermediary links between higher and lower brain regions. Finally, the telencephalon, the most advanced brain region (both phylogenetically and ontologically), consists of the entire cerebrum, including the neocortex, subcortical nuclear complexes, and the internal capsule. This subdivision therefore includes brain structures and regions that mediate functions as diverse as cognitive processing, emotional behavior, and motor movement. This classical scheme of structural organization has proven to be useful for describing and topographically categorizing the hard wiring of neuroanatomy. However, the clinician trying to design a rehabilitation program for a brain-injured patient will often have difficulty associating structural impairment with functional deficit. To understand the anatomic bases of complex behavior, it is more useful to consider a conceptual model of the human brain based on a functional paradigm.

In order to associate form with function, neurobiologist Paul Mac-Lean proposed a triunal model of brain and behavior in 1973 (2). This model emphasizes the notion that as the human CNS evolved, it increased in both size and complexity by *adding on* to more primitive, but extant brain structures. Hence, beneath a mantle of distinctly human neocortex, the modern human brain still retains the highly conserved archetypical patterns of structural organization that are reflections of its evolutionary past.

Based on this triunal model, the brain may be divided, both anatomically and functionally, into three basic components: reptilian, paleomammalian, and neomammalian (Figure 1.1). The reptilian component corresponds to the brainstem and consists not only of medulla, pons, and midbrain, but of the basal ganglia as well. Therefore, not only vegetative functions, but many volitional behaviors directed toward individual preservation and the propagation of the species, such as feeding, drinking, and sexual aggression, may be considered to be phylogenetic legacies of our cold-blooded ancestors. Correspondingly, the paleomammalian brain is characterized by the primitive cortex of the limbic lobe (first described by Paul Broca in 1878), the prominent convolution that surrounds the rostral brainstem of all mammalian brains

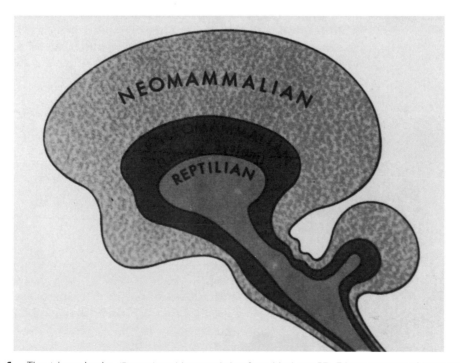

Figure 1.1   The triune brain. *(Reproduced by permission from MacLean PD. Triune concept of brain and behavior. Toronto: University of Toronto Press, 1973:9.)*

(*limbic* means "forming a border around"). Structures of the limbic cortex subserve primitive but distinctly mammalian behaviors such as hoarding and parental care of offspring. Finally, the outermost neo-mammalian brain, the neocortex, subserves the uniquely human behaviors such as cognition and speech that facilitate social behavior. The modern human brain, then, may be conceptually divided into three functional divisions: the brainstem, the limbic system, and the cerebral cortex.

The Brainstem

Both anatomically and physiologically, the brainstem marks a transitional zone between the brain and the spinal cord. In fact, much of the substance of the brainstem is devoted to ascending and descending tracts connecting these upper and lower divisions of the CNS, and, as such, it is densely packed with many vital structures. In addition to the long ascending and descending pathways, several specific nuclear groups, including the nuclei of the cranial nerves, are found there. The central core of the brainstem is occupied by the reticular formation, diffuse aggregations of cells surrounded by myriad interlacing fibers. Centers within the brainstem subserve not only the primary vegetative functions but also motor activities and mechanisms related to consciousness and sleep (Table 1.1).

Although the monoamine neurotransmitters (dopamine, norepinephrine, and serotonin) are widely distributed in the CNS, the cell groups from which the monoaminergic pathways arise are almost without exception located within the brainstem (3). The monoaminergic systems participate in the regulation of sleep-wake cycles, feeding

Table 1.1.   Localization of Brainstem Functions

Region	Nuclear Groups	Prominent Fiber Tracts
Medulla oblongata	Vagus, spinal accessory, & hypoglossal motor nuclei; trigeminal & vestibular sensory nuclei	Descending motor pyramidal & ascending sensory dorsal columns
Pons	Trigeminal, abducens & facial motor nuclei; sensory nuclei	Pontocerebellar tracts; corticopontine, corticobulbar & corticospinal tracts
Midbrain	Oculomotor & trochlear motor nuclei; reflex centers for vision & audition; substantia nigra	Medial longitudinal fasciculus; cerebral peduncles

behaviors, motor and neuroendocrine regulation, reward mechanisms, and probably many other functions.

The caudal portion of the brainstem is known as the *medulla oblongata*. At the level of the medulla, both the descending motor pyramidal tracts and the ascending sensory dorsal columns decussate, thereby producing the reason for the contralateral expression of many cortical lesions. In the dorsal medulla, the motor nuclei of the vagus (X), spinal accessory (XI), and hypoglossal cranial (XII) nerves lie medially, while portions of nuclei of sensory cranial nerves (trigeminal [V] and the vestibular complex [VIII]) lie laterally. The ventral surface of the medulla lies against the basilar portion of the occipital bone, while the dorsal surface (and the fourth ventricle) is lodged in a groove on the anterior surface of the cerebellum (Figure 1.2).

The *pons* ("bridge") of the brainstem is named for the massive bundles of transversely oriented fibers that originate in the pontine nuclei and enter the cerebellum via the middle cerebellar peduncles. These pontocerebellar fibers form the second link in a pathway between the cerebral cortex and the cerebellum. Longitudinally oriented pontine fiber bundles include the corticopontine, corticobulbar, and corticospinal tracts. Cranial nerve nuclei located in the pons include the trigeminal (V), abducens (VI), facial (VII), and superior vestibular (VIII). The pons occupies the central part of the ventral

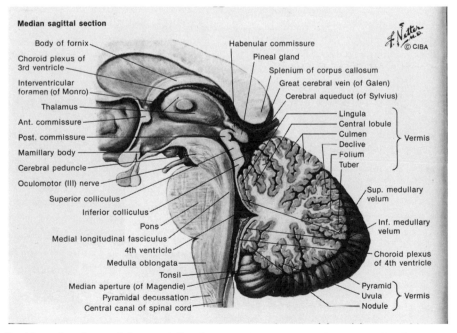

Figure 1.2   *Ventral surfaces of the medulla. (Reproduced by permission from Netter FH. CIBA collection of medical illustrations. Volume 1, Nervous system. Part 1, Anatomy and physiology, 1983:32. Reprinted with permission from the Ciba Collection illustrated by Frank Netter, M.D. All rights reserved.)*

brainstem, resting against the clivus of the occipital bone (see Figure 1.2).

The dorsal *midbrain* features reflex centers for visual and auditory impulses in the superior and inferior colliculi, respectively. Beneath the colliculi are the nuclei of the oculomotor (III) and trochlear (IV) cranial nerves. Running longitudinally through the area is the medial longitudinal fasciculus (MLF). This complex bundle of fibers, connecting the oculomotor apparatus with the vestibular nuclei and motor centers in the cervical cord, is essential for the coordination of eye and head movement. The ventral portion of the midbrain is dominated by the cerebral peduncles, parallel massive bundles carrying several ascending and descending tracts. The substantia nigra and red nucleus are deep to the peduncles.

The *reticular formation* is located in the central region of the brainstem, extending from the medulla to the rostral midbrain. It is characterized by diffuse aggregations of cells intermeshed among multidirectional fibers. Discrete populations of cells are grouped as either small, localized cells (the lateral parvicellular zone) or large arborizing cells that give rise to long ascending and descending pathways (the medial magnocellular zone) characterized by elaborate perpendicular interconnections. The extensive overlapping of these fibers facilitates the widespread convergence of afferent impulses.

The concept of the *ascending reticular activating system* (ARAS) is based on evidence of an arousal zone in the brainstem (4). It is a physiologic concept with anatomic correlates represented by discrete areas of the brainstem reticular formation as well as specific ascending pathways to the thalamus and cortex. The ARAS is critical for maintaining a state of wakefulness. The regulation of the conscious state, however, is an extremely complex function, in which many parts of the CNS are involved. In addition, areas of special importance for sleep have been identified in the ARAS as well as in the thalamus and the hypothalamus. The anatomic components of the ARAS lie in a narrow isthmus between the cerebellum in the infratentorial compartment and the cerebrum in the supratentorial compartment.

A number of neuron groups located primarily in the brainstem have been characterized according to their monoaminergic neurotransmitter: serotonin (5-hydroxytryptamine, 5-HT), norepinephrine (NE), and dopamine (DA) (Table 1.2). There are some notable anatomic differences among the three neurotransmitter systems. In the serotonin and norepinephrine systems, the cells of origin are located within or near the reticular formation, whereas their projections are widespread throughout the CNS. On the other hand, the dopamine-specific cells are located in the substantia nigra and nearby ventral areas of the midbrain, as well as in some hypothalamic nuclei. Axons of these cells project to specific areas of the CNS in a highly ordered topographic fashion.

Table 1.2.   Neurotransmitters of the Brainstem

Neurotransmitter	Location of Cells of Origin	Functional Modalities
Serotonin	Raphe nuclei of the reticular formation	Pain mechanisms; changes in mood, behavior, and sleep
Norepinephrine	Locus ceruleus of the reticular formation	Regulation of cerebral blood flow, alertness, mood, memory, and hormonal modulation
Dopamine	Substantia nigra, ventral tegmental area of the midbrain and hypothalamus	Motor control, mentation, and hormonal regulation

The cells of origin of the serotonin system are located primarily in the *raphe nuclei*, an extensive, continuous collection of cell groups close to the midline throughout the brainstem (5). Their axons project both caudally and rostrally, extending to the forebrain, the cerebellum, and the spinal cord. These pathways have been implicated in pain mechanisms, changes in mood and behavior (via projections to limbic structures), and sleep inducement.

Norepinephrine fibers arise from special cells in the pontine and medullary reticular formation, the nucleus *locus ceruleus*, located beneath the floor of the fourth ventricle (6). Projections from the locus ceruleus are characterized by widespread distribution of norepinephrine fibers via profuse branching of a limited number of neurons. This system participates in the regulation of cerebral blood flow, alertness, spinal cord locomotion, mood, memory, and hormonal modulation.

The majority of the dopaminergic cells are located in the substantia nigra or the ventral tegmental area of the midbrain. Traditionally, two dopaminergic systems are described (7). The nigrostriatal dopaminergic system originates primarily in the pars compacta of the substantia nigra and terminates in the dorsal striatum. Loss of neurons in this system results in parkinsonism. The mesolimbic dopaminergic system originates in the ventral tegmental area of the midbrain and projects to the striatum, septum, amygdala, and the frontal lobe. Some evidence suggests that excessive activity in the mesolimbic system may be involved in the genesis of psychosis. A dopaminergic pathway from the posterior hypothalamus to dorsal and intermediate cell columns of the spinal cord has also been identified.

The Limbic System

The term *limbic system* was coined by MacLean in 1952 to describe the limbic lobe and those anatomic structures with which it has primary connections. More often, however, this "system" is defined functionally rather than anatomically to include those regions associated with affective and motivational behaviors. The limbic lobe includes a large part of the basomedial telencephalon (Figure 1.3). Hence, its primary components, visible on the medial hemispheric surface, include the cingulate and the parahippocampal gyri (which together loop around the medial diencephalic components) and the septal region (which includes the midline septum pellucidum and the septal nuclei).

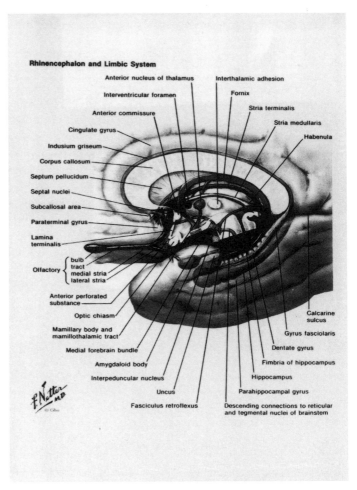

Figure 1.3   The limbic system. (Reproduced by permission from Netter FH. CIBA collection of medical illustrations. Volume 1, Nervous system. Part 1, Anatomy and physiology, 1983:27. Reprinted with permission from the Ciba Collection illustrated by Frank Netter, M.D. All rights reserved.)

In addition to the various regions of the limbic lobe, the primary components of the limbic system in a behavioral sense, include the amygdala and the hippocampal formation (Table 1.3). Both of these structures are located within the cerebral temporal lobe and are continuous with adjacent cerebral cortex. They also have extensive interconnections with other cortical and subcortical structures via numerous reciprocal pathways. In addition, these structures (as well as limbic lobe regions) are related to a considerable extent to the hypothalamus, the primary brain structure involved in the integration of various autonomic effects that accompany emotional expression (Figure 1.4).

The *amygdala* is actually a large heterogeneous nuclear complex that occupies the dorsomedial portion of the temporal lobe immediately deep to the uncus. It contains several different cellular subgroups that exhibit distinct cytoarchitectural and histochemical characteristics and connections. Bilateral ablation studies have implicated the amygdala in sensory-affective associations; that is, the relation of sensory information to experience. Thus, aggressive, sexual, and eating behaviors are specifically related to amygdaloid activities. In addition, a widespread system of amygdalocortical fibers allows the amygdala to modulate and influence the activities in cortical association areas, known to be of importance for higher order sensory functions such as storage of long-term memory. Because of close associations with the hypothalamus and other subcortical regions related to drive and motivation, the amygdala is likely to provide an emotional component to the learning experience.

The *hippocampal formation* is laid down embryonically when, on the medial wall of the hemisphere, the choroid plexus invaginates into the ventricle. The resultant fissure (the hippocampal sulcus) is carried downward and forward, forming an arch as the temporal lobe develops. The name hippocampus ("sea horse") derives from the convoluted appearance of the structure in coronal sections. The hippocampus appears immediately caudal to the amygdaloid complex in the temporal lobe. The primary components of the hippocampal formation

Table 1.3.   Localization of Limbic Functions

Limbic Lobe*	Amygdala	Hippocampal Formation
Elevation or depression of arterial blood pressure	Aggression Sexual behavior	Learning Memory
Inhibition or acceleration of respiration	Eating behavior Long-term memory Emotional component of learning	Spatial orientation

*Cingulate gyrus, parahippocampal gyrus, and septal region (septum pellucidum and septal nuclei).

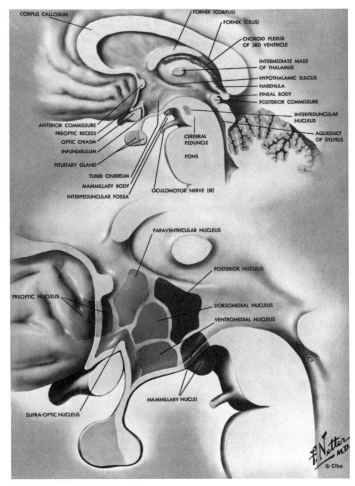

Figure 1.4   The hypothalamus. (Reproduced by permission from Netter FH. CIBA collection of medical illustrations. Volume 1, Nervous system, 1953:76. Reprinted with permission from the Ciba Collection illustrated by Frank Netter, M.D. All rights reserved.)

include the hippocampus, the parahippocampal gyrus, the dentate gyrus, and the fornix.

The hippocampus proper is traditionally divided into three fields (CA1, CA2, and CA3) based on cytoarchitonic differences (1). The dentate gyrus, which interlocks with the concave surface of the hippocampus proper, is characterized primarily by cells that project into the hippocampus. The fornix is the massive fiber bundle that connects the hippocampal formation with a variety of subcortical structures, including the septum, hypothalamus, and anterior thalamic nucleus.

Along with its extrinsic connections, the components of the hippocampal formation possess a complex intrinsic neuronal circuit. The dentate gyrus is richly innervated by projections from the parahippocampal gyrus, which has numerous connections with sensory cortical areas. The fibers of the dentate gyrus project, via interconnections with the hippocampus proper and the alveus, to the subiculum. The fornix, the subiculum, and the hippocampus itself send feedback projections to the sensory cortex.

Behaviorally, the hippocampus is traditionally implicated with learning and memory functions. In addition, physiologic studies of single hippocampal neurons indicate a critical involvement with spatial orientation mechanisms that permit recognition and prediction of environmental relationships and events.

Several other regions of the forebrain and the brainstem are frequently described as components of the limbic system, based on functional associations as well as extensive anatomic interconnections. These limbic system affiliates include neocortical areas in the basal frontotemporal region, the olfactory cortex, ventral parts of the striatum, the anterior and medial thalamic nuclei, the habenula, and parts of the medial midbrain. However, the inclusion of these structures under the aegis of the "limbic system" is variable (8).

The Cerebral Cortex

The human cerebral cortex, a convoluted mantle six cell layers (2–4 mm) thick, is densely and richly connected to most of the lower structures of the CNS. The numerous complex cortical projections reflect the degree of cortical influence, either directly or indirectly, upon practically every functional system of the entire CNS (Figure 1.5). In addition, the intrinsic circuitry of the cerebral cortex—the myriad interneurons, collateral pathways, and synaptic relationships—provides an almost unlimited number of possibilities for impulse transmission.

The cortex may be conceptually divided into motor, sensory, and association areas. Whereas primary motor and sensory function is generally localized to specific regions of the frontal or parietal cortex according to Brodmann's cytoarchitectural mapping scheme, association areas are represented by more general territories in the frontal lobe (the prefrontal cortex) and by extensive parietotemporal regions. Association cortex, then, is involved in associative functions such as the analysis and elaboration of sensory information.

Information about the localization of cortical functions in humans has depended historically on lesion or cortical stimulation studies. More recently, radiographic technologies have permitted the dynamic mapping of brain function based on measurements of cerebral blood flow or metabolic rate. General concepts correlating cortical regions with specific behavioral characteristics have been established, although the macroscopic boundaries by which hemispheric lobes and gyri are defined do not necessarily indicate strict functional boundaries (Table 1.4).

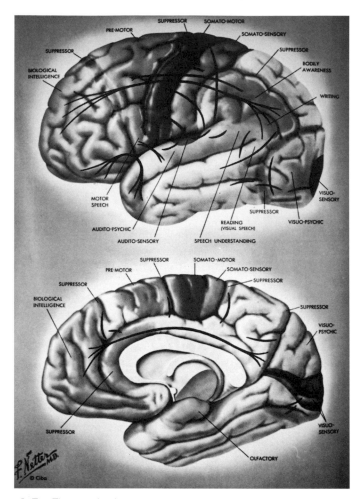

Figure 1.5   The cerebral cortex. (Reproduced by permission from Netter FH. CIBA collection of medical illustrations. Volume 1, Nervous system, 1953:74. Reprinted with permission from the Ciba Collection illustrated by Frank Netter, M.D. All rights reserved.)

That portion of the *frontal lobes* located immediately anterior to the central sulci is related to control of movement; this is true of all mammalian brains. However, the *prefrontal* cortex, occupying approximately a quarter of the total cerebral cortex, has increased dramatically in size and complexity in humans. Prefrontal cortical function is subtle and, therefore, difficult to describe with a high degree of specificity. Some insights have been gained, however, from studying patients who have experienced frontal lobe damage or psychosurgical procedures. Considering these analyses, the frontal lobe seems to be crucially involved in the integration and control of both the intellectual and the emotional factors of behavior. Many aspects of personality seem to be mediated by the prefrontal cortex, including self-awareness (Figure 1.6). In fact, via numerous connections with the major cortical and subcortical

Table 1.4. Localization of Cortical Functions

Frontal Lobe	Parietal Lobe	Temporal Lobe
Precentral gyrus Motor control	*Postcentral gyrus* Tactile sensation Proprioception	Olfaction Audition Language
Prefrontal cortex Organization and control of intellectual and emotional factors of behavior Self-awareness Appreciation of behavioral consequences Behavioral response to stimuli	Sensory associative area Integration of visual, somatosensory, and auditory stimuli	Memory Facial recognition

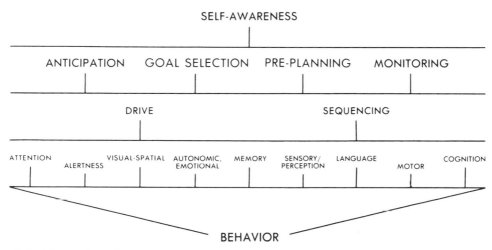

Figure 1.6 The prefrontal cortex. (Reproduced by permission from Stuss DT, Benson DF. The frontal lobes. New York: Raven Press, 1988:248.)

regions of the brain, the frontal cortex can continuously monitor internal and external stimuli; the close topographic association with motor control areas facilitates the behavioral response to such input.

In the *parietal lobe*, the postcentral gyrus has been well characterized as the terminal target tissue of ascending tactile and proprioceptive impulses. Most of the remainder of the lobe, the extensive posterior parietal association cortex, is generally considered to be a sensory association area for higher order processing such as the integration of visual, auditory, and somatosensory stimuli.

The *temporal lobe* contains receiving areas for the olfactory (in the region of the uncus) and auditory (deep to the lateral fissure) systems. In addition, the posterior temporal lobe, as well as nearby occipital and parietal areas, is involved with language functions. Interestingly, extensive areas on the underside of the temporal and occipital lobes are of special importance for facial recognition.

Due to the subcortical temporal loci of the amygdala and the hippocampal formation, the temporal lobe is considered to be intricately involved with memory functions. Not surprisingly, some of the cortical areas in the temporal lobe have been identified as neocorticolimbic associative areas.

The *occipital lobe* forms the most posterior boundary of the cerebral cortex and is principally devoted to visual capacities. As such, it contains the primary visual cortex that is surrounded by less specific visual association areas. There is point-by-point localization from the retina to the contralateral primary visual cortex via the optic radiations that have their origins in the lateral geniculate bodies. Pathways from the visual cortex to the temporal lobes appear essential for object recognition, while connections with the posterior parietal cortices are involved in visuospatial perception, visuomotor performance, and spatial attention.

In summary, several points warrant reemphasis: First, from a functional standpoint, the human CNS is hierarchically organized, with more primitive structures located medially and caudally, and more modern structures positioned more laterally and rostrally. Second, primitive structures tend to be excitatory; modern structures tend to be inhibitory or modulatory. Finally, most of the cerebral cortex is devoted to the regulation of social behavior, not the production of motor movement.

THE NEUROLOGIC MODEL OF REHABILITATION

The neurologic model of rehabilitation developed in this text is predicated upon two important constructs: diagnosis and prognosis (Table 1.5). In this context a meaningful *diagnosis* must extend beyond giving a label to the condition under consideration (e.g., head injury) and include an assessment of how this condition disrupts normal brain functioning and produces disability. Thus, it promotes an understanding of a patient's impairments in the context of a particular neuropathologic syndrome and accounts for other factors that interact with the CNS insult to produce a particular clinical profile in a given individual, for example, age, premorbid assets, and comorbid conditions. This process also permits more meaningful differential diagnosis to dis-

Table 1.5.   Neurologic Model of Rehabilitation

Diagnosis	Assessment of brain disorder is in relation to clinical impairments and disabilities. The *functional diagnosis* is placed in context of neurologic syndromes.
Prognosis	Projection of *course* and *outcome* probabilities in an estimated time frame based on *diagnosis, natural history,* and other personal, social, and environmental factors.
Treatment planning	Accounts for the interactive process of recovery (e.g., proportion of biologic vs. learning vs. psychological influences) and at what point the patient is in the recovery process.

tinguish which problems are directly attributable to the brain injury and which are not.

Prognosis takes the diagnostic information, viewed within the framework of *natural history,* and estimates an anticipated recovery profile for the patient. It also considers the trajectory of recovery, where the patient is currently, how long it took him or her to get there, and, based on those factors, estimates how improvement will progress. Thus, the observed impairments become understood in the context of a dynamic process, not simply as a static functional independence measure (FIM score). However, it must be explicitly stated that the confidence one places in delineating a patient's prognosis is dependent on the accuracy of the initial diagnosis. For some types of brain injury, direct diagnosis is difficult and information about the event or disease process causing the insult becomes of paramount importance. If this datum is unavailable or is distorted by misinformation, diagnostic reliability greatly suffers and accurate prognostication becomes nearly impossible. For some disorders, information on natural history is limited, presenting another challenge to precise prognostication.

This approach does not aver that all recovery is biologically driven. Rather it accepts that it is a complex interaction of biologic and other factors, including: constitutional diatheses, premorbid personality, new learning, directed treatment, and compensatory strategies (Figure 1.7). The relative influence of each of these factors changes with time. The biologic factors are most significant early in the course of recovery but wane with time, as psychosocial influences wax in importance. Following this line of reasoning, it becomes clear that early in the course of injury or illness, when biologic influences predominate, rehabilitative interventions may have little, if any, direct influence on recovery. On the other hand, as time progresses and the dominance of biologic processes diminishes, directed, restorative treatment can influence the outcome of deficits that are known to be responsive to therapy.

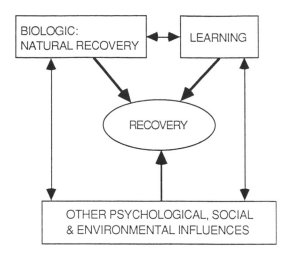

Figure 1.7 *Interaction of factors that contribute to recovery from neurologic disorders. Biologic factors are proportionally more important earlier in recovery and less important later in recovery.*

Finally, the natural history of the disorder dictates when deficits become fixed and the benefits of therapy directed at the remediation plateau. Therapy directed at teaching patients compensatory strategies for impairments is not limited to the natural recovery time period and can be of value many years post illness. Thus, the neurologic model of rehabilitation attempts to be clear about which impairments spontaneously improve, regardless of treatment, which can benefit from directed treatment and when, and which are fixed and therefore unresponsive to restorative therapeutic interventions, despite their continuing existence.

Traditional Rehabilitation Approaches

The neurologic model of rehabilitation differs in several respects from the way assessment and treatment are traditionally approached in clinical rehabilitation. Rehabilitation diagnoses are usually framed according to deficits and their functional consequences. The neurologic diagnosis is usually limited to a diagnostic label and perhaps some clinical consequence, for example "stroke with right hemiparesis." Other medical diagnoses may be listed, but syndromic understanding of the underlying conditions is rarely appreciated. The assessment may conform to the useful system of distinguishing impairments, disabilities, and handicaps (Table 1.6). Nevertheless, these assessments rely on evaluating the surface manifestations or phenotype, if you will, of the patient's disorder at a single moment. This diagnostic process usually lists impairments and disabilities without attention to how these problems relate to the underlying brain disorder (the genotype) or where

Table 1.6. *Traditional Rehabilitation Model*

Functional assessment	Based on the patient's *impairments* (organic dysfunction), *disabilities* (difficulty with tasks), and *handicaps* (social disadvantage) at time of assessment.
Diagnosis	Functional diagnosis is usually the diagnosis. Neurologic diagnoses or syndromes usually unelaborated. The patient assessment is an amalgam of team members' assessments.
Treatment planning	Treatment plans are developed for enumerated functional problems at time of assessment. The prognosis and natural history is less emphasized during planning.

they occur within the recovery process. The underlying assumption suggests that the brain is an inaccessible "black box" and that only the "output" (the surface manifestations) is accessible for evaluation and treatment planning.

For instance, when a clinician encounters a patient with a weak and spastic arm, he or she may perform an evaluation, develop a treatment plan, and set goals using clinical experience and empiric treatment choices based on the observable impairments seen in the patient during the initial consultation (e.g., strength, tone, range of motion, function). Although in many situations this approach may be adequate, it does not consider how that person's arm will function as the natural history of the underlying neurologic condition evolves. Further, it does not consider that based on the underlying neuropathology, the problem might not be spastic paresis, but, perhaps, another disorder masquerading as weakness, such as hypokinesia or lack of initiation.

Central to traditional rehabilitation is the team approach. Accordingly, assessment and treatment planning are usually an amalgam of what all the members of the team bring to the process. Each discipline brings their assessment and treatment plan, and the overall plan may be more or less shared or interdisciplinary. This approach to assessment assumes that somehow the "sum of the parts" will lead to a complete diagnosis and that treatment will be directed toward all the discovered impairments. The neurologic model presented here takes exception to this assumption. First, not all individual assessments may be essential or appropriate for all disorders or at all times post-onset. Individual assessments should be guided by the larger picture of neurologic diagnosis and natural history. For instance, patients who are still in a confusional state after traumatic brain injury (TBI) should not have elaborate neuropsychological evaluations or language assessment batteries. Although data can be gathered, they will invariably lead to the conclusion that the patient is still in a confusional state. Therefore, these efforts are at best redundant and at worst improvident.

Diagnosis in the Neurologic Model

This model incorporates the principles of neurologic diagnosis and applies them to rehabilitation. Neurologic diagnosis in the rehabilitation setting is somewhat different from diagnosis in the acute setting. Acute neurologic diagnosis begins with recognizing clusters of clinical signs and symptoms to formulate a syndromic, anatomic diagnosis, followed by an etiologic or pathologic diagnosis. The functional diagnosis is a later, secondary issue. For patients in rehabilitation, the process is somewhat reversed. The etiologic diagnosis is generally established, and the aim is to create a functional diagnosis framed in the context of the syndromic, neuroanatomic, and pathologic diagnoses. The clinical and pathophysiologic formulations will likely be more elaborate than in the acute setting, when etiology was the primary concern, in order to understand the functional diagnosis and to establish prognosis.

Neurologic diagnosis is based on the premise that brain pathology largely, although not exclusively, determines the clinical manifestations of the disorder and its course of recovery. Determining the type, location, and severity of damage is a vital step to understanding a patient's clinical problems. Further, an understanding of how certain neurologic syndromes relate to particular patterns of brain injury promotes appropriate interpretation of clinical signs. It cannot be overemphasized that a diagnostic label such as "traumatic brain injury" or "encephalitis" does not provide this information. Further elaboration is necessary; for example, "traumatic brain injury, with severe diffuse axonal injury and a large, left, orbital frontal contusion with secondary transtentorial herniation." The complete neurorehabilitation diagnosis also consists of some assessment of severity (e.g., "duration of unconsciousness 3 days, post-traumatic amnesia 4+ weeks") and a summary of the clinical signs and symptoms (e.g., "ongoing confusional state, right motor hypokinesia").

The Pathophysiology of Brain Injury

Two distinct components contribute to the pathophysiology of brain injury: 1) the immediate consequences resulting from the biomechanical or pathophysiologic perturbations to the cranial contents; and 2) the secondary complications that develop from the subsequent metabolic disturbances. The first component is a function of the neuropathologic event and generally cannot be affected by currently available treatments, although this is an area of promising and active clinical research. On the other hand, prompt and appropriate medical or surgical intervention often plays a key role in alleviating secondary complications and improves the potential for recovery.

Neuropathologic Factors

The three cardinal neuropathologic dimensions to consider in diagnosis are the distribution, severity, and type of pathology (Table 1.7), recognizing that severity parameters vary depending on the distribution and type of pathology. The questions regarding distribution include whether brain damage is focal, multifocal, or diffuse.

For *focal lesions*, such as stroke, the main diagnostic and prognostic elements in determining severity are the location, size, depth, and secondary effects (Figure 1.8). Small differences in location of lesions can be associated with very different clinical problems, especially when occurring in deeper brain structures where there is significant convergence of subcortical white matter pathways. Furthermore, lesions usually interrupt multiple overlapping functional neurologic systems or networks. Thus, the particular presentation of a neurologic syndrome in a patient depends on which and how many of these distributed neurologic systems are affected. Prognosis is also affected by size and depth of the lesion; as might be anticipated, large lesions produce

Table 1.7. Important Neuropathologic Parameters

Distribution	Severity Factors	Type (Pathologic Process)
Focal lesion	Location Size (big lesions worse than small) Depth (deep lesions worse than superficial) Secondary effects	Hemorrhage Infarct Tumor Abscess Trauma Demyelinating secondary effects (edema, mass effect, neuronal degeneration)
Multifocal lesions	Same as focal + number (the more lesions the worse) Simultaneous vs. staged (simultaneous worse) Unilateral vs. bilateral (bilateral worse)	Hemorrhage Infarct Tumor Abscess Trauma Demyelinating secondary effects (edema, mass effect, neuronal degeneration)
Diffuse	Density or quantity (the more the worse) Locations (structures and neural elements involved, e.g., axonal vs. neuronal vs. myelin)	Traumatic Hypoxic-ischemic Inflammatory Metabolic Degenerative Secondary processes

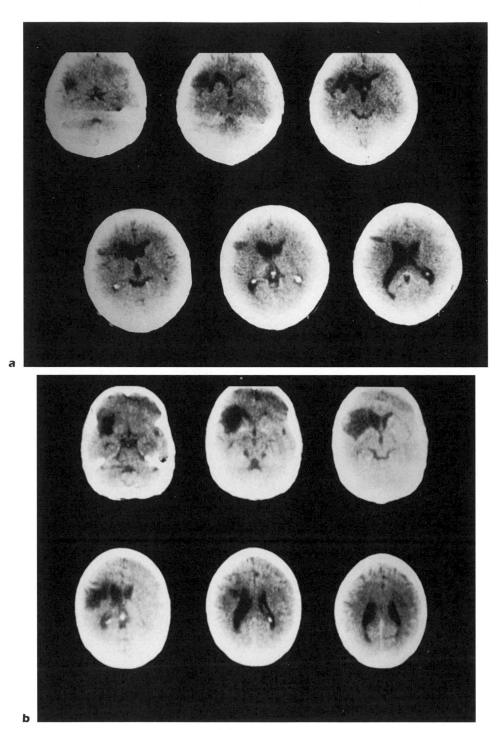

Figure 1.8   Small differences in the size and depth of a lesion may have profound effect on outcome. Both CT scans demonstrate a lesion in Broca's area, but the lesion in **a** extends less deeply than the one in **b** to the anterior periventricular white matter pathways, considered critical for recovery of fluency (10). Although both patients initially had a nonfluent Broca's aphasia, the patient with the lesion in **a** recovered fluent language and the patient with **b** did not.

worse outcomes than small ones. Depth of lesion refers to the extent that a lesion extends from the cortical surface into so called "deeper" subcortical structures. As alluded to above, these deep lesions are worse because they affect a wider array of primary pathways and secondary connections.

For *multifocal* lesions, additional elements are important. Recovery may be different depending on whether the lesions occur simultaneously or at separate times, allowing some recovery and reorganization after the first lesion. Involvement of both hemispheres, especially in homologous regions, is another important prognostic issue. Bilateral lesions usually preclude reorganization of the lost brain functions in the intact area of the contralateral hemisphere and therefore are always associated with poorer prognosis and worse functional outcome.

For *diffuse* pathology, the diagnostic and prognostic elements that determine severity are the *quantity* or *density* of pathology and the structural components involved. For instance, does the pathology primarily affect neurons (as in the case of anoxia, encephalitis, or the metabolic encephalopathies), axons (as in trauma), myelin (as in multiple sclerosis), or small blood vessels (as is characteristic of vasculitis and autoimmune disorders)? Location is secondarily important. Some diffuse pathologies preferentially affect certain areas of the brain; for example, anoxic damage occurs principally in cortex, basal ganglia, hippocampus, visual cortex, and cerebellum; diffuse axonal injury after trauma occurs in a superficial to deep gradient; while in multiple sclerosis, demyelinated plaques are typically dense in periventricular areas.

Along with distribution and severity, the *type* of pathology is central in determining prognosis and natural history. A lesion in the same anatomic location will have very different effects and patterns of recovery depending on whether it involves hemorrhage, infarct, tumor, infection, or some other process. It is well recognized, for instance, that tumors, especially slow-growing ones, can expand to a large size before manifesting a clinical effect. The same size lesion involving infarction, which occurs rapidly, has sudden, catastrophic effects. Similarly, an acute hemorrhagic lesion that is of similar size and clinical presentation to an acute ischemic lesion may ultimately leave a smaller area of residual damage when the hemorrhage is resorbed, leading to a better long-term outcome.

Clinical Neurologic Syndromes

The location, type, and severity of neuropathology associated with acquired brain disorders have a reasonably predictable relationship with disturbed behavior and function. The specificity of the relationship varies depending on a number of factors including the following:

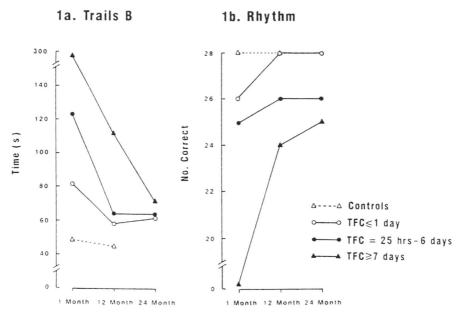

Figure 1.9   *Results from a study by Dikmen and colleagues illustrates that recovery is a function of the severity of the injury and the nature of the task. Note that recovery curves plateau earlier and at higher levels for patients with less severe injuries. Recovery rates also vary depending on the task (Trails B and Rhythm) for the same severity levels. (Reprinted with permission from [9].)*

1. The extent of localization, distribution, and lateralization of particular brain functions
2. The focality of the lesion or simultaneous effect on multiple neurologic systems
3. The ability to recognize and measure certain clinical problems
4. The degree of current knowledge of the brain-behavior relationship under consideration
5. The obscuring of focal clinical signs by overwhelming global impairments (e.g., low arousal, confusion)
6. The extent that plasticity and recovery has altered the usual clinical-anatomic relationship.

Despite these limitations, there are numerous, well-recognized neurologic syndromes associated with particular diseases or regions of brain dysfunction. Identification of these syndromes helps to put impairments and disabilities into an understandable framework that can help the clinician to focus evaluation, identify appropriate treatment priorities, and formulate prognosis. Thus in this model, behavioral dysregulation and loss of executive cognitive capacity are conceptualized in the context of a "frontal lobe syndrome," or as a component of left neglect, visuospatial dysfunction, and unawareness of hemiplegia as part of a "right hemisphere syndrome." Some syndromes have a highly specific anatomic correlate, but others have multiple loci that produce their phenotype.

Prognosis in the Neurologic Model

Establishing prognosis is the next important step in this model. For rehabilitation patients, it is essential to relate prognosis to functional outcome. By that we mean: What is that patient going to be able to do, and when? Will he or she be independent? And if so, in what setting?

When discussing prognosis, the clinician is considering probabilities—a kind of actuarial or statistical analysis of the facts at hand. As alluded to previously, the certainty of prognosis will vary depending on the accuracy of the diagnosis, the nature of the disorder, other premorbid, comorbid, and postmorbid factors, and the knowledge base for that disorder. The ability to conclusively project recovery beyond the short term is particularly limited early during recovery. As the pattern of recovery develops, it is easier to plot its trajectory, and prognostication becomes more meaningful and reliable.

There are two components of prognosis: *course* and *outcome*. The former includes a projection of the recovery process placed in an estimated period. The process of recovery is conceptualized as a *recovery curve*. The nature of these curves is highly dependent on the measure employed. A typical recovery curve usually illustrates an early period of accelerating recovery, followed by a decelerating rate of improvement that eventually reaches a plateau or asymptote (Figure 1.10). In projecting such recovery curves, one considers the natural history of

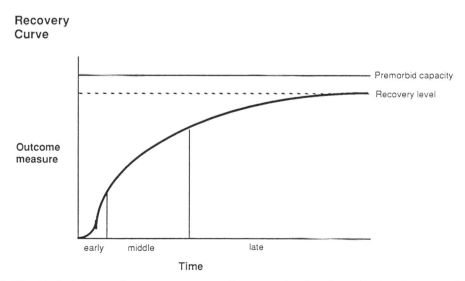

Figure 1.10 *Typical shape of a recovery curve with an accelerating then decelerating rate of improvement that reaches a plateau or asymptote at or below premorbid level.*

the disorder and particular issues of severity, time post-onset, and other elements in that patient. In evaluating a patient's impairments, it is essential to consider where the patient is on the curve (early, middle, or late phase) and what clinical phenomena are expected at different stages of recovery along the curve.

There are several factors that may distort these recovery curves. Clearly, with increasing severity, the course of recovery is more prolonged and the expected outcome is diminished. (Figure 1.11) The distribution of the lesion may be critically important, not only for clinical presentation as already discussed, but for recovery. Again, small differences in lesion location, affecting one or more distributed functional networks, can have a major impact on recovery. Another factor that alters the recovery curve is the complexity of the function measured. Recovery curves for less demanding tasks will tend to plateau earlier, while more complex ones may demonstrate a more protracted course (Figure 1.12).

The pathologic process also affects the course of recovery. Two patients with the same impairment profile (phenotype) at a given time post injury may have a very different course of recovery depending on the underlying neuropathologic process (genotype). For instance, patients with focal traumatic brain injury have a more rapid, but less complete recovery than patients with diffuse injury for similar impairments in a particular function, (e.g., frontal lobe functions or hemiparesis) (Figure 1.13). Hemorrhagic and ischemic lesions of similar size and distribution with similar early clinical effects may have different recovery curves. In general a patient with a hemorrhagic lesion has a better prognosis if, as the hemorrhage is resorbed, it leaves a smaller residual lesion.

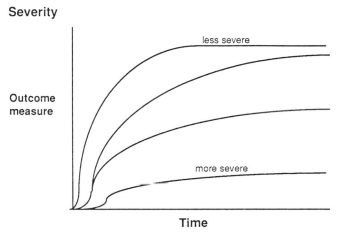

Figure 1.11   *Recovery curves vary with severity of the injury: the less severe the injury, the faster the recovery.*

Task Difficulty

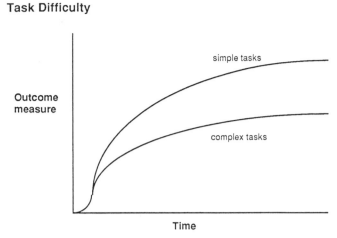

Figure 1.12   *Recovery as a function of task difficulty. Recovery on simpler tasks occurs at a faster rate than for complex tasks.*

Focal vs. diffuse

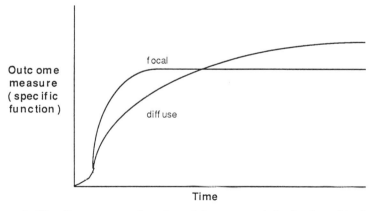

Figure 1.13   *Recovery as a function of the type and distribution of brain damage (e.g. focal vs. diffuse). Recovery occurs more quickly with focal pathology than diffuse pathology (after TBI). Patients with diffuse pathology from TBI may have a more protracted recovery, eventually achieving similar or better levels of recovery than patients with focal injury.*

Finally, age is another well-recognized factor that has a negative influence on the course of recovery, with older age groups demonstrating slower progression toward improvement and poorer outcome at its completion (Figure 1.14).

Age

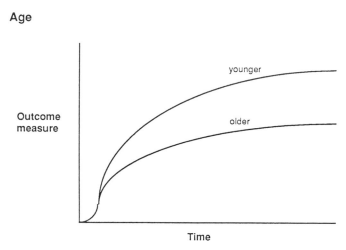

Outcome
measure

younger

older

Time

Figure 1.14 *Recovery as a function of age. In general, younger patients recover faster than older patients with the same severity of injury.*

CONCLUSION

In conclusion, the neurologic model of rehabilitation proposes fundamental changes to current rehabilitative practice. Changes that center on the natural history of a disorder or a disease process dictate treatment, rather than the converse. The remaining chapters will develop these constructs and provide clinical examples that demonstrate its application in various rehabilitative settings.

References

1. Carpenter MB. Human neuroanatomy. Baltimore: Williams & Wilkins, 1976.
2. MacLean PD. A triune concept of the brain and behavior. Toronto: University of Toronto Press, 1973.
3. Langman J. Medical embryology. 3rd ed. Baltimore: Williams & Wilkins, 1975.
4. Moruzzi G, Magoun HW. Brainstem reticular formation and activation of the EEG. Electroencephalogr Clin Neurophysiol 1949;1:455–473.
5. Azmitia ED. The CNS serotonergic system: progression toward a collaborative organization. In: Meltzer HY, ed. Psychopharmacology, the third generation of progress. New York: Raven Press, 1987:61–73.

6. Janowsky A, Sulser F. Alpha and beta adrenoreceptors in brain. In: Meltzer HY, ed. Psychopharmacology, the third generation of progress. New York: Raven Press, 1987:249–256.

7. Creese I. Biochemical properties of CNS dopamine receptors. In: Meltzer HY, ed. Psychopharmacology, the third generation of progress. New York: Raven Press, 1987:257–264.

8. Broca P. Anatomic comparee circonvolutions cerebrates. Le grad lobe limbique et la scissure limbique dans la serie des mammiferes. Rev Anthopol 1978;1:384–498.

9. Dikmen S, Machamer J, Temkin N, McLean A. Neuropsychological recovery in patients with moderate to severe head injury: 2 year follow-up. J Clin Exp Neuropsychol 1990;12:507–519.

10. Alexander MP, Naeser MA, Palumbo CL. Correlations of subcortical CT lesion sites and aphasia profiles. Brain 1987;110:961–991.

Medical, Neurologic, and Functional Outcome of Stroke Survivors

Michael P. Alexander

This chapter is intended to provide clinicians in stroke rehabilitation with a guide to anticipating the rate and extent of natural recovery of neurologic deficits after stroke, but some expansion of the purpose will also provide some helpful context for clinical management. The Appendix to this chapter has a synopsis of definitions of causes and types of stroke for the novice reader.

Patients who have survived a stroke for 1 week have four distinct horizons in front of them. The first horizon is medical. Most stroke survivors are elderly, and the occurence of a stroke strikingly reduces likely subsequent life span. Some patients with severe vascular disease may have high probability of recurrent stroke or heart disease. A practical rehabilitation plan aims to move directly to considerations to improve quickly the quality of life when medical prognosis is poor.

The second horizon is neurologic: To what extent do neurologic deficits improve, with or without treatment? A realistic rehabilitation plan recognizes constraints produced by deficits that are permanent.

The third horizon is functional: For any given residual deficit profile, we attempt to bring a patient to functional independence. The view of this horizon often determines whether patients get home. Improving function is, in many ways, the product of rehabilitation programs. It is what we measure, attempt to predict, and hope translates into a better quality of life. We have little or no evidence to tell us which services that we provide are most critical for functional improvement. A modern rehabilitation program will measure improvement across as many dimensions as possible and document the cost-efficiency of producing improvement.

The fourth horizon is quality of life after survival. At present, we know that improving function has a high probability of allowing discharge home, and we know that home discharge, as opposed to nursing home discharge, increases quality of life. Beyond that linkage, rehabilitation has no direct therapeutic influence on an individual patient's quality of life, but a sympathetic rehabilitation program will always set patient goals and measure their own accomplishments by focusing on this horizon, no matter how distant.

To meet the primary goal of this chapter and also the stretched goals of context, there are three sections to follow. First is a brief summary of the mortality and morbidity expectations of stroke survivors, considered in aggregate and in various clinical subsets. Second is a lengthier, but still skeletal, review of the prevalence rates, recovery profiles, and, in some cases, treatments of the individual neurologic deficits common after stroke. Finally, there is a brief consideration of the contribution to understanding recovery when patients are characterized by syndromes or by their computed tomography and magnetic resonance imaging (CT/MRI) lesions.

MORTALITY, MORBIDITY, AND FUNCTION IN STROKE SURVIVORS

Analyses of consecutive stroke cases to determine vascular subtype are quite common. Outcome measures, however, are usually limited to recurrence of stroke and mortality. It is uncertain if specification of stroke subtype carries much prognostic information about the level of function of survivors. On the other hand, knowledge of recurrence rates has direct practical importance for construction of rehabilitation programs.

Acute mortality (<28 days after stroke) can only be established in studies that enter patients from first medical contact, and mortality will be influenced by population demographics. Several large series from the United States and Europe report an overall acute mortality of at least 20% (1–3). Mortality is highly related to stoke etiology. Patients with intracerebral hemorrhages have the highest acute mortality (30%) and that mortality correlates with intraventricular rupture of blood on acute CT and with hemorrhage size (1). Lacunar infarcts have essentially no acute mortality. For the remainder (nonlacunar) of ischemic lesions, mortality is related to infarct size, with alteration of consciousness being a particularly bad acute prognostic sign (3). Acute mortality of nonlacunar ischemic stroke is approximately 15%, and cumulative mortality is approximately 30% at 1 year. The common causes of late mortality are recurrent stroke and myocardial infarction.

The risks of recurrent stroke are also related to etiology of the first stroke. Acute noniatrogenic recurrence (<30 days) is seen in approximately 2% of cases, but early recurrence is greatest after initial atherothrombotic stroke (2) and least for lacunar stroke (4). A potential cardioembolic source may be a particularly high risk for early recurrence. The risk of recurrent stroke in patients with nonrheumatic atrial fibrillation is 1% each day for the first 20 days (5).

By 3 months post onset, the overall risk of recurrence among survivors is approximately 5%, and the presence of a cardioembolic source carries the highest risk. By 2 years post onset the cumulative risk of recurrence among survivors is 14%, and risk is greatest in patients whose initial stroke was atherothrombotic (2). The clinical predictors of recurrent stroke are hypertension, diabetes, and an abnormal electrocardiogram (ECG), but even together they are only modestly precise predictors. The Stroke Data Bank investigators concluded that because the general, multifactorial risk of recurrent stroke is so high after first stroke, no single risk profile will have much predictive power (6).

An additional complication in calculations of recurrence and of the effect of stroke type on functional outcome is the occurrence of "silent strokes" (7). Because they are "silent," the incidence is not known. In the Framingham study, 10% of patients presenting with a clinical first stroke had CT evidence of prior, "silent" stroke. The "silent" strokes were an equal mix of capsulostriatal lacunar lesions and small cortical strokes. In a large autopsy series, 6% of brains had lacunar infarctions, and over 50% of the brains with lacunes had more than one; only 15% to 26% of the first lacunes had been symptomatic (4). These "silent" lesions probably are major contributors to multi-infarct dementia and may be factors in unexpectedly poor functional improvement.

Finally, it must be recognized that clinical metrics to establish a definitive stroke type are not terribly strong. Despite impressive efforts to establish broadly inclusive criteria for specific stroke types, 40% of the cases entered in the Stroke Data Bank were considered infarctions of unknown cause. Two very focused assessments of agreement (and presumably reliability) of clinical diagnosis of stroke subtype offer little encouragement that the diagnosis is certain enough to carry broad predictive power (8). Given only history and examination data, agreement will be low. Given all clinical data (ECG, carotid noninvasives, CT/MRI, etc.) agreement is substantial but not certain enough to use as a predictive variable.

In summary, stroke subtype information and vascular risk factors do provide coarse predictive capacity about mortality and recurrence. Any sensible rehabilitation system should consider medical prognosis with current functional status and *functional* prognosis to establish plans for treatment type and treatment intensity. For most patients (at least 60%), precise stroke etiology can be established (8). Even if vascular etiology is unclear, coarse prognostic distinctions certainly exist between patients who might all have comparable hemiparesis but some from a small single lacune, some from a large lenticulostriate infarct, and some from a larger cortical-subcortical infarct. Lesion etiology is critical for expectations of mortality and recurrence, but distinctions between anatomic locations and lesion sizes are critical for functional outcome, whatever the lesion etiology. Medical prognoses are always actuarial, that is, there is a 14% risk of recurrence over 2 years in a *group* of patients (5). Functional prognosis may be much more individualized; that is, lesions of a particular size, in a particular location, in a patient with particular prior neurologic events may have a specific functional prognosis (1).

PREVALENCE AND RECOVERY OF SPECIFIC NEUROLOGIC DEFICITS

Rehabilitation programs focus on correction and compensation of functional impairments based on the presumption that improved function leads to less disability and less handicap. Functional impairments after stroke are caused by neurologic deficits and their interactions, and much of the treatment in rehabilitation actually aims at the deficit as much as or more than at the functional impairment. Thus, patients receive therapy aimed at reducing deficits in arm power, balance, visual neglect, auditory comprehension, etc. Everyone involved in these therapeutic endeavors should have a clear understanding of the probabilities of improvements; that is, the natural history of recovery of deficits with treatment should be known. There are two reasons why every clinician should have this information at her or his fingertips: 1) patients and families will want to know the prognosis of the deficit—"Will he ever (talk, understand, walk, move his arm, etc)?" and 2) addressing functional deficits requires realistic assessment of how much any underlying deficit is likely to improve. This section will provide estimates assembled from the extensive literature on recovery that can guide clinicians' expectations for treatment. All studies reviewed were from rehabilitation centers, so the recovery figures cited assume adequate treatment of any deficit. Notice that this assumption does not mean that there is any proof that "adequate treatment" influences recovery from basic neurologic impairment.

For all of the deficits reviewed, there are important methodologic issues. If a study is community-based, it will include mild cases that might not come to a tertiary hospital center. If a study is hospital-based, there are admission biases that make conclusions only partly suitable for generalization. If a study begins with stroke onset, there will be large numbers of deaths and large numbers of good outcomes with minimal impairment. If a study begins with admission to rehabilitation, there will be a much narrower range of outcomes, the deaths and minimal deficit cases never entering the study. The most informative studies are community-based and come from Europe. Nevertheless, an American clinician can focus on the middle range of those studies to form an image of the typical rehabilitation population.

Another problem with this review is the necessity of surveying studies that have used dramatically different assessment tools. If one study has two levels of outcome—walks or doesn't walk—and another study has seven levels of outcome—walks, doesn't walk, and five grades of walks with assistance—how are the studies added together?

A corollary effect of the type of study is a difference in time post onset that the initial assessment is made. If the examination that sets baseline impairment is done in the first few days, subsequent assessments of recovery will demonstrate much greater improvement than if the initial evaluation is performed 2 to 3 weeks after onset. Thus, in all studies, time post onset of initial assessment and initial severity will have potent effects on the apparent "natural" history and on the possible effects of any treatment. Despite all of these impediments to interpretations of the literature, all of the major impairments of stroke are open to rough sketches of natural history with predictive, prescriptive, and even proscriptive lessons.

Ambulation

Impaired walking is both a deficit state and a functional problem. Stroke can damage brain mechanisms for ambulation (deficit state), but stroke can also cause leg weakness or ataxia—(deficit state) that secondarily disrupt walking (the functional disturbance). All studies of ambulation can be viewed, however, as tabulations of the prevalence of impaired walking at any point post stroke, thus providing a nearly natural history of recovery rates.

Approximately 30% to 40% of patients diagnosed with a stroke (but remember the "silent" strokes) can walk independently at the outset of symptoms (9). A small number will worsen and become nonambulatory. The majority either have small strokes with rapid recovery or large strokes in nonmotor portions of the brain. They typically present with visual, cognitive, or behavioral signs. Most will not be referred to inpatient rehabilitation units.

The group of patients unable to walk at outset includes more patients with large strokes. This group has a high mortality (at least 33%), and approximately 50% of survivors will not be able to walk even at the end of a typical intensive rehabilitation hospitalization (9). Furthermore, few patients not ambulatory at discharge will walk even with ongoing out-patient therapy.

There are several easily applied clinical predictors. Survivors who could not walk at all on admission have only a 15% probability of *independent* walking after rehabilitation (9). Survivors who could take a few steps with assistance at admission have a 60% probability of independent walking and nearly a 100% probability of walking at least with assistance. Patients with hemiplegia, hemisensory loss, and hemianopia (or cognitive deficits) as opposed to just one or two of those deficits at 1 month after stroke have only a 3% probability of independent ambulation at discharge from rehab (10). There are three potent correlates of retained or recovered walking: independent sitting balance, leg power, and wheelchair maneuverability. Patients who cannot maintain independent sitting balance will not walk independently even if leg power and cognition are normal. Proximal leg power is absolutely necessary, but not sufficient, to regain walking. Very few severely weak stroke patients can even manage to ambulate with a long leg brace. For patients unable to walk 3 weeks after a stroke, inability to maneuver a wheelchair 30 feet down a corridor 6 feet wide, through a $4^1/_2$ foot doorway, and then turn around and reverse the course has an almost perfect correlation with failure to regain walking (11).

Numerous studies have demonstrated that recovery of independent ambulation, if it occurs, will occur in the first few months (9,12). Some studies suggest that 95% of walking will be accomplished as early as 11 weeks after stroke. Others have found no increase in the proportion of survivors that can walk after 2 months post stroke. No studies suggest that routine therapy will increase the number of independent ambulators after 6 months post stroke. Very intensive and prolonged therapy might increase the percentage of patients able to walk short distances.

Arm Paresis

Several features of motor recovery of the arm are known (13–17):

1. Functional recovery of the arm is highly correlated with the *initial* deficits in power and tone.
2. Arms that will eventually be well recovered begin recovery quickly, perhaps within 48 hours, and recovery is well established by 7 days.
3. At least two thirds of the good recoveries will occur by 4 weeks.
4. Most recovery occurs within 6 weeks although statistically significant changes occur up to 3 months.
5. For patients with severe weakness at 1 to 2 weeks, no more than 2% will be completely recovered at 3 months although 15% will have enough recovery that the arm is functional.

6. As many as 20% to 40% of arms impaired at 3 months will show continued functional improvement up to 1 year, but no changes in neurologic capacity are seen.
7. For patients with severely impaired arms, over 95% will show spasticity at some time in the course. As recovery progresses, spasticity decreases.
8. Even patients with arms that have full return of power may have reduced dexterity.
9. Functional capacity of the arm is correlated with power *and* sensation (18). Barthel scores correlate with both arm power and functional dexterity.

The neural mechanisms of recovery are unknown. Good recovery is not simply return to prestroke functional relationships (19). There is physiologic evidence that even well recovered hands achieve recovery through entirely novel neural reorganizations (20). There is no evidence that any specific program of treatment is particularly efficacious in accelerating or extending recovery. Whatever school of treatment is used (facilitation, reeducation, electromyogram [EMG] biofeedback, etc.), recovery is the same. The best predictors of arm function are initial severity and time post onset of testing (14). It is possible that more intense therapy does facilitate better recovery in patients with initially milder paresis, but probably not in severe cases.

Sensory Recovery

There are many fewer studies of the course of recovery of sensation than of power, perhaps because of the difficulty of objective assessment. One study suggested that recovery, if it occurs, will be within 2 months, but the assessment was quite coarse (21). Other studies have demonstrated that persistent sensory loss is a bad prognostic sign for recovery of arm function.

Visual Fields

Presumably because of the difficulty of assessment of visual fields in patients with aphasia, confusion, or obtundation, there are few studies of the evolution of visual field deficits. One attempt, using only coarse confrontation fields and not attempting to distinguish between field loss and neglect, reached two interesting conclusions (22). Fields were first examined 3 days post stroke in 149 patients. Of 81 patients with complete hemianopia, 50% were dead at 1 month. Among survivors, recovery of normal visual fields had occurred by 10 to 14 days post stroke if it was going to occur. A much more elegant study by Zihl and von Cramon complements that finding (23). Very thorough perimetry and visual field mapping was performed in 55 patients with deficits at 2 weeks post onset. When testing was repeated 3 weeks later, only four cases had shown any improvement. Delayed follow-up at least 9 weeks post stroke demonstrated *no* further improvement.

Recovery of visual neglect has been investigated somewhat more intensively than visual field defects, but variation in neglect measures selected makes a comprehensive summary of the literature difficult. Furthermore, there is not complete theoretical agreement about the elements of comprehensive assessment of neglect.

Few investigations begin with comprehensive assessment in the acute stage. One study compared the rate of recovery in neglect after left or right hemisphere lesions (n = 68) first examined 3 days after onset with a battery of six tasks (24). They found the most rapid recovery occurred in the next 7 days for lesions of either hemisphere. Continued recovery from 10 days to 3 months post onset was significant but less striking. Persistent severe neglect was uncommon (only 8 [24%] of 34 patients with right sided strokes). All of their test instruments were equally effective. Another study examined patients (n = 41) within 7 days of onset, but much less objectively. They also found that improvement continued until approximately 4 months post onset, but they made the additional observation that sparing of the frontal lobe was correlated with faster recovery of neglect (25,26).

If most recovery is early, then studies that commence at admission to rehabilitation will not find as much improvement and may find a high incidence of neglect. An analysis of the evolution of numerous neurologic and functional deficits from rehabilitation admission to 12 weeks later (unknown time post onset) in a small group of patients (n = 31) found the following (27). The neglect assessment was limited, but 8 (57%) of 14 patients with right stroke had visual neglect. All improvement occurred within 4 weeks of admission. There was no significant improvement from 4 weeks to 12 weeks, but in a subsequent long-term report on 28 of the cases, 50% were said to show some additional improvement. This was one of many reports to demonstrate that neglect has a significant negative correlation with ADL measures at every stage of rehabilitation. Denes and colleagues measured neglect at rehab admission (n = 48), on average 8 weeks post onset, and then in follow-up 2 months and 4 months later (28). Visual neglect was found in 8 (28%) of 29 patients with right sided strokes, but showed improvement in only 1 of those 8 at follow-up. Neglect was a major factor in poor restitution of independent ADLs.

In summary, unilateral visual neglect is common after large right brain strokes. It apparently recovers quickly in most patients and, if still present, at 1 to 2 months post onset, is not likely to improve greatly thereafter. Persistence of hemianopia (either side) or unilateral left neglect both have negative implications for functional recovery. For hemianopia, this probably reflects lesion size. For neglect, the poor prognosis may be due to implications for capacity to perform ADLs.

Treatment of visual field defects has only rarely been suggested. Zihl has demonstrated that functional fields can be increased through drills that focus on visual attention and simple signal detection (22).

On the other hand, several programs have been proposed for treatment of neglect. Most require teaching patients explicit verbally mediated strategies of search and scanning. Patients can learn the strategies and seem to improve, but the specifity of treatments is unknown.

Continence

Among hospitalized patients with stroke, approximately 50% will be incontinent of urine 1 week post onset (29). As a group, the incontinent patients will be older and have more severe neurologic deficits (30). If they have left brain strokes, they will be more aphasic. Whichever hemisphere is involved, they will have more cognitive deficits. At 1 month post onset, approximately 35% of survivors will still be incontinent. This figure continues to drop to a lowest frequency of 14% at 6 months (30). The best predictors of eventual continence are age <70, mild motor deficits, and clear mental status in the first week post onset (31). Patients with persistent incontinence are those with severe initial incontinence and persistent abnormal mental state. They also have had severe strokes and are the most impaired in ADLs.

There seem to be two mechanisms of incontinence. In many patients, it is due to profound impairment in mobility and communication of need. In others, it is due to a basic neurourologic deficit, usually detrusor hyperreflexia. This mechanism is readily recognized with cystometrogram and may be treated with anticholinergic medication.

When incontinence is used as an independent variable, it serves as a powerful predictor of outcome (29). Patients incontinent at 1 week are much likelier to die or to be profoundly impaired in ADLs at 6 months post stroke. The predictive power is true for men and women and for all ages. Continence usually precedes functional independence.

Fecal incontinence is present in 31% of patients with hemiparetic stroke at some point in the first 2 weeks (30). It is seen almost exclusively in patients with severe deficits in mobility and communication of need to toilet (cognitive or aphasic). Persistent fecal incontinence at 2 weeks is correlated with left hemiparesis and bilateral Babinski's signs.

Aphasia

Of patients with acute stroke, approximately 25% are aphasic (32). Of patients who survive the first few days and who are conscious and assessable, 33% are aphasic. At 6 months post onset, at least 20% of survivors are aphasic, divided evenly among severe and mild cases (33).

Of patients with aphasia at 1 month post onset, 33% to 50% will remain substantially aphasic at 6 months and 25% at 1 year. Initial severity predicts long-term severity (34,35).

The most common aphasia syndrome at onset is global aphasia (36). Most global aphasias improve rapidly and over time tend toward persistent severe nonfluent aphasias (either global or Broca) or anomic aphasia of no specificity (35,37). The *patterns* of recovery are reasonably predictable. Patients with severe nonfluent aphasia at 1 month overwhelmingly stay severely nonfluent although they may improve somewhat. Milder nonfluent patients become fluent, usually within a few weeks. Recovery of comprehension is fastest over the first few months, but may continue for at least 1 year (35,38).

The patterns of recovery are partly constrained by lesion site and lesion size. The constraints are all on probabilities of recovery and are not absolute predictors. Two examples suffice. First, recovery of some, even telegraphic, speech output is unlikely if the lesion includes extensive damage to the deep periventricular white matter extending up into the supraventricular white matter including the anterior callosal region. Second, recovery of auditory comprehension is unlikely if all of the posterior superior temporal gyrus is damaged, and the white matter deep to it or the adjacent temporoparietal cortex are also damaged. If incompletely damaged, overall recovery of comprehension is most rapid in the first 3 to 4 months and then slows dramatically.

Despite considerable investigation, the value of specific treatment of aphasia is still uncertain. Most, but not all, group studies have demonstrated some overall value to language therapy (39–41). In some, the methodology is unconvincing—unspecified treatments, noncomparable control groups, and an apparent need for many months of therapy before an effect is seen (40). Other studies have suggested that language therapy is useful but need not be delivered by highly trained therapists (41). In group studies that have failed to demonstrate a benefit of therapy, the patients did not receive much therapy (42,43). All of these studies are of heterogeneous groups, and even when therapy types are specified, there is little control over actual therapies utilized. Perhaps only a subset of the therapies are effective in a subset of the patients. In other investigations, smaller, more homogeneous groups or single patients are given specific, usually theoretically driven, treatments. These studies are quite convincing that language can be stimulated and improved, even if only narrowly, but it remains unclear how much the narrow areas of improvement generalize in natural language settings.

When aphasia becomes an independent variable in outcome studies, several potent consequences are noted for patient and family. Few previously employed patients with aphasia manage any return to work. Those who do remain dependent, in part, on others to work and remain reduced in capacity. Furthermore, even those who return to work are frequently socially isolated. Compared to other stroke survivors, aphasic patients have particular reduction in social contacts. They also have more marital problems (44). Spouses of aphasic patients report more loneliness, boredom, and decreased sexual satisfaction than spouses of nonaphasics. These changes are equally true of husbands or wives of survivors. Almost 50% of spouses are depressed, and problems seem to increase over time post onset. Depression in the aphasic patients themselves is very common; this is addressed in the section on depression.

Apraxia

The methodologic variability in the study of apraxia has been so extreme over the past 10 years that it is virtually impossible to reach any overall conclusions. For purposes of this review, only limb (actually arm) apraxia will considered. *Ideomotor apraxia* is the inability to carry out familiar actions (e.g., waving, combing) in response to a stimulus that should elicit the correct movement (i.e., being told to wave or to comb, or being shown through gesture to wave or to comb). *Ideational apraxia* is the further inability even to use the implements (e.g., comb) correctly. Ideomotor apraxia is frequent (approximately 50% incidence) after large left brain lesions (45). Ideational apraxia is less common and, again, only after large left brain lesions (46). Large parietal lesions are the most common anatomic correlate of ideomotor apraxia and ideational apraxia, but ideomotor apraxia apparently has a more distributed neural basis, as lesions of deep central structures (corona radiata) are also likely to cause ideomotor apraxia (47). Ideomotor apraxia has a high co-occurence with (but is *not* caused by) aphasia and right hemiparesis. Ideational apraxia also has a high co-occurence with both agraphia and spatial deficits.

Both ideomotor apraxia and ideational apraxia have obvious implications for recovery and particularly for restitution or remediation of ADLs. There is, however, remarkably little known about the natural history of recovery of apraxia. One small, but systematic study demonstrated the high frequency of recovery but not the precise time course (45). From the first examination at 2 to 4 weeks post onset (coincidentally, at about the time of admission to rehabilitation in this country) to 5 months post onset, 50% of the patients with ideomotor apraxia recovered. With continued follow-up, over 50% of the remainder also recovered. Recovery is likelier if left parietal regions are partially spared. There is no correlation of recovery of ideomotor apraxia with recovery of aphasia (47). Ideomotor apraxia is primarily a problem for therapists and nurses who may mistake as comprehension impairment a patient's failure to do some requested action. Most patients with ideomotor apraxia actually use objects correctly in context. There are, however, no existing treatment models or programs of any recorded validity.

Rate of recovery of ideational apraxia is unknown. It may be apparent as long as 3 years after stroke. In many patients, ideational apraxia may be a critical impediment to recovery of ADLs, but no report based on sound definitions has proposed any compensatory or treatment strategies.

Disorders of Cognition and Mood After Stroke

A review of this topic would be virtually a review of twentieth century behavioral neurology. Patients with stroke have been the medium in which almost all current knowledge of brain-behavior relationships has been painted. Regional brain damage, whether cortical or subcortical, has quite specific consequences for cognitive function. These cognitive impairments appear to have substantial impact on self-care and subsequent functional independence when they involve language and hemispatial neglect (reviewed above). Other and less common focal cognitive impairments have self-evident domain specific effects on function. Left occipital damage causes alexia and thus work, school, and recreational problems. Frontal damage causes impaired problem solving and thus finances, work, and unsupervised living problems and so on. This is not the setting to review the numerous claims on focal brain regions for specific cognitive operations.

Memory Deficit

Substantial memory deficit would be, however, one cognitive deficit with profound implications for independent function. Persistent severe amnesia has been reported after bilateral anterolateral thalamic infarcts, bilateral medial temporal (hippocampi, parahippocampal gyri, enterorhinal regions, retrosplenial gyri, or white matter of collateral sulcus) infarcts, and bilateral basal forebrain infarcts (usually after anterior communicating artery aneurysm rupture). Unilateral left-sided infarcts in any of those regions may also produce substantial functional memory difficulties. Otherwise, the side of damage is correlated with predominantly verbal (left) or nonverbal (right) memory deficits. Learning impairments have been demonstrated in up to 40% of stroke survivors (aphasics excluded) at least 3 months post onset, but the possible causes of these problems are numerous and not well elucidated (48). There is, however, an obviously high potential prevalence of disabling memory problems in stroke survivors. Treatment would require clarification of underlying mechanisms. There is no evidence that severe amnesia can be treated by any direct rehabilitation strategy. Milder memory problems may be managed by establishing systems of compensatory reminders.

Dementia

Dementia is a pervasive decline in mental abilities, not restricted to a single cognitive domain (e.g., aphasia, amnesia). Many stroke survivors meet strict criteria for dementia. Most patients with left-sided stroke, for instance, in addition to aphasia, may have apraxia, may have constructional deficits, and surely have verbal memory problems. Nonetheless, it is customary to restrict the diagnosis of vascular dementia to patients who are not made aphasic by stroke. One mechanism for vascular dementia is straightforward: patients with bilateral large strokes, particularly in temperoparietal regions. The other causes of vascular dementia are less clinically obvious: frontal strokes only or small, deep strokes only (Figure 2.1). Stroke as the cause of dementia can be easily overlooked or mistaken as the dementia of the Alzheimer's type (DAT) in a predominantly elderly population in some clinical settings.

Patients with multiple lacunar infarcts have a high prevalence of dementia when seen for stroke and a high risk of developing dementia (over 20%) with follow-up at 4 years (49). Because lacunar lesions are most common in capsular-striatal regions, the dementia profile is dominated by "frontal" features and is associated with frontal changes on metabolic imaging studies. The commonly used brief screens for dementia are not as sensitive to frontal deficit profiles as they are to language, spatial, and memory deficits. This confusion between frontal *deficit patterns*, frontal (and striatal) *systems*, and actual frontal *lesions* underlies some of the controversy about the dementia diagnosis.

Depression

There is a high incidence of depression after stroke. A summary of 11 investigations reveals 388 (36%) of 1078 patients experienced depression after stroke. This is higher than the frequencies of visual impairments, aphasia, apraxia, amnesia, and dysphagia. When specifically indicated, this number is approximately equally split between major and mild depression (50,51). The frequency is equal for right- and left-sided strokes (52), although there may be a higher proportion of severe depression in the left sided cases, particularly with deep frontal lesions (53). No other demographic or neurologic factor correlates consistently with depression.

Whatever the anatomy, depression does have consequences beyond those of the stroke on patients' recovery. While not a universal finding, most reports have found that depression after stroke is correlated with greater deficits in motor function and ADLs. Of even greater concern has been the observation that when patients with depression are discharged from rehabilitation, their functional status may decline in the

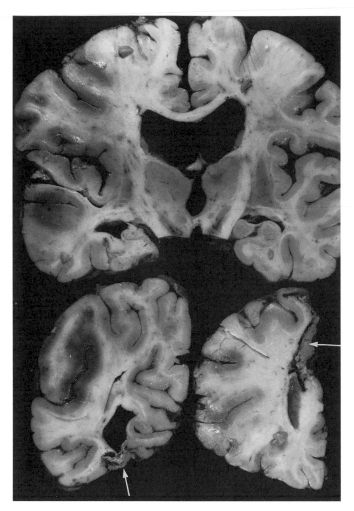

Figure 2.1   Cerebral hemisphere slices from a case of multi-infarct dementia. Old infarcts (arrowed) are present in the left superior frontal gyrus (below right) and left fusiform gyrus (below left). There is also ischemic atrophy of the left hippocampus (top), and a terminal infarct in territory supplied by the left middle cerebral artery. Lateral ventricles are dilated. (Reprinted from Esiri MM, Oppenheimer DR. Diagnostic neuropathology: a practical manual. Oxford: Blackwell Scientific, 1989:268.)

next several weeks (52). The direction of causality is not, however, always clear. Are depressed patients more impaired functionally because they are depressed or are they depressed because they are more impaired? In one report the correlation of mood with functional capacity was as robust as those for lesion size or mental status. After discharge, patients who were depressed had declining mental state scores for up to 6 months, while other patients' scores improved. This suggests that, at least in part, depression contributes to functional impairment. The impact of depression may be more telling on left-sided stroke patients (54). When controlled for lesions, depressed patients with left brain damage are more impaired on tests of language and verbal memory than nondepressed patients with left brain damage and all patients with right brain damage. Depression may be a different disorder when it complicates left-sided lesions.

Diagnosis of depression in this population is difficult. There are methodologic obstacles to use of standard depression questionnaires in this population. Many of the behavioral items, and even vegetative symptoms, are invalidated by physical infirmity. Severe aphasia precludes detailed interviews, and all of the surveys summarized above excluded severe aphasics. Right-sided strokes with anosognosia may leave patients unaware of their own emotional state. One comprehensive comparison (55) of the validity of various diagnostic instruments concludes that the Zung has the highest overall usefulness in the geriatric stroke population (56). This test cannot be given to patients with severe aphasia, so staff observations and an external rater may be required for those patients. It is probably correct to assume that fearfulness, withdrawal, and resistant behaviors are adequate diagnostic markers for major depression in the population with global or Wernicke's aphasia.

Whatever the uncertainties of diagnosis and anatomy and even of the neurobiology of depression in stroke, the consequences of depression on function seem to require that patients should be referred for possible treatment, but treatment seems to be rarely considered. A retrospective review of all stroke admissions to one rehabilitation hospital over 10 years revealed that only 5% had had a psychiatric referral! At most, only 30% of clearly depressed patients receive referrals for treatment even when hospitalized; particularly few depressed outpatients seem to be offered treatment.

As the neurobiology of depression after stroke might include damage to the brain regions critical for response to drug treatment of depression, it cannot be assumed that treatment of depressed patients with brain damage is informed by the literature in patients without brain damage. There is, however, little evidence from the stroke literature demonstrating unequivocal response to medication. Studies carried out at rehabilitation centers have been too methodologically flawed to illuminate the value of treatment. In a small double-blind, placebo-controlled study with nortriptyline, the treated group was better than the placebo group on every depression measure and on measures of ADL independence and social functions (58). In the drug-treated group, there was a 30% dropout rate due to side effects including several cases of agitated delirium, always reversible with cessation of drug. The peripheral anticholinergic side effects of many antidepressants are also frequently limiting in this population. Recent reports indicate that new serotonin-specific reuptake inhibitors may be effective for poststroke depression (59). Clinical experience suggests precipitation of agitated states may be a limiting factor in use of these drugs.

NEUROLOGIC SYNDROMES AND OUTCOME

Even if stroke etiology cannot be successfully used as a functional prognostic indicator, it remains possible that there are specific clusters of neurologic signs—presumably representing specific regional damage—that do illuminate the prognosis. In part, this is a trivial supposition and is discussed throughout the prior sections. For instance, the syndrome of global aphasia with right hemiplegia clearly has a worse prognosis than the syndrome of conduction aphasia with no hemiparesis. Any measure—initial ADLs, CT lesion size, or neurologic findings—would differentiate the prognosis for these two patient groups. It is unknown if functional outcome is satisfactorily predicted by coarse groupings.

In one study from England of 137 acute strokes, patients were classified by neurologic deficits rather than functional deficits; that is, as hemiparesis alone, hemiparesis and hemianopia, cognitive alone, hemiparesis and cognitive, and so on, irrespective of side of lesion (60). The outcome measures were an overall functional rating and a coarse division of transfer status at 6 months post onset. Not surprisingly, patients with the combination of hemiparesis, hemianopia, and cognitive deficits did much worse than those with hemiparesis alone or cognitive deficits (probably largely aphasias) alone.

Similar relationships emerge from U.S. studies (10). Of patients with only motor deficits, 90% had independent ADLs and were ambulating by 14 weeks. For patients with both motor and sensory deficits, only 80% were ambulating and only 25% were independent in ADLs. Among patients with motor, sensory, *and* visual field impairments, only 45% were ambulating at 14 weeks and only 2% had independent ADLs. It is likely that these neurologic differences were accompanied by CT lesion size differences, by different prevalence of cognitive deficits, and by different initial functional measures. Thus, it is not clear that this type of principled neurologic cluster adds anything to prognosis beyond the functional assessment.

Neither of these approaches considers side of stroke, and finer grained analyses may provide more specific functional predictions (61). In a study of 226 admissions to a rehabilitation service, patients were classified into one of 11 clinical syndromes, respecting side of hemiparesis and lateralized specifics of the cognitive deficits. The outcome measure was ADL function. Patients with pure left hemiparesis did the best, and patients with left hemiparesis plus spatial/constructional deficits did the worst. Patients with left temperoparietal ("fluent") aphasias did well; those with right parietal spatial/neglect syndrome did not.

The overall impression drawn from these few studies is that clustered neurologic findings will have reasonable prognostic value, but it remains unclear if these coarse clusters have better prognostic power than functional measures. It is likely that they are interchangeable because patients with hemiparesis, hemisensory loss, and cognitive deficits *or* visual field deficits will certainly have larger lesions and worse ADL function than those who have only one or two of those problems.

If identification of different neurologic profiles (regardless of stroke type) has prognostic information, distinct CT profiles may have similar predictive power, regardless of stroke type. There are, however, few convincing data on this question.

One study from Denmark claimed that the only correlation between acute CT lesion site and mortality was that involvement of the temporal lobe increased mortality (62). The authors offered no plausible explanation for this finding. Furthermore, lesion location was done in a crude manner, which, it was unfairly suggested, represented a "rehabilitation point-of-view." When CT lesion site and size are added to other independent variables, they seem to add essentially no predictive power about functional outcome. Nevertheless, all functional outcome measures show a significant negative correlation with lesion size.

Two studies have analyzed CT's value in prognosis of functional outcome for rehabilitation admissions. In one study of 40 infarcts, CT was performed at some point after the first few days, lesions were classified as large or small, cortical or deep, and outcome was ADL status at 6 months, either good or bad (63). Cases with normal CT or small cortical lesions had nearly uniform good outcome; patients with large deep lesions did badly. In the other study of 41 mixed strokes, CT was performed at various times in the acute illness. Lesions were classified as large, medium, small, or absent (64). Lesion site was grossly specified, and outcome was ADL status at discharge in three categories. In a multiple regression analysis, both lesion size and site were significant, but the main two independent variables to emerge with predictive power were initial ADL status and patient age. Only two examples are provided. One CT shows a partly resolved hemorrhage, and the other shows multiple infarcts, but the authors never state how they handled either of these issues (etiology or multiple lesions) in their analyses.

In summary, CT provided reasonable prognostic information. Large strokes do less well than small strokes, and cases with normal CT do best of all. It is obvious, however, that neurologic profiles or functional measures will generally reflect these differences. Patients with large deep lesions will surely have hemiparesis, hemisensory deficits, and hemianopia or cognitive deficits as their neurologic profile and severe

ADL limitations as their functional measure. As with neurologic profiles, perhaps the wrong question is being asked of CT in the rehabilitation setting. It is also possible that CT has not been properly assessed.
Etiologies have been mixed, and CTs have routinely been performed
too early to be definitive. None of the studies reviewed would meet
even the most generous criterion of adequacy for any standard localization study.

CONCLUSION

Rehabilitation services for stroke have proliferated in the last 30 years.
Intensive, multidisciplinary, hospital-based rehabilitation became the
norm despite relatively little compelling evidence for any particular
interventions. Too often treatment goals have been to "maximize" or
to "optimize" some function with little sober consideration of how
much improvement can actually be expected in a paretic arm, a laterally biased gait, a severe nonfluent aphasia, etc. Treating clinicians
should learn to incorporate reasonable expectations into their inten-
tions and goals. The clinical recovery guidelines reviewed here should
be some help.

References

1. Jørgensen HS, Nakayama H, Raaschoy HO, Olsen TS. Intracerebral
   hemorrhage versus infarction: stroke severity, risk factors and prognosis.
   Ann Neurol 1995;38:45–50.
2. Hier DB, Foulkes MA, Swiontoniowski M, et al. Stroke recurrence within
   2 years after ischemic infarction. Stroke 1991;22:155–161.
3. Allen CMC. Predicting the outcome of acute stroke: a prognostic score.
   J Neurol Neurosurg Psychiatry 1984;47:475–480.
4. Tuszynski MH, Petito CK, Levy DE. Risk factors and clinical
   manifestations of pathologically verified lacunar infarctions. Stroke
   1989;20:990–999.
5. Wolf PA, Dawber TR, Thomas HE Jr, Kannel WB. Epidemiologic
   assessment of chronic atrial fibrillation and risk of stroke: the
   Framingham study. Neurology 1978;28:973–977.
6. Hier DB, Foulkes MA, Swiontoniowski M, et al. Stroke recurrence within
   2 years after ischemic infarction. Stroke 1991;22:155–161.
7. Kase CS, Wolf PA, Chodosh EH, et al. Prevalence of silent stroke in
   patients presenting with initial stroke: the Framingham study. Stroke
   1989;20:850–852.

8. Madden KP, Karanjia PN, Adams HP, et al. Accuracy of initial stroke subtype diagnosis in the TOAST study. Neurology 1995;45:1975–1979.
9. Jørgensen HS, Nakayama H, Raaschoy HO, Olsen TS. Recovery of walking function in stroke patients: the Copenhagen study. Arch Phys Med Rehabil 1995;76:27–32.
10. Redding MJ, Potes E. Rehabilitation outcome following initial unilateral hemispheric stroke. Life table analysis approach. Stroke 1988;19:1354–1358.
11. Blower PW, Carter LC, Sulch DA. Relationship between wheelchair propulsion and independent walking in hemiplegic stroke. Stroke 1995;26:606–608.
12. Friedman PJ. Gait recovery after hemiplegic stroke. Int Disabil Stud 1991;12:119–122.
13. Parker VM, Wade DT, Langton Hewer R. Loss of arm function after stroke: Measurement, frequency, and recovery. Int Rehabil Med 1986;8:69–73.
14. Gray CS, French JM, Bates D, et al. Motor recovery following acute stroke. Age Ageing 1990;19:179–184.
15. Duncan PW, Goldstein LB, Matchar D, et al. Measurement of motor recovery after stroke: outcome assessment and sample size requirements. Stroke 1992;23:1084–1089.
16. Bonita R, Beaglehole R. Recovery of motor function after stroke. Stroke 1988;19:1497–1500.
17. Wade DT, Langton Hewer R, Wood VA, et al. The hemiplegic arm after stroke: measurement and recovery. J Neurol Neurosurg Psychiatry 1983;46:521–524.
18. Kusoffsky A, Wadell I, Nilsson BY. The relationship between sensory impairment and motor recovery in patients with hemiplegia. Scand J Rehabil Med 1982;14:27–32.
19. Twitchell TE. The restoration of motor function following hemiplegia in man. Brain 1951;74:443–480.
20. Weiller C, Ramsay SC, Wise RJS, et al. Individual patterns of functional reorganization in the human cerebral cortex after capsular infarction. Ann Neurol 1993;33:181–189.
21. Yekutiel M, Gutman E. A controlled trial of the retraining of the sensory function of the hand in stroke patients. J Neurol Neurosurg Psychiatry 1993;56:241–244.
22. Gray CS, French JM, Bates D, et al. Recovery of visual fields in acute stroke: homonymous hemianopia associated with adverse prognosis. Age Ageing 1989;18:419–421.
23. Zihl J, von Cramon DY. Visual field recovery from scotomata in patients with post geniculate damage. Brain 1985;108:335–365.
24. Stone SP, Patel P, Greenwood RJ, Halligan PW. Measuring visual neglect in acute stroke and predicting its recovery: the visual neglect recovery index. J Neurol Neurosurg Psychiatry 1992;55:431–436.
25. Hier DB, Mondlock J, Caplar LR. Behavioral abnormalities after right hemisphere stroke. Neurology 1983;33:337–344.
26. Hier DB, Mondlock J, Caplar LR. Recovery of behavioral abnormalities after right hemisphere stroke. Neurology 1983;33:345–350.
27. Kinsella G, Ford B. Hemi-inattention and the recovery patterns of stroke patients. Int Rehabil Med 1985;7:102–105.
28. Denes G, Semenza C, Stoppa E, Lis A. Unilateral spatial neglect and recovery from hemiplegia. Brain 1982;105:543–552.

29. Barer DH. Continence after stroke: useful predictor or goal of therapy? Age Ageing 1989;18:183–191.
30. Brocklehurst MD, Andrews K, Richards B, Laycock PJ. Incidence and correlates of incontinence in stroke patients. J Am Geriatr Soc 1985;33:540–542.
31. Wade DT, Langton Hewer R. Outlook after an acute stroke: urinary incontinence and loss of consciousness compared in 532 patients. Q J Med 1985;56:601–608.
32. Wade DT, Langton Hewer R, David RM, Enderby PM. Aphasia after stroke: natural history and associated deficits. J Neurol Neurosurg Psychiatry 1986;49:11–16.
33. Enderby PM, Wood VA, Wade DT, Langton Hewer R. Aphasia after stroke: a detailed study of recovery in the first 3 months. Int Rehabil Med 1987;9:162–165.
34. Knopman DS, Selnes OA, Niccum N, Rubens AB. Recovering of naming in aphasia. Neurology 1984;34:1461–1470.
35. Kertsz A, McCabe P. Recovery patterns and prognosis in aphasia. Brain 1977;100:1–18.
36. Scarpa M, Colombo A, Sorgato P, DeRenzi E. The incidence of aphasia and global aphasia in left brain-damaged patients. Cortex 1987;23: 331–336.
37. Knopman DS, Selnes OA, Niccum N, et al. A longitudinal study of speech fluency in aphasia. Neurology 1983;33:1170–1178.
38. Demeurisse G, Demol O, Derouck M, et al. Quantitative study of the rate of recovery from aphasia due to ischemic stroke. Stroke 1980;11: 455–458.
39. Shewan CM, Kertesz A. Effects of speech and language treatment on recovery from aphasia. Brain Lang 1984;23:272–299.
40. Mazzoni M, Vista M, Geri E, et al. Comparison of language recovery in rehabilitated and matched non-rehabilitated aphasic subjects. Aphasiology 1995;9:553–563.
41. Wertz RT, Weiss DG, Aten JL, et al. Comparison of clinic, home and deferred language treatment for aphasia. Arch Neurol 1986;43:653–658.
42. Hartman J, Landau LM. Comparison of formal therapy with supportive counselling for aphasia due to acute vascular accident. Arch Neurol 1987;44:546–549.
43. Lincoln NB, Mulley GP, Jones AC. Effectiveness of speech therapy for aphasic stroke patients. Lancet, 1984:1197–1200.
44. Williams SE, Freer CA. Aphasia: its effect on marital relationships. Arch Phys Med Rehabil 1986;67:250–252.
45. Basso A, Capitani E, Della Salla S, et al. Recovery from ideomotor apraxia. Brain 1987;110:747–760.
46. DeRenzi E, Lucchelli F. Ideational apraxia. Brain 1988;111:1173–1185.
47. Alexander MP, Baker E, Naeser MA, et al. Neuropsychological and neuroanatomic dimensions of ideomotor apraxia. Brain 1992;115:87–107.
48. Wade DT, Parker V, Langton Hewer R. Memory disturbance after stroke: frequency and associated losses. Int Rehabil Med 1986;8:60–64.
49. Tatemichi TK, Foulkes MA, Mohr JP, et al. Dementia in stroke survivors in the Stroke Data Bank cohort. Stroke 1990;21:858–866.
50. Ebrahim S, Barer D, Nouri F. Affective illness after stroke. Br J Psychiatry 1987;151:52–56.
51. Sinyor D, Jacques P, Kaloupek DG, et al. Poststroke depression and lesion location. Brain 1986;109:537–546.

52. Robinson RG, Bolduc PL, Price TR. Two-year longitudinal study of poststroke mood disorders: diagnosis and outcome at one and two years. Stroke 1987;18:837–843.

53. Starkstein SE, Robinson RG, Price TR. Comparison of patients with and without poststroke major depression matched for size and location of lesion. Arch Gen Psychiatry 1988;45:247–252.

54. Bolla-Wilson K, Robinson RG, Starkstein SE, Price TR. Lateralization of dementia of depression in stroke patients. Am J Psychiatry 1989;146:627–634.

55. Agrell B, Dehlin O. Comparison of six depression rating scales in geriatric stroke patients. Stroke 1989;20:1190–1194.

56. Zung WWK. A self rating depression scale. Arch Gen Psychiatry 1965;12:63–70.

57. Finklestein SF, Benowitz LI, Baldessarini RJ, et al. Mood, vegetative disturbance and dexamethasone suppression test after stroke. Ann Neurol 1982;12:463–468.

58. Lipsey JR, Robinson RG, Pearlson GD, et al. Nortriptyline treatment of post-stroke depression: A double-blind study. Lancet 1984;1:297–300.

59. Dam M, Tonin P, DeBoni A, et al. Effects of fluoxetine and maprotiline on functional recovery in post stroke hemiplegic patients undergoing rehabilitation therapy. Stroke 1996;27:1211–1214.

60. Allen CMC. Predicting the outcome of acute stroke: a prognostic score. J Neurol Neurosurg Psychiatry 1984;47:475–480.

61. Gordon EE, Drenth V, Jarvis L, et al. Neurophysiologic syndromes in stroke as predictors of outcome. Arch Phys Med Rehabil 1978;59:399–403.

62. Rasmussen D, Køhler O, Worm Petersen S, et al. Computed tomography in prognostic stroke evaluation. Stroke 1992;23:506–510.

63. Miller LS, Miyamoto AT. Computed tomography: its potential as a predictor of functional recovery following stroke. Arch Phys Med Rehabil 1979;60:108–109.

64. Hertanu JS, Demopoulos JT, Yang WC, et al. Stroke rehabilitation: correlation and prognostic value of computerized tomography and sequential functional assessments. Arch Phys Med Rehabil 1984;65:505–508.

Appendix: Definitions

INTRODUCTION

Stroke is a general term that covers all brain injuries caused by diseases of the blood vessels to the brain or in the brain. The injury may be permanent or transient. It may be caused by too little blood flow in the brain (*ischemia*) or by bleeding into or around the brain (*hemorrhage*). It may be localized to one part of the brain, or it may affect the brain in multiple locations. Stroke is one of the three major neurologic causes of death and disability with traumatic brain injury and dementia of the Alzheimer's type. It is the third leading cause of death in the United States, the leading cause of rehabilitation hospitalization, and, because 25% of stroke patients are less than 65 years old, a major cause of lost productivity.

CAUSES AND TYPES OF STROKE

The terminology on stroke can be confusing. *Stroke* is a generic term for all vascular injuries to the brain. *Cerebrovascular accident* (CVA) is synonymous with stroke. Most strokes are caused by inadequate blood flow to a portion of the brain; this is *ischemia*. If ischemia lasts long enough (5 minutes), brain cells are irreversibly damaged, and the ischemic portion of brain dies; this is *infarction*. If ischemia is reversed, brain cells function again. An episode of temporary impairment due to ischemia is called a *transient ischemic attack* or TIA. By convention, TIAs last less than 24 hours although most are actually less than 15 minutes. Some infarctions clear almost completely over days or weeks, and the patients are said to have a *residual neurologic disability* (RND) state.

There are many causes of infarction, but three are dominant. Blockage of one of the large arteries supplying the brain can reduce blood flow sufficiently to cause infarction (Figure 2.2). If blockage is complete, the vessel is *occluded*. If incomplete, the artery is *stenosed*, usually described by a percentage. The arteries most commonly involved are the internal carotid arteries at their origin from the common carotid arteries in the neck (Figure 2.3). The most common cause of blockage is *atherosclerosis* with or without a local blood clot on the area of atherosclerosis. Other large arteries that can be occluded are the vertebrals (usually at their origins in the neck), the basilar (anywhere along its course), and the middle cerebral artery (at its origin at the circle of Willis). The anterior and posterior cerebral arteries are also possible sites of occlusive disease. Atherosclerosis is a gradual process of large vessel narrowing due to a buildup of cholesterol and blood components on and in the vessel wall. Risk factors for atherosclerosis are high blood pressure, smoking, diabetes, various disorders of lipid/cholesterol metabolism, a complex genetic factor, and perhaps obesity and sedentary life style. Large vessels are sometimes blocked by a tear in their inner surface—a *dissection*—that allows blood to move into the wall of the vessel and block the normal arterial passage. Dissections can occur spontaneously, but they often seem related to extension trauma to the neck, such as whiplash injuries, and prolonged dental procedures. There are a few inherited disorders that predispose to dissections.

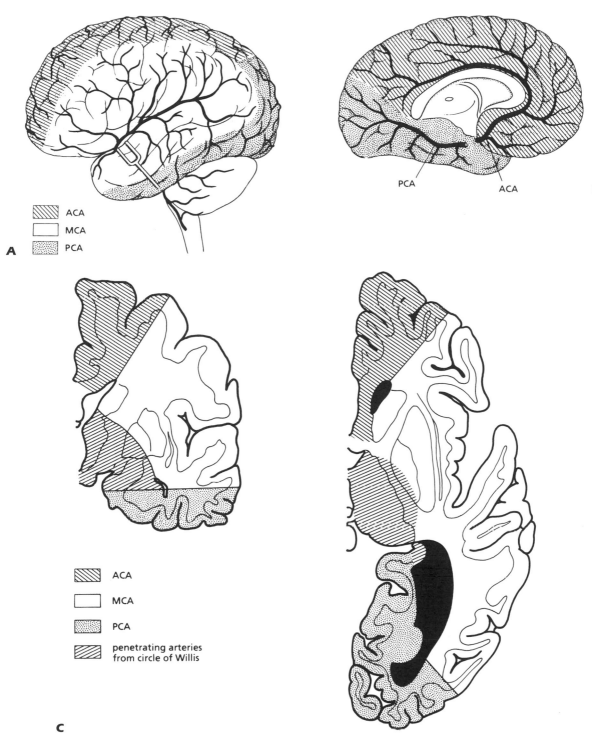

Figure 2.2 (A) The superficial distribution of the left middle cerebral artery. (B) The distribution of the anterior and posterior cerebral arteries on the medial surface of the right cerebral hemisphere. (C) The territories of the anterior, middle, and posterior cerebral arteries (left) in a coronal slice at level A1 and (right) in a horizontal slice at mid-thalamic level. (Reprinted from Esiri MM, Oppenheimer DR. Diagnostic neuropathology: a practical manual. Oxford: Blackwell Scientific, 1989:113–114.)

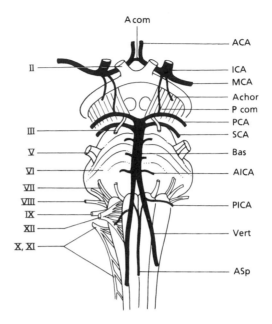

ACA	Anterior cerebral artery
Acho	Anterior choroidal artery
A com	Anterior communicating artery
AICA	Anterior inferior cerebellar artery
ASp	Anterior spinal artery
Bas	Basilar artery
ICA	Internal carotid artery
MCA	Middle cerebral artery
PCA	Posterior cerebral artery
P com	Posterior communicating artery
PICA	Posterior inferior cerebellar artery
SCA	Superior cerebellar artery
Vert	Vertebral artery

Figure 2.3 The basal arteries of the brain. The circle of Willis comprises the proximal parts of the anterior and posterior cerebral arteries, and the anterior and posterior communicating arteries. (Reprinted from Esiri MM, Oppenheimer DR. Diagnostic neuropathology: a practical manual. Oxford: Blackwell Scientific, 1989:113.)

A second cause of infarction is a cerebral *embolus*. An embolus is a piece of debris (blood clot or atherosclerosis plaque) within the arterial system that travels with blood flow until it reaches a vessel too small to allow its passage. It stops and prevents blood flow to the brain beyond it. Emboli may be small and cause minor infarctions or even break up and cause only a TIA. Emboli may also be large and block a major vessel such as the internal carotid or middle cerebral or one of the smaller branch arteries. There are many causes of emboli, but two are most important. First, atherosclerotic plaques in the aorta, the carotids, or the vertebrobasilar system may cause clots to form a fragile

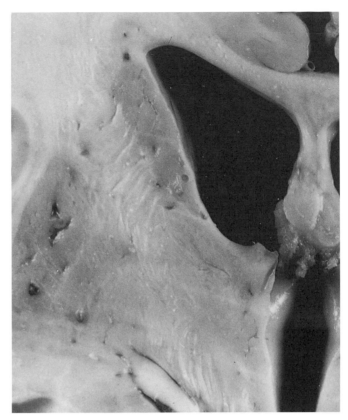

Figure 2.4   *Rarefactions ("lacunes") in the corpus striatum. Man, aged 65, with long-standing hypertension (heart weight, 500 g) and 18 months' progressive dementia. (Reprinted from Esiri MM, Oppenheimer DR. Diagnostic neuropathology: a practical manual. Oxford: Blackwell Scientific, 1989:117.)*

attachment to the vessel wall. The clot is dislodged by the normal blood flow. Thus, the embolus is *artery to artery*, and a search for embolic source must start downstream in the affected artery. The second main source of embolic strokes is the heart; these are *cardiogenic* emboli. Atrial fibrillation can lead to emboli because blood flow is stagnant in the left atrium. Acute myocardial infarction can lead to emboli, probably through temporarily rendering a piece of heart wall immobile and flaccid, allowing blood to collect along that piece of heart wall. Aortic and mitral valve diseases, endocarditis, and cardiomyopathies are other causes of cardiogenic emboli.

The third cause of infarction is a specific degeneration of small blood vessels in the brain. This has been called *lipohyalinosis*, and the blockage of these small vessels causes minor infarctions called *lacunar infarcts* (Figure 2.4). Lipohyalinosis is caused by hypertension. The vessels affected are small arteries that branch directly off large arteries. These include, most prominently, the lenticulostriate branches of the middle

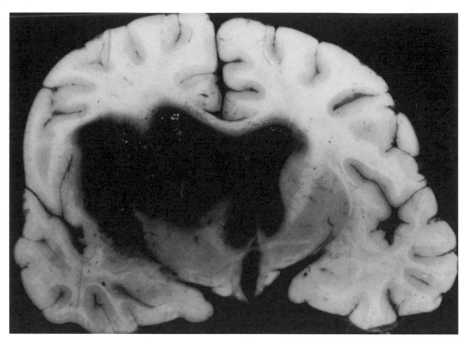

Figure 2.5 Acute hemorrhage into the lentiform nucleus, erupting into the ventricular system, in a 60-year-old woman. (Reprinted from Esiri MM, Oppenheimer DR. Diagnostic neuropathology: a practical manual. Oxford: Blackwell Scientific, 1989:102.)

and anterior cerebral arteries, the thalamic branches of the posterior communicating arteries, the basilar and posterior cerebral arteries, and the pontine branches of the basilar arteries.

To be sure, small emboli and atherosclerosis of a large vessel that happens to block the origin of small vessels can also cause *lacunes*. Thus, lacune describes a type of infarction—small and deep—whatever the vascular mechanism. Large vessel occlusion and embolus describe vascular mechanisms of ischemia whatever the resulting infarction pattern.

Strokes that are not ischemic are caused by hemorrhage—bleeding into or around the brain. There are two clinical classes of hemorrhage, based on the primary location of bleeding. *Intracerebral hemorrhages* are strokes caused by rupture of a blood vessel with bleeding directly into the substance of the brain (Figure 2.5). *Subarachnoid hemorrhages* are strokes caused by rupture of a blood vessel with bleeding directly into the subarachnoid space. Intracerebral hemorrhages often track into the subarachnoid space, and subarachnoid hemorrhages sometimes dissect into the brain, but, by convention, the strokes are described by the presumed origin of bleeding.

There are many potential causes of intracerebral hemorrhage (ICH). *High blood pressure* is a major risk for ICH. Lipohyalinosis (see above) produces weak spots in the walls of small vessels through which blood

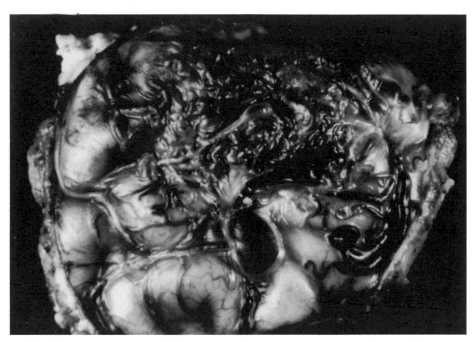

Figure 2.6 *Arteriovenous malformation. Operation specimen from the right frontal lobe of a boy aged 12, who presented one month earlier with an epileptic fit. (Reprinted from Esiri MM, Oppenheimer DR. Diagnostic neuropathology: a practical manual. Oxford: Blackwell Scientific, 1989:261.)*

can burst. The arteries at greatest risk are exactly the same as for lacunes (see above). Another cause of ICH is rupture of congenitally abnormal blood vessels—arteriovenous malformations (AVM) (Figure 2.6) or cavernous hemangiomas. These often cause ICH in younger patients and may be in any vessel territory. A third cause of ICH is *amyloid angiopathy*, a degenerative disorder of blood vessels. Amyloid angiopathy is a disease of the elderly. It is often associated with dementia of the Alzheimer's type. When it causes ICH, the bleeding is often in cortical regions and particularly in the posterior cerebral cortex. Hemorrhages may be recurrent. A fourth cause of ICH is impaired blood clotting. This can be due to congenital impairments (such as hemophilia), to acquired disorders (such as chronic liver disease), or to medications (coumadin or aspirin).

Subarachnoid hemorrhage (SAH) also can have many causes. The most common is ruptured *aneurysms* (Figure 2.7). These are weak spots in the walls of large vessels. The tendency to form aneurysms is inherited and accentuated by high blood pressure. Common sites of aneurysms are the junctions of vessels, particularly the posterior communicating and internal carotid arteries, the anterior communicating and anterior cerebral arteries, and the origin of the middle cerebral artery. Aneurysms can be located anywhere and can be multiple. A

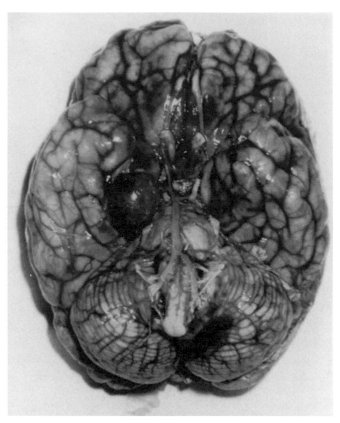

Figure 2.7 *Aneurysm of the posterior cerebral artery in a 15-year-old (an unusual finding at this stage). (Reprinted from Esiri MM, Oppenheimer DR. Diagnostic neuropathology: a practical manual. Oxford: Blackwell Scientific, 1989:100.)*

second cause of SAH is AVMs. Because AVMs are often on the surface of the brain when they rupture, the bleeding is into the subarachnoid space. The third cause is impaired blood clotting as described above. Subarachnoid hemorrhages may dissect into the brain and cause neurologic damage directly. The presence of blood in the subarachnoid space may induce vasospasm in the large arteries at the base of the brain. The vasospasm can be so severe that blood flow is reduced, causing infarction. Blood in the subarachnoid space can also block the flow of spinal fluid, causing hydrocephalus. All of these phenomena cause neurologic disability.

There is not complete agreement about the relative proportions of the causes of stroke. Most studies agree that approximately 85% are infarctions and 15% hemorrhages. Large vessel occlusions and embolic strokes are each approximately 33% of all strokes, and lacunes the remaining 20%. Some strokes could be counted twice. If the stroke is a lacune but the cause is a small embolus, or if a large vessel occludes due to clot or atherosclerotic plaque but the stroke occurs because the clot becomes an embolus, how should these be counted? Clinical criteria alone do not establish stroke mechanism with high reliability.

VASCULAR TERRITORIES

It is customary to describe stroke syndromes by either the presumed vascular territory of the stroke or the general brain region involved; thus, the terms *middle cerebral artery stroke* or *capsulostriatal hemorrhage* or *lenticulostriate stroke*, etc. The vascular territory or brain region designated are not synonymous with the vascular mechanism. An internal carotid artery occlusion may cause a lenticulostriate territory stroke, a middle cerebral territory stroke, or any of several other regional infarcts or only a TIA or nothing at all. The stroke area will inform us about likely impairments and disabilities. The stroke mechanism will inform us about medical treatments and prognoses.

MORTALITY

Stroke is the third leading cause of mortality in the United States. Most mortality is directly neurologic and within the first 30 days of stroke. A small number of patients die of secondary causes such as pneumonia or pulmonary emboli. With infarctions, mortality is directly related to size and best predicted by level of consciousness 12 hours after onset. With ICH, mortality is related to size and location. Deep ICH that ruptures into the ventricles and pontine ICH have very high mortality. For more superficial ICH, size is the prideomotor apraxiary factor leading to increased intracranial pressure, secondary ischemia, more increased pressure, and so on, until fatal brainstem compression occurs. Subarachnoid hemorrhages also have high mortality: 20% for first SAH and 60% with rerupture. Overall 30-day mortality for stroke is about 20% to 30%.

Specific Stroke Syndromes

Mark D'Esposito

Stroke is a common cause of brain injury that is encountered on neurorehabilitation units. It is imperative that clinicians who care for these patients recognize that stroke does *not* cause a single unified group of clinical manifestations. However, there are similar patterns of clinical symptoms and signs that can be recognized and classified into stroke syndromes. Each stroke syndrome will produce a unique constellation of deficits affecting cognitive, behavioral, motor, and sensory systems. These various stroke syndromes produce a wide range of deficits that are due to damage in numerous locations throughout the brain. Understanding the different manifestations of the most common stroke syndromes is critical for diagnosis, treatment, management, and rehabilitation of stroke patients.

Rehabilitation clinicians who encounter neurologically impaired patients caused by diverse etiologies such as closed head injury and encephalitis will recognize that many stroke syndromes have neurologic deficits that share many surface manifestations with these other neurologic disorders. These shared clinical features are outlined in other chapters of this book and should be compared and contrasted to the stroke syndromes presented below. In this chapter, I will first review the clinical pathophysiology of stroke in order to provide a foundation for the clinician to understand the approach one should take toward making a neurologic diagnosis. Several specific stroke syndromes have been chosen to illustrate the range of clinical manifestations that can result from damage to different regions in the human brain. The group of syndromes chosen is not meant to be exhaustive, but is merely meant to represent several syndromes that are commonly encountered on neurorehabilitation units. This group was chosen especially to illustrate classical neurobehavioral syndromes such as aphasia, neglect, amnesia, and dementia. Certainly, there are other stroke syndromes that neurorehabilitation clinicians will encounter. However, it is my intention that the principles reviewed in this chapter can be applied to other stroke syndromes. The reader who wishes to learn about other neurobehavioral syndromes caused by strokes is directed to either of the following textbooks: *Behavioral Neurology and Neuropsychology* (1) or *The Neurology of Thinking* (2).

The clinical description of each stroke syndrome will be followed by a representative clinical case presentation that is typically encountered on neurorehabilitation units. A comprehensive evaluation of a stroke patient includes a mental status examination as well a full neurologic examination. In these presentations, a full examination will be described in order to acquaint the reader with an appropriate assessment as performed by a behavioral neurologist. The prognosis of each stroke syndrome will be reviewed since all strokes do not follow a similar path of recovery. The management and strategies for remediation of the most prominent clinical manifestation of each syndrome will also be reviewed. Thus, it is the aim of this chapter to provide a guideline for a rational clinical approach toward the assessment and rehabilitation of patients who have suffered a stroke.

OVERVIEW OF THE CLINICAL PATHOPHYSIOLOGY OF STROKE

Strokes can be classified into two main categories based on their underlying mechanism of injury: ischemic and hemorrhagic. Ischemic infarcts account for the vast majority of strokes, approximately 80%, while the remaining 20% are hemorrhagic (3). Ischemia refers to a reduction of blood flow to a particular region of the brain, leading to an infarction. Reduced blood flow may be caused by an embolus, usually from the heart of thrombosis of an artery, usually due to atherosclerosis of the carotid arteries, the large vessels that supply blood to the brain. If the reduction of blood flow is prolonged, a neurologic deficit will occur. Ischemic strokes will produce deficits depending on the vascular territory that has interrupted blood flow.

The brain is supplied by an anterior and posterior circulation (Figure 3.1). The anterior circulation derives from the internal carotid artery, which divides into the anterior cerebral artery (ACA) and middle cerebral artery (MCA). The ACA supplies the medial portions of each cerebral hemisphere, which includes the medial and orbital portions of the frontal lobes and the medial portion of the parietal lobes. The MCA

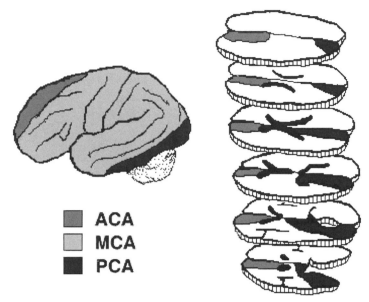

Figure 3.1 *Schematic drawing of the territories of the brain supplied by the major arteries (only the left hemisphere is shown). ACA = anterior cerebral artery; MCA = middle cerebral artery; PCA = posterior cerebral artery.*

supplies the lateral portions of each cerebral hemisphere. This includes the lateral frontal, parietal, and temporal lobes. There are also proximal branches of the MCA before it reaches the cerebral hemisphere, the lenticulostriate arteries, which supply the basal ganglia (i.e., caudate, putamen, globus pallidus), and the internal capsule. The MCA distribution is the most common site for strokes. This chapter will focus on two syndromes in this territory: left hemisphere strokes that cause aphasia and right hemisphere strokes that cause neglect.

The posterior circulation originates from two vertebral arteries that form the basilar artery, which then divides into two posterior cerebral arteries (PCA). The PCAs supply the entire occipital lobes and the medial and inferior parts of the temporal lobes. Branches of the PCA also supply the thalamus. Another syndrome discussed in this chapter is that caused by an infarction of the thalamus. The thalamus is the main relay station of most neural pathways to the cerebral cortex. Both the anterior and posterior circulation have a similar predisposition to embolic and thrombotic stroke. The territory supplied by the three major vessels of the brain, the anterior, middle, and posterior cerebral arteries, are illustrated in Figure 3.1.

There are a number of factors common to all ischemic strokes that may influence the clinical manifestations, prognosis, and remediation of these stroke syndromes. First, patients with a new stroke may have had a stroke in the past and are clearly at an increased risk for having another stroke in the future. On admission to a neurorehabilitation unit, a careful review of the patient's previous stroke history should be performed. If the patient's or family's account of the history is unclear, previous hospital records should be obtained and reviewed. Another method of determining the possibility of previous strokes is to review the most recent CT or MRI scan with a neurologist or radiologist for the presence of old strokes. In this way, detection of old strokes can be factored into the overall rehabilitation plan.

Previous strokes may affect recovery in several ways. Accumulation of strokes in both the right and left hemispheres can worsen the recovery of specific functions such as speech, swallowing, or urinary incontinence. Often, a lack of recovery in one of these functions as noted by the clinicians can be accounted for by determining that the patient has bilateral strokes. Accumulation of multiple strokes over time can lead to dementia, called *multi-infarct dementia*, which can also adversely affect recovery of cognitive function. For example, a patient with a mild conduction aphasia that in general would make an excellent recovery may not because of other cognitive deficits due to the effects of adding a new lesion to the overall lesion burden.

There are several secondary complications that can occur following an ischemic stroke. In the days to weeks following an acute stroke, patients are at risk of extending their recent stroke or developing a new one. Any apparent change in the patient's neurologic status, even if it appears subtle, warrants immediate evaluation by a neurologist. Within the first week following a stroke, patients are at risk for developing cerebral edema. Patients with large MCA-territory strokes are probably at the greatest risk. The signs of cerebral edema include a decreased level of arousal, enlargement of the pupil on the side of the stroke, and upper motor signs (i.e., increased motor tone, increased deep tendon reflexes, a Babinski's sign) on the same side as the stroke. Massive cerebral edema can lead to herniation where the brain is forced downward, causing compression on the brainstem (Figure 3.2). Herniation syndromes can be fatal if compression of respiratory centers in the medulla occur. Downward herniation, or *uncal herniation*, can also cause compression of the PCA leading to an ischemic stroke in that distribution. Of course, patients during the course of recovery of a stroke can develop new strokes. All rehabilitation clinicians should be aware of these secondary complications of ischemic strokes so that they can be acted on promptly. Understanding the outcome of these complications will help in goal setting for these patients, since they alter the outcome of a patient without complications.

Hemorrhages can occur within the brain substance itself (intracerebral hemorrhage) or beneath the coverings of the brain (subdural or subarachnoid hemorrhage). Intracerebral hemorrhage (ICH) is usually due to rupture of the small, deep penetrating arteries of the brain. The most common cause of ICH is hypertension. ICH can occur early after a patient is discovered to have hypertension because of leaking of vessels exposed to high pressure. Alternatively, after patients have had

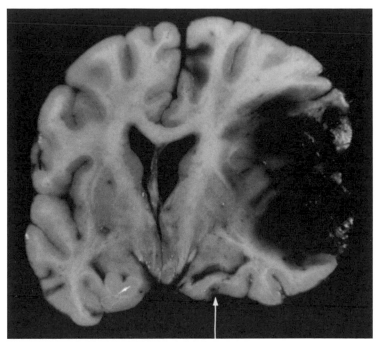

Figure 3.2   Downthrust in a case with a right-sided hemorrhagic infarction due to phlebothrombosis. Note the midline shift to the left, herniation of the right cingulate gyrus, and bruising and grooving of the right parahippocampal gyrus (arrowed). (Reprinted from Esiri MM, Oppenheimer DR. Diagnostic neuropathology: a practical manual. Oxford: Blackwell Scientific, 1989:23.)

hypertension for a prolonged period of time, the small arteries of the brain undergo significant wear and tear due to the prolonged increased pressure. Such damage makes these vessels more vulnerable to rupture. There are many other causes of ICH, including being on anticoagulation drugs or having a disease that causes a coagulopathy (e.g., leukemia), suffering a closed head injury, or harboring an arteriovenous malformation, which is a congenital and abnormal bundle of arteries and veins.

It is important to note that ICH, unlike ischemic stroke, does not usually occur in traditional vascular territories such as the MCA, ACA, or PCA territory. Most ICHs are in the deeper structures of the brain. The most common sites for ICH include the basal ganglia, pons, thalamus, and cerebellum (e.g., basal ganglia, brainstem). Lobar hemorrhages can also occur, but are less common. However, when a hemorrhage within the MCA, ACA, or PCA territory takes place, the hemorrhage itself can extend well beyond the traditional boundaries of these large arteries. This observation explains why hemorrhages can produce clinical syndromes that are quite different from the ischemic stroke syndromes. An ICH may cause clinical signs that combine many of the signs seen in ischemic syndromes from different vascular territories. For example, a deep ICH affecting the basal ganglia can track into the overlying white matter and cortex and cause a significant aphasia.

In general, hemorrhages have a better outcome than ischemic strokes because hemorrhage, unlike permanent ischemia, will resorb over time. If there is no underlying damage to the brain, patients may make a miraculous recovery. For example, a patient may have a significant nonfluent aphasia that resolves completely whereas a similar ischemic lesion would have left the patient with a permanent deficit. Sometimes after a hemorrhage has resolved, there is underlying permanent damage that can lead to a persistent deficit. It is important to review a neuroimaging study after a hemorrhage has resorbed, usually within a few months, to determine if there is an underlying lesion. In summary, hemorrhages provide a more diverse group of clinical manifestations than ischemic strokes. The latter will have a fairly consistent pattern of deficits depending on the vascular territory that is affected.

Subarachnoid hemorrhages (SAH) are due to rupture of cerebral saccular aneurysms, which are caused by congenital weakening of the arteriolar walls. SAH forces blood throughout the base of the brain and can be easily diagnosed with an MRI or CT scan or a lumbar puncture which will reveal the presence of red blood cells. Aneurysms exist in at least 5% of the population and most commonly rupture between the ages of 40 to 70 years of age, an earlier onset than typically seen with ischemic strokes (4). A SAH is a serious medical illness; it is estimated that at least 30% of patients will die before reaching the hospital and another 20% will die in the hospital or not recover (3). The patient's clinical state is often classified into five grades according to the Hunt and Hess system (5). Grade 1 is asymptomatic; grade 2, severe headache without a neurologic deficit; grade 3, drowsy, confused, and mild neurologic deficit; grade 4, stuporous and neurologic deficit; and grade 5, coma. In general, patients with a high grade on presentation have a worse prognosis. Aneurysms tend to occur on the circle of Willis, a group of arteries at the base of the brain, and often exist where these arteries bifurcate. The most common saccular aneurysm is on the anterior communicating artery (ACoA), one of the vessels of the circle of Willis (see Figure 2.3). ACoA aneurysms are the most common aneurysms of the circle of Willis and occur in at least 30% of SAH patients. Aneurysm clipping remains a major challenge for neurosurgeons despite the advent of the operating microscope, but microscopic surgery has greatly enhanced survival.

There are several causes for permanent brain injury following aneurysm rupture. First, infarction can occur as a result of vasospasm, which causes a constriction of arteries. Typically, the arteries that come in contact with subarachnoid blood are vulnerable to this effect and are most vulnerable in the first week following the SAH. The aneurysm clipping surgery can also cause vasospasm and infarction. In the case of ACoA aneurysm, the ACoA, ACA, and the recurrent artery of Heubner, which is a branch of the ACA, are the arteries usually affected. Thus, constriction will cause infarction in the areas of the brain supplied by these arteries. The ACoA has several branches that supply a region of the brain called the *basal forebrain*. The basal forebrain includes two important structures, the septal nuclei and the nucleus basalis of Meynert, both of which are critical for memory function. The ACA supplies the medial and orbital frontal lobes, and the recurrent artery of Heubner supplies the head of the caudate, part of the basal ganglia. Second, the SAH can be massive, causing extension of blood into the overlying brain tissue, potentially causing permanent damage. Third, in the acute stage, massive cerebral edema can occur as well, leading to hydrocephalus or increased ventricular size. Later, following repair of aneurysms, hydrocephalus can occur as the subarachnoid blood absorbs, since it may cause blockage of the arachnoid granulations that resorb cerebrospinal fluid. Acute hydrocephalus can be fatal if it causes brainstem herniation. Chronic hydrocephalus usually manifests itself as a decrease in arousal, although any other subtle change in the neurologic status could be caused by hydrocephalus and should be attended to immediately.

In summary, ischemic stroke will cause damage to the brain that is supplied by specific vascular territories, and the clinical manifestations may be consistent across patients. Intracerebral hemorrhages do not occur in traditional vascular territories and may have a unique constellation of clinical symptoms from patient to patient. Subarachnoid hemorrhage, when it occurs secondary to an ACoA rupture, may cause persistent deficits as a result of vasospasm and subsequent infarction.

SPECIFIC STROKE SYNDROMES

Left Hemisphere Infarction (Wernicke's Aphasia)

Clinical Profile

A stroke in the distribution of the left MCA territory causing damage to the frontal, temporal, and/or parietal lobes will usually cause aphasia. *Aphasia* is defined as a disturbance of *language*, that is, the set of symbols that humans use as a means for communication. In contrast, *speech* is defined as only the mechanical process of language, such as articulation and phonation. The major difference is the neural substrate for these disorders is that impairments in language are generally caused by a lesion in the left hemisphere of the brain, whereas damage to any component of the motor system for vocalization can cause an impairment in speech. For example, a motor neuron disease such as amyotrophic lateral sclerosis or a muscle disease such as myasthenia gravis can cause a speech disturbance that leaves language intact.

A language disturbance, or aphasia, is specifically due to cortical or subcortical brain damage. In approximately 99% of right-handers and 70% of left-handers, language is subserved by the left hemisphere, and a stroke on that side will cause aphasia. Since more than 90% of the population reports themselves as right-handed, the vast majority of patients encountered in rehabilitation hospitals with aphasia will be due to strokes in the left hemisphere. In contrast, a very small percentage of right-handers, less than 1%, and approximately 30% of left-handers have language subserved by the right hemisphere and can develop an aphasic syndrome from a stroke in the right hemisphere. Since aphasias due to right-hemisphere lesions are uncommon, they have not been studied extensively; however, a few clinical observations have been made. First, right-hemisphere lesions can cause two types of aphasia. One type of aphasia shows the same clinical manifestations it would have if it was due to damage in the left hemisphere. Alternatively, aphasia due to a right-hemisphere lesion can appear quite anomalous. For example, anterior lesions may cause a fluent aphasia.

Although language is sometimes subserved by the right hemisphere, especially in left-handers, right-hemisphere functions such as directed attention and visuospatial skills often are retained on that side. As one can envision, a large lesion in the right hemisphere in some left-handers can cause a profound cognitive disorder. For further reading about aphasia due to right-hemisphere damage, or *crossed aphasias*, the reader is referred to the work of Alexander and colleagues (6).

The left hemisphere contains an organized distributed network for language function. Lesions in anterior portions of the brain, the frontal lobes, will cause impairments in ability to produce fluent output, yet auditory comprehension of language is relatively preserved. The classic anterior aphasia is called *Broca's aphasia*, which results in patients with telegraphic utterances and good comprehension. Alternatively, damage to posterior portions of the brain, in the temporal and parietal lobes, will not cause a problem with producing fluent output but will cause a significant deficit in auditory comprehension of language. The classic posterior aphasia is called *Wernicke's aphasia*. Large lesions that extend both anteriorly and posteriorly result in *global aphasia*, that is, patients who are nonfluent and have a significant comprehension impairment. For a more comprehensive description of the clinical aphasia syndromes and related disturbances, the reader is referred to a review by Alexander and Benson (7). For the purposes of illustrating one of the aphasic syndromes, Wernicke's aphasia will be reviewed.

Wernicke's aphasia is due to a stroke that causes extensive damage to the posterior region of the left temporal lobe (Figure 3.3). This region of the superior temporal gyrus is called *Wernicke's area*. A purely subcortical lesion can also cause a classic Wernicke's aphasia when such a

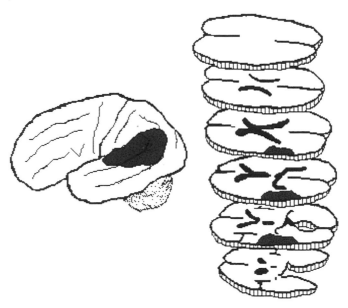

Figure 3.3 *Schematic drawing of the lesion site—the posterior region of the left temporal lobe—that causes Wernicke's aphasia.*

lesion undercuts and interrupts fibers that are on their way to Wernicke's area. A stroke extensive enough to cause Wernicke's aphasia usually also interrupts visual pathways as they course through the temporal lobe on their way to the visual cortex. This is manifested clinically as a visual field deficit in the right upper quadrant of space. It rarely causes a significant functional deficit and often goes unnoticed by both the patient and persons that are initially in contact with the patient. Since the lesion is in posterior portions of the brain, motor and sensory functions are usually spared. Therefore, unlike most patients with stroke, especially those with Broca's aphasia, patients with Wernicke's aphasia usually do not manifest a hemiparesis or hemisensory deficit.

Wernicke's aphasia consists of fluent output with poor comprehension and poor repetition of spoken language. In contrast to their language impairment, Wernicke's aphasic (WA) patients have normal articulation and prosody, and can produce sentence length phrases effortlessly. Their spontaneous speech can be filled with *neologisms* (nonsense words, e.g., "platin"), *phonemic paraphasias* (sound substitutions, e.g., "scoon" for "spoon"), or *semantic paraphasias* (word substitutions, e.g., "knife" for "spoon"). Comprehension of spoken language is impaired. This deficit may be mild (e.g., the patient only has difficulty at the sentence level) or severe (the patient cannot even understand single words). Interestingly, even aphasics with severe spoken language comprehension deficits may understand an examiner's gestures. Also, the patient may retain many pragmatic skills that are involved in everyday conversation, such as knowing when to speak and when to pause and listen. These preserved abilities in a WA patient can sometimes lead to an underestimation of the severity of the patient's comprehension deficit. Finally, in the evaluation of language, it is important to evaluate writing and reading in addition to spoken language. It is typical for comprehension of written material to be as impaired as spoken language in most WA patients. However, some patients, especially those with more anterior lesions to the classic Wernicke's area, may have relatively preserved reading comprehension. Finding this dissociation between oral and written comprehension may provide an alternative means of communication—an avenue for therapeutic remediation.

On the surface, the WA patient will appear confused, since these patients will not be making any sense when they speak and will not understand what other people are saying to them. This is a common misinterpretation of the patient's clinical problem, especially among family members or friends who are the first to encounter the patient at the time of the stroke. Acute confusional states are due to a deficit in attention, rather than a deficit in language, the salient feature of Wernicke's aphasia. Unfortunately, it is not uncommon for a WA patient to be brought to a police station or to be admitted to a psychiatric unit, only later to be discovered that the patient had a stroke. Limited knowledge of the manifestations of aphasia and a lack of any motor or sensory signs in the patients leads to such outcomes.

Unlike many patients with nonfluent aphasia, fluent aphasic patients can have several profound behavioral impairments. First, they often seem quite unaware (anosognosic) of their language deficits. It is common during an attempted conversation between the examiner and the patient, the patient is frustrated that the examiner does not understand him. This can lead to the patient becoming anxious, agitated, and even overtly paranoid. Patients are often markedly perseverative and it is sometimes difficult to get the patient to stop talking and get set for the clinical exam. A combination of these behavioral symptoms as well as speech output that is uninterpretable can lead to a difficult clinical examination.

In summary, Wernicke's aphasia syndrome consists of a fluent aphasia with poor comprehension, a right-sided visual field deficit, and a lack of sensorimotor deficits. Several accompanying behavioral deficits, including anosognosia, perseveration, and agitation can occur. The clinical manifestation of Wernicke's aphasia are outlined in Table 3.1.

Recovery and Prognosis

Grouping all aphasic syndromes together, one study found that 28% of patients made a poor recovery, 19% fair, 13% good, and 40% excellent

Table 3.1. Clinical Profile of Wernicke's
Aphasia Syndrome

Cognitive impairment
- Fluent aphasia with poor comprehension
- Abundant neologistic "jargon" output
- Markedly perseverant

Behavioral impairment
- Appears "confused"
- Unaware (anosognosic) of their language deficits
- Can become anxious, agitated, and even overtly paranoid

Neurologic impairment
- Motor and sensory deficits are uncommon
- Right visual field deficit may occur

(8). However, the extent and pattern of recovery will depend on the specific aphasic syndrome. Several clinical factors will affect these recovery patterns. First, the greatest amount of improvement in language occurs in the first 3 months following the onset of the patient's stroke (9). At this time, the patient's clinical condition may closely approximate what the patient will be like permanently. However, this does not mean that patients cannot show some improvement in specific components of language, such as comprehension, even years after the onset of the stroke. A corollary to this rule is that patients with the most severe aphasia at the onset generally have the worst outcome.

Second, of the two most devastating language deficits caused by stroke—poor speech output and poor comprehension—comprehension is more likely to show a greater degree of recovery (10). This may be because the right hemisphere may also participate in processing the meaning of spoken words, whereas speech output seems more strictly lateralized to the left hemisphere (7). Thus, recovery of auditory comprehension seen in WA patients may depend on the integrity of homologous regions in the right hemisphere.

Third, although it has been observed by clinicians that lesion *size* is proportional to recovery (e.g., larger lesions have a worse outcome), evidence is accumulating that lesion *location* is a critical factor for determining language recovery. For example, the extent of damage to Wernicke's area correlates with language recovery (11). Patients with a lesion greater than half of Wernicke's area will have a poor recovery of auditory comprehension. Damage to the subcortical white matter structure called the *temporal isthmus* (the site of projections that carry auditory information from the medial geniculate to primary auditory cortex) also correlates with recovery of auditory comprehension. In general, lesions in this subcortical region will have a better outcome than a patient with a cortical lesion. Extension of the lesion from Wernicke's area to surrounding posterior structures, such as the supramarginal and angular gyrus, are more likely to lead to persistent deficits in language comprehension (8).

Finally, there are two other factors that likely influence recovery of aphasia, although the evidence is not as strong. The first is age. An aphasia that is acquired before the age of 10 or 12 usually has an excellent prognosis, presumably due to the ability of the right hemisphere to take over language functions. Such "plasticity" is not as evident after this age period (12). Second, there is a clinical impression that left-handers recover better from aphasia than right-handers. This impression may be because left-handers are more likely to have language function distributed in both hemispheres.

Clinical observation has revealed that the language deficit of WA patients generally recovers along two paths. In one path, the abundant neologistic or phonemic jargon evolves into semantic paraphasias, eventually demonstrating only word-finding pauses and periods of circumlocution. Concurrent improvements are noted in repetition and auditory comprehension, leaving the patient classified as an anomic aphasic (13). In a second path of recovery, significant improvement is observed only in auditory comprehension. The patient has only a persistent deficit in repetition and can be classified as a conduction aphasic. Each of these recovered language profiles is compatible with functional language, and patients can lead relatively normal lives, communicating effectively with others.

Therapeutic Remediation

Unfortunately, since most WA patients do not have a sensorimotor deficit, the allowance for an inpatient rehabilitation stay for these patients is likely to be short. Many other patients will be discharged from acute-care hospitals directly home for outpatient rehabilitation. Patients with WA who are noted to have a behavioral disturbance clearly should receive inpatient rehabilitation since such a disturbance can be difficult to manage at home by family members. Moreover, behaviors such as agitation can impede progress of aphasia therapy. In the hospital, pharmacologic therapy can be initiated for behavior disturbances if necessary. Low dosages of benzodiazepines or neuroleptics may be necessary to help a patient adjust to their illness. Anosognosia, although probably not amenable to cognitive remediation, must be recognized by the clinician and family. Some untoward behaviors exhibited by WA patients may be due to their unawareness of the fact that they are not being understood in day-to-day conversations. Recognition of this problem can be alleviated with a calm reassuring interaction. Such interactions are aimed at preventing behaviors that can escalate to a situation that is out of control and not appropriate for rehabilitation.

Another important goal during an inpatient rehabilitation stay is for family members to be educated as to the nature of the language disturbance in patients with Wernicke's aphasia. Family members must become aware of the extent of the patient's auditory comprehension deficit so that an appropriate level of communication can occur. An overestimation of the patient's ability to comprehend spoken language by family members can lead to frustrating interactions. The ability of WA patients to use gestures in a manner that seems appropriate for a conversation can often fool family members into believing that WA patients have a greater understanding of spoken language than they actually do. A complete assessment of the range of the patient's language abilities and behavioral status can be conveyed to family members in order to allow them to participate in an intelligent manner during the course of the patient's recovery.

Most patients will not exhibit a significant behavioral disturbance, and aphasia rehabilitation will be their only need. There are many aphasia therapy programs that are implemented by speech pathologists depending on the specific type of aphasia being treated (14). A comprehensive review of the details of these programs is beyond the scope of this chapter. There are several approaches that have been attempted for the remediation of Wernicke's aphasia. Specifically, the main goal is to improve the predominant deficit, auditory language comprehension. Such therapy aimed at remediating a specific component of language can also be utilized for patients classified under the taxonomic categories of global aphasia (i.e., an additional impairment in fluency) and transcortical sensory aphasia (i.e., lacking an impairment in repetition).

Two current speech therapies, called "deblocking" and "reauditorization," use spoken language as a carrier for remediation. *Deblocking* is a method to stimulate impaired auditory comprehension skills by using a different modality for communication, one that is presumably not impaired. For example, comprehension of spoken language may improve if the speech therapist predominantly trains the patient's reading and writing skills. In this way, written stimuli are used to reinforce auditory stimuli. In another example of deblocking, speech therapists will train patients to use gestures, which WA patients often do well, to represent objects. Again, a technique that does not require spoken language is used to improve impaired auditory processing skills.

Reauditorization is a process of trying to improve auditory comprehension by improving the patient's ability to repeat words and phrases. This approach is based on the hypothesis that the ability to repeat spoken language may be linked to the ability to understand spoken language. Support for this hypothesis was the observation that in aphasic patients, there was a relationship between repetition ability and certain types of auditory comprehension (15). Thus, concentration on improving repetition is the mainstay of reauditorization.

Ultimately, the speech therapist will try many methods, such as the ones described, to create a comprehensive aphasia therapy program.

One such program that combines both deblocking and reauditorization is the "Treatment for Wernicke's Aphasia," developed by Helm-
Estabrooks and Fitzpatrick (14). This treatment program begins with
the development of written language skills, including reading comprehension and oral reading. Next, oral repetition is trained. Finally,
auditory comprehension skills are addressed. This program and others
(16) have shown good treatment effects.

Speech therapy should take advantage of several clinical observations of aphasic patients. First, it is unusual for a patient to have
absolutely no ability to comprehend spoken language. Interestingly,
many patients can answer appropriately to such commands as "close
your eyes"; the exact underlying mechanism and brain regions
involved in this phenomenon are not known. Thus, most patients will
have some limited comprehension ability that can be used as an anchor
for therapy. Second, in many WA patients, reading comprehension is
better than auditory comprehension. This avenue, as outlined above,
is used in many therapy programs. In fact, relatively preserved single
word reading comprehension is a prerequisite for being a good candidate for the Treatment for Wernicke's Aphasia program.

Although there are a limited number of studies that have critically
investigated the effectiveness of speech therapy, most clinicians believe
it is warranted in most aphasic patients under the appropriate guidelines (17). Speech therapy keeps both the patient and family engaged
and, hopefully, confident that everything is being done to help promote
recovery. Aphasia therapy should have practical goals and not just be
a means to improve a specific component of language. What may be
most important is knowing when to stop therapy. If a patient is not
showing signs of improvement or 2 to 3 months have passed, therapy
should be stopped and reevaluated (7).

Clinical Case Presentation

J.W. is a 62-year-old, right-handed male who was sitting in a neigh-
borhood diner on a weekend morning. After returning from the bathroom, he appeared to the waitress as confused. His speech was fluent,
but he was rambling in a fashion that did not make any sense. He was
refusing to pay his bill, which was brought to the attention of a police
officer in the diner. He seemed agitated and resisted the request of the
police officer to step outside the diner. He was subsequently brought
to the police station and held overnight in a detoxification cell. The next
day his behavior had not changed and he was brought to the local
emergency room (ER) for evaluation.

It was determined by a family member who was eventually contacted that he had a history of an intermittently irregular heartbeat for
which he was not being treated with any medications. It was also determined that he was a high school teacher and had never had any similar

problems to what he was having at the current time. He also never drank alcohol.

A neurologic examination was performed in the ER; it revealed that the patient was fully alert but was agitated and did not want to remain on the stretcher. Cranial nerve examination revealed that the patient was not detecting visual stimuli in the right superior quadrant of his visual field. Motor strength and tone was symmetric and normal. Sensory exam was difficult to assess because the patient did not understand the instructions, but it appeared normal as well. His deep tendon reflexes were slightly brisker on the right as compared to the left, and his right toe was extensor in response to plantar stimulation of his feet. He seemed to have normal coordination. He could stand and walk normally.

A mental status examination was also performed. The patient's speech was fluent with normal volume and well articulated. The patient spontaneously uttered numerous phonemic paraphasias and neologisms. For example, a typical utterance was "every batin is crunny and it niffin hasn't been benny well." The patient would speak for long periods of time, resisting interruption. When asked a question directly, he would either continue speaking or frown. His speech carried little meaning and often had few content words (e.g., "I think but it somehow I don't that it is"). He could not repeat simple sentences. He had tremendous difficulty naming familiar objects that were shown to him, such as a pencil for which he replied, "Oh, you know, that thing that you use to do things with . . . you use it to do stuff . . . you know, that thing." He was not able to point to objects that were placed in front of him. He could follow some commands that involved his midline, such as closing his eyes or looking behind him. He could not get in set to test praxis. His writing and reading were as impaired as his spoken language. After about 10 minutes of questioning, he got agitated, would not participate further in the exam, and had to be physically restrained temporarily.

An EKG performed in the ER revealed that he was in atrial fibrillation. A CT scan of the brain showed some early evidence of a left-hemisphere stroke. The patient was admitted to the neurology service and started on anticoagulation for a presumed embolic stroke. Several days later an MRI was performed that showed a left MCA stroke (Figure 3.4). After 1 week on the acute care service, he was transferred to the rehabilitation unit.

Right-Hemisphere Infarction (Neglect Syndrome)

Clinical Profile

A stroke in the distribution of the right MCA territory, causing damage to the frontal, temporal, and/or parietal lobes will cause a constella-

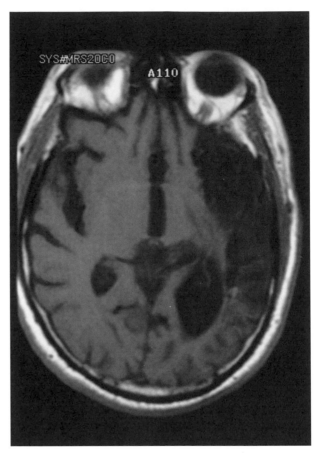

Figure 3.4 MRI scan from a patient with a left-hemisphere infarction that demonstrates damage to Wernicke's area (left temporal lobe).

tion of cognitive and behavioral impairments that reflect the functions subserved by the right hemisphere (Figure 3.5). Although the left hemisphere is often considered the "dominant" hemisphere because it subserves language functions in most individuals, the right hemisphere is "dominant" for several other cognitive processes. The most important function subserved by the right hemisphere is the ability of individuals to direct their attention into their environment. It is postulated that the right hemisphere can direct attention into both the left and right half of space, whereas the left hemisphere mostly directs attention into the right half of space. Thus, damage to the right hemisphere will cause a deficit directing attention into the left visual space. This deficit is known as *neglect*, the inability to respond to or acknowledge stimuli present in the left hemispace. Although neglect can also occur after left-hemisphere lesions, it is much more common and more severe after right-hemisphere damage. For a more comprehensive review of this topic, the reader is referred to the work by Heilman and colleagues (18).

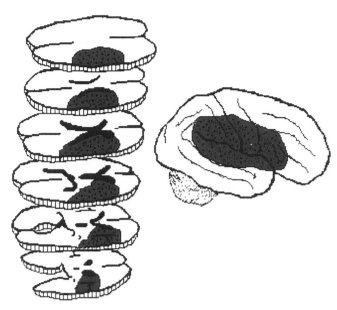

Figure 3.5 Schematic drawing of the lesion site—the right middle cerebral artery territory—that causes the right hemisphere syndrome.

Recent research of patients with right-hemisphere damage has demonstrated that there are at least three forms of neglect: attentional, representational, and intentional (18). *Attentional neglect* is the failure to attend to stimuli in the left hemispace. This type of neglect is easily demonstrated on the clinical examination. The patient seems to ignore people on his or her left side or will not eat items on the left side of the plate. On formal mental status testing, the patient shows marked rightward deviation when attempting to bisect a line. Another easy test for attentional neglect is to place a number of lines on a blank page and ask the patient to cross off all of the lines. The patient with attentional neglect will only cross off lines on the right side of the page and fail to acknowledge the lines on the left side of the page. It is vital that the clinician be able to recognize the difference between left visual neglect and *left visual hemianopia*, that is, the inability to see in the left visual field. The latter is due to damage to the visual system, usually at the level of the optic radiations in the temporal and parietal lobes or primary visual cortex in the occipital lobes. When the line bisection or line cancellation test is given to patients with neglect or a visual field deficit, performance may be identical. One way to distinguish between these two possibilities is to move the piece of paper with target stimuli into the right visual field of the patients. The patient with left visual field deficit should now be able to see the targets and bisect or cross them off. Patients with neglect will continue to avoid the left side of the page regardless of where the target stimuli is in their field of view. Unfortunately, there will be some patients with extensive right hemisphere damage that will demonstrate both neglect and a visual field deficit. In these patients, it may be impossible to disentangle these two phenomena. Another important point for clinicians to be aware of is that neglect may not be limited to the visual modality. When visual stimuli are presented simultaneously in opposite visual fields, patients with neglect will "extinguish" stimuli presented in the left visual field. That is, patients will fail to acknowledge stimuli in the left field only under simultaneous conditions, not during single presentation in the left field. This same phenomenon can occur with simultaneous presentation of auditory or tactile stimuli. The most common site of damage causing attentional neglect is in the posterior parietal lobe. However, attentional neglect can also occur after subcortical lesions, such as in the posterior thalamus.

A second type of neglect is called *representational neglect.* This type of neglect is manifested as a loss of the internal mental representation of the space opposite the side of the lesion. For example, when a group of patients with right hemisphere lesions were asked to imagine that they were facing a well known cathedral in a square in Milan, they were unable to recall details regarding the left side of the square. However, when they were asked to imagine themselves facing away from the cathedral they were able to recall those left sided details that were now on their right (19). Like patients with "attentional" neglect, patients with representation neglect also tend to have posterior lesions.

A third type of neglect, *intentional neglect*, is a unilateral deficit of motor program activation that causes reduced and delayed movements to the contralesional side (20). Thus, despite being aware of stimuli in the left side of space, patients will fail to respond to stimuli on the left side. For example, if a patient was blindfolded and asked to find all items spread across a table, they would be reluctant to move their right hand into the left side of the table for exploration. Intentional neglect is most common after frontal (or anterior) lesions.

In summary, the probable areas of organization for neglect are the parietal cortex for attentional-representational aspects (including attention to stimuli) and frontal-striatal structures for exploratory-motor (intentional) aspects. Several case reports have documented that the neural basis of these different behavioral components of neglect (exploratory-motor vs. perceptual sensory) corresponds to anterior vs. posterior right-hemisphere strokes (21). Patients with anterior lesions (frontal-anterior subcortical) exhibit neglect predominantly on tasks that emphasize exploratory-motor components of directed attention. Conversely, patients with posterior lesions (parietal) exhibit neglect on tasks that emphasize perceptual-sensory components. However, in most patients with right-hemisphere damage, clinical neglect probably represents an interaction of multiple mechanisms.

Other cognitive processes are likely lateralized to the right hemisphere; thus, damage to this hemisphere will cause additional impairments that accompany neglect. *Visuospatial skills* are often markedly impaired, especially following posterior lesions. Patients have significant difficulties with drawing copies of simple geometric figures or judging spatial relationships such as by matching lines with the same angle of orientation. Of course, patients with neglect will often only draw the right side of a figure (e.g., a flower or a house). *Motor impersistence*, the inability to maintain a posture, may also be present, especially after anterior lesions. Postures such as closing one's eyes or sticking out one's tongue cannot be maintained even for a few seconds. When motor impersistence is severe, almost any command that is asked by the physician or therapist will not be maintained, leading to a frustrating experience for patient and clinician. Language function, although subserved by the left hemisphere, can be impaired in a special way after right hemisphere damage. The resulting language deficit is called *aprosody*, or the inability to produce intonation required for adequate speech. Thus, patients will sound monotonous and are unable to place inflections in their voice to present a question, sound surprised, or sound angry. They may also have the inability to understand the inflection in other people's language, resulting in difficulty grasping the meaning of conversation. This type of language problem can be misinterpreted as depression.

Behavioral impairments following right-hemisphere damage are also common. One of the hallmark behaviors is *anosognosia*, the unawareness or denial of a deficit. This symptom can be one of the most striking phenomena in clinical neurology. For example, patients may deny that their hemiplegic arm is actually their own. These patients will often make many excuses for their inability to move their left arm or leg, yet never acknowledge that there is any deficit on the affected side. Right-hemisphere damage can lead to agitation, confusion, and mania. The severity of these symptoms can escalate to a point where the use of neuroleptics is necessary.

In summary, the right-hemisphere syndrome is a constellation of symptoms that include neglect, visuospatial impairments, aprosody, motor impersistence, and anosognosia. It is common for large lesions of the right hemisphere to cause hemiparesis or hemiplegia, sensory loss, and hemianopia. The clinical manifestations of the right hemisphere syndrome are outlined in Table 3.2.

Recovery and Prognosis

There is an empirical notion among rehabilitation clinicians that patients with right-hemisphere infarction in general have a poorer outcome than patients with left-hemisphere infarctions. That is, even with comparably sized lesions, right-hemisphere patients are less likely to walk out of the rehabilitation hospital and live with minimal assistance whereas it is not uncommon for patients with aphasia, even global aphasia, with comparable hemiparesis, to return to the physi-

Table 3.2. Clinical Profile
of Right-Hemisphere Syndrome

Cognitive impairment
- Neglect
- Visuospatial impairment
- Aprosody
- Motor impersistence

Behavioral impairment
- Denial of illness (anosognosia)
- Variety of behavioral deficits, including agitation and delusions

Neurologic impairment
- Motor, sensory, and visual deficits are common

cian's office for follow-up walking independently. This may not seem intuitive; one may have thought that the aphasia and apraxia that accompany left-hemisphere strokes would have more deleterious effects on motor recovery than visual neglect.

This clinical observation has baffled clinicians and has been substantiated in a study of patients recovering from left- and right-hemisphere strokes (22). It was found that after 6 months, patients with left hemiplegia (right-hemisphere strokes) had a lesser degree of independence and social adjustment as compared to patients with right hemiplegia (left-hemisphere strokes). Thus, patients with right-hemisphere strokes showed much less improvement in activities of daily living. This difference could not solely be accounted for by less motor recovery in patients with left hemiplegia. The presence of unilateral spatial neglect seemed to be the most important clinical factor that had a major role in deterring recovery of patients with right-hemisphere strokes. Other factors such as anosognosia, impaired intellectual performance, and global attentional disturbance were not important. This study emphasized the critical point that strategies for improving patients' overall functioning at home are not only dependent on their sensorimotor abilities but on their cognitive abilities as well.

The various deficits that occur after right-hemisphere infarction—inattention, neglect, anosognosia, aprosody, extinction of sensory stimuli, and hemiplegia—may recover at different rates. Extinction to simultaneous sensory stimuli can persist long after there are no signs of right-hemisphere damage or can be the only sign after a small right-parietal infarct. This phenomenon is often not tested for but can be critical. For example, after apparent recovery, one of my patients still showed evidence of extinction to double simultaneous visual stimuli. Although there were no other signs of neglect, this subtle deficit prevented him from immediately returning to driving, for if he was in the center lane of a highway, he may not see a car on his left if there was a car passing him simultaneously on the right. However, these issues have never been studied systematically. In light of the vital role of neglect in predicting functional outcome, this cognitive deficit may be the most important to study.

The overall incidence of neglect may be as high as 82% of patients with right-hemisphere stroke (23), and anosognosia may be as high as 28% (24). The rate of recovery from visual neglect appears to be similar to that for other neurologic deficits caused by stroke. Most recovery seems to occur in the first 10 days and reaches a plateau by 3 months (25). Overall, most patients with neglect make a good recovery, and many have no or a little neglect at 3 months. In a study of 34 patients with left-sided neglect, only 7 patients (21%) had significant neglect at 3 months (25). In this study, it was determined that three factors—the severity of neglect, anosognosia at 2 to 3 days, and the patient's age—could predict the extent of recovery of neglect and regaining of functional independence. Another study has shown that patients with larger right-hemisphere lesions and greater premorbid cortical atrophy showed the least recovery of neglect. Interestingly, lesion location did not correlate with recovery of neglect. Thus, it seems that recovery of neglect may depend on the extent and integrity of remaining undamaged brain tissue (26).

Therapeutic Remediation

Therapeutic remediation of unilateral spatial neglect remains a significant challenge for rehabilitation specialists. In general, neglect has been difficult to treat. As a first step, family members and others who will be interacting with these patients should be educated regarding the manifestations of the neglect syndrome. Neglect is a striking disorder and its manifestations are not always obvious. For example, it is a common misconception of family members of neglect patients that they cannot see out of their left "eye," rather than the patient being unable to attend to objects on the left side of their "world" that is being perceived by *both* eyes. Therefore, family members need to be taught that initially, in the acute stages when neglect is severe, it may be necessary to interact with the neglect patient on his or her right or non-neglected side. Although anosognosia is often transient, family members should understand that patients are not consciously denying the extent of their illness, but rather the denial is a manifestation of their brain damage.

A number of approaches toward treating neglect have been investigated. The studies from which the strongest conclusions can be drawn are those that have tested a specific type of experimental therapy against a standard course of rehabilitation that served as a control. For example, one group tested the hypothesis that a major part of the problem of patients with neglect is that these patients fail to adequately scan their environment (27). Patients were extensively trained to compensate for their impaired visual scanning through several strategies: 1) by utilizing tasks that compel patients to turn their heads to the left so that they could see the stimuli in their non-neglected right visual field; 2) by utilizing tasks that provide a target on the left side of space to serve as an anchoring point; 3) by utilizing tasks that do not have a high density of stimuli; and 4) by pacing the patient's visual scanning behavior to slow down impulsive tendencies to gaze toward the right side of space. After 1 month of training 1 hour per day, patients with this experimental treatment program showed significantly less visual neglect than the group that received standard rehabilitation. In a follow-up study, neglect patients were also trained to overcome other components of neglect behavior, which the investigators termed *sensory awareness* and *spatial organization* (28). Training in sensory awareness consisted of teaching the patient to locate on the back of a mannequin the spot on the patient's back that was touched by the examiner. Training in spatial organization consisted of learning to estimate the size of rods of various lengths. Again, patients that received this experimental therapy improved on measures of neglect to a greater degree than those receiving standard rehabilitation.

Another type of neglect therapy is based on the observation that limb movements on the side contralateral to the lesion can cause improvement in neglect (29). In this procedure, patients are trained to place and hold their left arm at the left margin of any activity they are engaged in. This therapy has the advantage of relying on a stimulus for an anchor, the left arm that is always present, unlike other scanning training procedures. The disadvantage is that the patients often have a profound left hemiplegia, making it difficult to use the left arm as an anchor. Interestingly, the left limb movement does not have to be visualized by the patient; that is, even when the left arm is placed behind a screen, improvement is seen. Thus, this method does not rely on visual cues. Another therapy shown to improve visual neglect is the use of Fresnel prisms fitted to the inside of a patient's glasses, intended to shift a peripheral image in the neglected visual field into the center of the retina. This treatment improved neglect as compared to controls, but there was no improvement noted in activities of daily living (ADL) function (30).

Although the above findings appear encouraging, there are a number of issues that must be considered. These studies have not shown that the effects of training to reduce neglect can improve performance on ADLs, which is a predominant goal in any type of cognitive rehabilitation. A possible reason for a lack of generalization of such neglect therapy may be due to the general attentional deficits that patients with right-hemisphere damage often suffer, limiting their ability to learn strategies and utilize them in real-life situations. It also appears that the effects of these therapies are not long lasting. In a follow-up study that utilized several of the neglect therapies described above, it was found that training could result in greater participation in daily activities, but by 4 months the performance of patients who underwent experimental therapy was equivalent to those who had standard rehabilitation (31). This suggests that patients who are trained in these types of procedures may learn compensatory strategies at a faster rate but their final level of performance is not affected.

Approaches other than compensatory strategies have been attempted to increase orientation to the neglected side; these strategies attempt to alter the neural system subserving directed attention. For example, it is hypothesized that neglect following a cortical lesion in the right hemisphere may be due to reduced activation of subcortical structures, specifically the superior colliculus on the right side. Thus, treatments designed to increase the activation of the right (ipsilesional) superior colliculus—a brain region that receives direct visual input from both eyes—may reduce left neglect. How does such treatment work? First, it is known that transient visual stimuli that move in a jerky motion are potent activators of the superior colliculus. When these type of stimuli were presented in the neglected (left) visual field in patients with right-hemisphere damage, it was found that their neglect was substantially reduced, presumably due to increased activation of the right superior colliculus (32). An interesting point to note about this study is that patients could benefit from this therapy even though they were unaware of the visual stimuli being presented in their neglected left visual field. This therapy does not require that the patient learn or remember a strategy because it is used automatically and unconsciously.

A second possible reason for unilateral neglect is that rather than the right superior colliculus being underactive and preventing orientation leftward, the left superior colliculus may be overactive, driving orientation predominantly to the right. Thus, treatments that would reduce activation to the left superior colliculus may also reduce neglect. It was proposed that if the right eye was patched (i.e., the eye ipsilateral to the lesion causing neglect), neglect would be reduced because the left superior colliculus (which gets most of its input from the right eye) would be less active. Also, the right superior colliculus would function more effectively because it would no longer be inhibited by the left colliculus. When the right eye was patched in neglect patients, they showed significant improvement in their performance on a line bisection task (33). The reduction of the neglect was noted to occur only when the patch was worn. An advantage of this second strategy is that it does not require the patient to remember a learned compensatory strategy. It was also found that combining monocular patching with presenting dynamic stimuli in the neglected left visual field were more effective at reducing neglect than either therapy alone (33).

Finally, pharmacologic therapy has also been attempted. Based on evidence from work with animals showing that the dopaminergic system is present in pathways involved in directed attention, dopaminergic agonist therapy using a drug called bromocriptine in two patients produced a statistically significant, yet mild, improvement in neglect. When the medication was removed, neglect worsened (34). However, to date, no double-blind controlled study has been performed to determine if this type of therapy is warranted.

Clinical Case Presentation

R.K. is a 62-year-old female with a history of hypertension and diabetes who presented to the hospital with a sudden onset of left-sided weakness. On presentation to the ER, she had an elevated blood pressure of 195/100 and a normal sinus rhythm on EKG. On neurologic examination, she demonstrated extremely poor attention and was markedly distractible. Her speech was hypophonic and monotonous, but there were no obvious paraphasic errors in spontaneous conversation. She had a difficult time staying in focus to follow verbal commands. Her head was turned to the right and she didn't seem to acknowledge anyone who stood on the left side of her bed. She responded to *threat* by eyeblink in her left visual field, but she didn't appear to acknowledge objects held in that visual field. Her left arm and leg were markedly hemiplegic. She vehemently denied that there was anything wrong with her and wanted to go home. She was admitted to the neurology service. An angiogram was performed, which documented that the etiology of her stroke was a complete occlusion of her right carotid artery. An MRI scan done 4 days after presentation revealed a large right MCA territory stroke (Figure 3.6). After a short course of anticoagulation, she was placed on aspirin and transferred to a rehabilitation hospital 7 days after the onset of her stroke.

On presentation to the rehabilitation hospital she underwent another neurologic examination. She did not appear distractible and seemed to have a depressed affect. She had difficulty with tasks of mental control such as counting backward from 20 or saying the months backward. She would get lost during these tasks as well as perform them very slowly. Her speech was aprosodic. When asked to repeat the sentence "John took Peter to the store?" as if she was asking a question, she was unable to place a terminal rise in her voice. When she sang the song "Happy Birthday," the words were correct but no melody was produced, despite her having been in her church choir. Her language was fluent with normal naming, repetition, and simple comprehension. Her reading demonstrated that she often did not read the first few letters of compound words (e.g., replying only "ball" for "baseball"). When asked to write several lines, they all deviated to the right side of the page. She had evidence of significant neglect when bisecting lines and was unable to cross off lines on the right side of the page. She could not close her eyes or stick out her tongue for more than a few seconds despite being told to do so several times. Her copy of a geometric

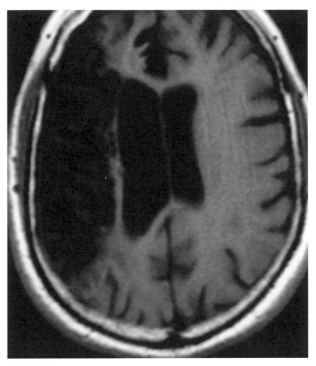

Figure 3.6   *MRI scan from a patient with a right hemisphere infarction affecting the frontal and parietal lobes.*

design lacked details on the left side. When asked why she was in the hospital, she replied, "I had to come here for an operation on my hip, it has been bothering me lately." When asked if she had ever had a stroke she replied, "Not that I am aware of." She was shown her left arm and asked whose it was. She replied, "Is it yours?" Even after feeling it with her right hand and tracing it back up to her right shoulder, she denied it was her arm.

On the rest of her neurologic exam, visual field testing revealed that she could sometimes detect finger movement in her left visual field but she always extinguished left-sided stimuli with double simultaneous stimuli. She also extinguished to tactile stimuli. She had left-face weakness, no movement of her left arm, and relatively good extensor strength in her left leg. Her tone and reflexes were increased on her left side. A positive Babinski's sign was found in her left foot.

During the hospital stay, she eventually acknowledged that she had indeed had a stroke and that it had affected her left side. However, even several weeks later, she still underestimated the extent of her deficit. Her global attention improved dramatically, but she still showed evidence of visuospatial neglect upon discharge 5 weeks after her stroke. Despite gaining almost full motor function in her left leg, she left the hospital requiring a wheelchair and home services.

Anterior Communicating Artery Aneurysm Rupture (ACoA Syndrome)

Clinical Profile

Rupture of an anterior communicating artery (ACoA) aneurysm commonly leads to cognitive and behavioral deficits, usually in the setting of minimal neurologic impairments (35). The resulting neurobehavioral deficits—referred to as the *ACoA syndrome*—are not due to nonspecific factors related to subarachnoid hemorrhage, such as diffuse vasospasm or an overall toxic effect of the bleed itself. Rather, the clinical manifestations of ACoA syndrome are caused by damage to specific locations in the anterior portions of the brain. As previously discussed, the ACoA syndrome results from infarction secondary to vasospasm of the arteries near the site of aneurysm rupture. Since the arteries involved are the ACoA, the ACA, and recurrent artery of Heubner, the areas of the brain involved are the basal forebrain, orbitomedial frontal lobes, and caudate nuclei, respectively (Figure 3.7).

Any combination of lesion sites can occur after an SAH due to an ACoA, which can lead to a wide range of deficits that includes amnesia, executive dysfunction, behavioral changes, and confabulation (36). The patient with the full syndrome may demonstrate all of these deficits. Alternatively, each of these deficits can occur in isolation. That is, the patient may have predominantly executive function impairments or an isolated amnesia. Finally, all these cognitive and behavioral impair-

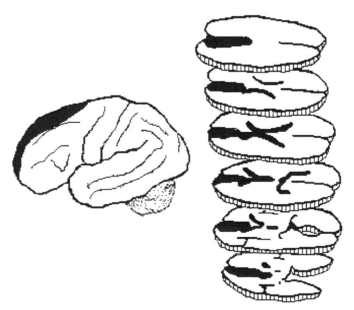

Figure 3.7 *Schematic drawing of the lesion site that causes the ACoA syndrome.*

ments can occur to varying degrees of severity. Several investigators have explored specific aspects of these impairments in detail in small groups of patients. For example, Irle et al (37) described a spectrum of *anterograde amnesia* (i.e., the ability to learn new information) in ACoA patients ranging from a severe deficit comparable to that seen in global amnestics (i.e., Korsakoff's syndrome) to no memory deficit at all. Likewise, Gade et al (38) described a pattern of *retrograde amnesia* (i.e., the ability to recall past information) in ACoA patients as a group that was similar to Korsakoff's syndrome. They observed a temporal gradient of remote recall with information from earlier decades being retrieved better than information from more recent decades. The memory deficits are thought to be due to damage of the basal forebrain, which is the location of the septal nuclei. These nuclei are directly linked to the hippocampus, one of the most important structures for learning and memory (39).

The executive function impairments commonly present following ACoA rupture have only been characterized in a small number of patients (40,41), and a clear understanding has not emerged. Executive dysfunction encompasses a wide variety of deficits including the inability to solve problems, poor organization and planning, inability to inhibit actions, and perseveration (42). These deficits are often referred to as the "frontal lobe syndrome" since they most commonly occur after frontal lobe damage, as with ACoA aneurysm rupture. Along with these cognitive impairments, the behavioral disturbance of the ACoA syndrome is consistent with that seen after frontal lobe damage. That is, patients can appear unconcerned and lack initiative and spontaneity.

Many, but not all, patients with ACoA rupture confabulate. In those who do, confabulation ranges from spontaneous and fantastic to confabulations that are only obtained when provoked. Spontaneous confabulations are often not based on factual information and may not even be compatible with general world knowledge. For example, a patient may tell her physician that over the previous weekend she was on vacation in the mountains with her family even though she was actually in the hospital. Provoked confabulations are often related to factual information and are usually in response to direct questioning. For example, patients may acknowledge that they have had an operation when asked about their stitches, but they may state that it was because they hit their head rather than for aneurysm repair. Recent research is beginning to identify the underlying mechanisms for confabulation (43). It has been observed that patients with severe amnesia or severe executive function impairment alone do not necessarily confabulate. However, patients with a combination of severe amnesia and executive dysfunction will markedly confabulate. Thus, confabulation is not solely due to amnesic patients who cannot fill in gaps or dysexecutive patients who cannot monitor their responses, rather it results from the interaction of the these two impairments. Since this combination of deficits is often seen after ACoA rupture due to combined lesions of the frontal lobes and basal forebrain, confabulation in these patients is commonly observed.

In summary, the ACoA syndrome may consist of a variable degree of amnesia, executive dysfunction, confabulation, and behavioral changes. Motor, sensory, or visual deficits are uncommon. Sometimes patients can exhibit motor akinesia; that is, despite good motor strength they will fail to initiate responses in the arm or leg contralateral to the side of their medial frontal lesion. Bilateral lesions of the frontal lobes can also lead to urinary incontinence and an abnormal gait that is described as "magnetic" since it appears as though the patient's feet are stuck to the floor. The clinical manifestations of the ACoA syndrome are outlined in Table 3.3.

Recovery and Prognosis

A number of studies have examined the prognosis of patients with ACoA rupture. It is critical to remember that a large number of patients who suffer subarachnoid hemorrhage do not survive. This is unlike ischemic stroke, where the risk of mortality is quite low but the high morbidity becomes a tremendous burden to society. Studies of unselected ACoA rupture patients have found persistent cognitive deficits present in a large percentage (59% to 83%) of patients (44,45). The occurrence of vasospasm seems to be the most consistent predictor of long-term cognitive deficits (45). This is logical since vasospasm will cause a stroke in the territory of the artery involved, accounting for the resulting neurologic disability. In the first few months following injury, the deficits that comprise the ACoA syndrome correlate with the extent of frontal and basal forebrain infarction. As previously mentioned, the ACoA syndrome reflects a wide range of deficit profiles, due to the

Table 3.3. *Clinical Profile of ACoA Syndrome*

Cognitive impairment
Executive function impairment
• Variability in degree and extent of deficit
Memory impairment
• Anterograde amnesia
• Retrograde amnesia
Behavioral impairment
• Confabulation ("spontaneous" and "provoked")
• Apathy, unconcern, disinhibition
Neurologic impairment
• Motor, sensory, and visual abnormalities are uncommon

combination of lesions in the basal forebrain and frontal lobes, and thus the patterns of recovery will also be variable.

Memory is the only cognitive function that has been studied in great detail in terms of recovery. One study demonstrated a relationship between lesion site and severity of anterograde amnesia. Patients with combined lesions in the basal forebrain and striatum or basal forebrain, striatum, and frontal lobes had a severe memory deficit, whereas patients with lesions in the basal forebrain or striatum alone showed essentially no deficit (37). Recovery of retrograde amnesia may depend on the extent of concurrent executive impairments. In another study, retrograde amnesia, but not anterograde amnesia, improved in a group of ACoA patients in parallel with recovery of executive function (46). Executive dysfunction can also persist. In the early stages of recovery, patients with the most significant frontal lobe damage have the most severe executive dysfunction. However, the factors that lead to poor recovery of executive function in ACoA patients have not been elucidated. Since the behavioral impairments in the ACoA syndrome are related to frontal lobe damage, it is likely that such impairments will improve in parallel with executive dysfunction. Also, since confabulation results from the interaction of executive and memory impairments, it will also recover along with these functions. It has been my experience that spontaneous confabulations are usually only noted during the acute stages following recovery, whereas the more limited and provoked confabulations may persist if executive and memory deficits persist.

Therapeutic Remediation

The most significant and persistent cognitive deficit in patients with ACoA syndrome is memory dysfunction. Cognitive remediation approaches to memory rehabilitation have developed along three general lines: 1) retraining a damaged memory system through exercises and drills, 2) using compensatory strategies such as memory aids and mnemonics, and 3) tapping residual learning abilities. The notion that practice improves memory is pervasive, yet there is no scientific evidence that such repetitive practice effectively generalizes to real-life situations despite numerous hours of intensive training (47,48). An illustration of this important point is an individual who increased his digit span from 7 to 80 by repetitive practice, but when switched to a memory-span task using letters, his performance dropped back to 7 items—the standard span performance (49).

Unlike a weakened muscle, damaged memory processes show little recovery through repetition training. The proliferation of inexpensive software for personal computers that allows endless memory drills increases the likelihood that patients will be exposed to memory rehabilitation paradigms that have no therapeutic value and that will ultimately lead to continued failure (50,51).

The alternative to repetition retraining is to develop strategies to compensate for impaired memory abilities. The goal of memory rehabilitation is not to restore the unrestorable but to produce improvements that will allow amnesic patients to understand and cope with these difficulties in ways that will lead to a more normal life (52). Several compensatory strategies for improving amnesia can be used, such as training patients to perform more elaborate encoding during the learning of new information or to use visual imagery to organize information during the time of learning in order to facilitate later recall. Unfortunately, any optimism that is generated from these techniques must be tempered by several limiting factors that likely prevent their practical use outside the laboratory. First, elaborate encoding by visual imagery or other mnemonics places excessive demands on brain-damaged patients who have limited processing capacities (53). Second, even if amnesic patients were capable of using these strategies, many patients are unaware of their memory deficits and thus unmotivated to use the strategies spontaneously. Third, it is not clear that even individuals with normal memory use these types of mnemonics when attempting to recall past learned information (50). Finally, mental imagery may help amnesic patients learn a short shopping list, but why not just teach the patient to write the items down on a piece paper—the ultimate compensatory strategy (54)?

A simple compensatory technique that can be highly effective in helping amnesic patients compensate for their difficulties is the use of memory prostheses. External memory aids reduce reliance on defective memory. Notebooks, diaries, name tags, posted signs containing useful information in critical areas around a person's living environment, or simply relying on a spouse all have been useful (55). Patients and families are often given too little instruction in the use of these aids; patients may then reject these memory aids or not use them correctly. Memory rehabilitation programs must be designed to train amnesic patients to use these external aids. One well-designed program takes at least 2 months to train patients to use a memory book spontaneously (56). ACoA patients with poor motivation due to frontal lesion may be poor candidates for external aids. It is our impression that external aids are only valuable for "forgetful" patients and not for the densely amnesic.

As a complement to memory aids, several investigators have developed "memory manuals" written for patients with a mild memory disturbance. They address typical day-to-day problems that patients will likely face and strategies for dealing with them (57,58). Many centers that treat patients with memory disorders also provide memory support groups to emphasize and reinforce the strategies. These groups may reduce anxiety and depression rather than improve memory performance, but this aspect of memory rehabilitation is also critical, and the efficacy of these groups is affirmed by the continued participation of its members (59).

Another type of compensation for memory difficulties is attempting to use residual memory capacities. The aim is to teach amnesic patients complex domain-specific knowledge that can be used to enhance their day-to-day functioning. Glisky et al (60) were able to teach dense amnesiacs the vocabulary necessary to use a personal computer and carry out simple programs. In this procedure, a definition is presented and the patient provided with as many letters as are needed to elicit the correct word. In subsequent learning trials, letters are gradually withdrawn from the cues until the patient can produce the correct word without the letter cues. The amnesic patients were eventually able to generate the definitions of each word in the absence of letter cues, and this was retained across a 6-week interval. This technique of "vanishing cues" produced faster learning and better retention than techniques without cues given.

In a follow-up study using the same technique, memory-impaired patients were taught the knowledge necessary to manipulate information on a computer screen and execute simple computer programs (61). Further, this knowledge was retained for up to 9 months (62). Finally, a severely amnesic patient with encephalitis was taught how to perform data entry into a computer and was able to demonstrate her skills in the workplace (63).

For amnesia, this technique has a profound limitation; the knowledge learned is "hyperspecific." That is, the knowledge is only accessible when the original conditions are reintroduced. This suggests that neither the information nor the procedure of learning generalizes to other situations. When the patients who were successful in the workplace were presented with novel situations, learning slowed dramatically (51). As a practical treatment matter, there are additional problems with implicit memory techniques. First, they take an inordinate amount of time and effort for a result with little generalization. Second, the patient is not prevented from making errors during learning, so errors can be endlessly repeated and inadvertently primed (52). Recent studies have shown that errorless learning paradigms are substantially better when the subject is not allowed to guess during the learning process (52). Despite these potential limitations, utilization of intact implicit memory systems in amnesic patients seems to have potential, but must be investigated further before it can be used clinically.

In summary, a theme for effective memory rehabilitation is beginning to emerge. Efforts to restore memory function are probably futile, thus efforts should be directed toward *compensating* for memory impairments. An important adjunct to these cognitive remediation therapies are "behavioral" therapies aimed at modifying a patient's attitude or beliefs concerning their condition (64). There is a single acid test for the value of any proposed memory therapy: Does treatment generalize to daily living? Little evidence exists that the various memory rehabilitation strategies previously discussed are effective in the real-life situations of these patients. Wilson argues that generalization should not be expected to occur and should be specifically taught in memory rehabilitation programs (64). Future work should be aimed at systematically evaluating the outcome of these programs.

Pharmacotherapy offers another potential approach toward improving memory dysfunction. The neurotransmitter most closely linked to memory function is acetylcholine. Early studies observed that healthy young subjects developed impairments on immediate and delayed free recall of word lists following the administration of the anticholinergic preparation scopolamine (65,66) and that these memory deficits could be alleviated by physostigmine, a cholinesterase inhibitor, which prolongs acetylcholine action within the synapse (67,68). This observation led to numerous investigations of acetylcholine replacement and augmentation therapy as a means of improving memory function in patients with dementia, especially Alzheimer's disease, in which a dominant cognitive impairment is amnesia. Overall, clinical trials with cholinergic medications in Alzheimer's disease have been disappointing since improvement in memory function has not been dramatic or sustained (for review, see 69). There have also been a handful of single case studies in which cholinergic drugs were administered to patients with memory impairments due to acute brain injury. A patient with temporal lobe damage from herpes simplex encephalitis HSE and another from a penetrating injury showed improvement on long-term memory tasks after administration of cholinergic agonists (70,71). A third patient with a lesion limited to the diagonal band of Broca in the basal forebrain after surgical resection of a low-grade glioma had modest improvement in supraspan immediate recall during treatment with physostigmine during the dose-finding phase. However, no benefit was found during a 6-day double-blind placebo-controlled trial (72). SPECT showed decreased blood flow in the medial temporal region ipsilateral to the lesion during baseline and increased blood flow in this region after a physostigmine dose. Placebo-controlled clinical trials of neurotransmitter drugs are necessary to determine their ultimate effect in patients with acute brain injury.

These pharmacologic studies have focused on episodic long-term memory. Much less work has addressed short-term memory. As mentioned, patients with ACoA rupture will have impairments in both short-term and long-term memory. The neurotransmitter most closely linked to short-term memory function is dopamine. The frontal lobes, damaged in ACoA rupture, and the structure that supports short-term memory contain the highest concentration of dopaminergic receptors in nonhuman primate cortex (73). Preliminary studies in humans have recently demonstrated that a dopaminergic agonist, bromocriptine, improves performance on short-term memory tasks when given to normal young subjects (74,75). Future studies will be necessary to determine if this medication will also help patients with impaired short-term memory.

In summary, acetylcholine may be one neurotransmitter that is critical for episodic long-term memory, and dopamine appears to modulate short-term memory. However the picture is probably much more complex. Many other neurotransmitters such as γ-aminobutyric acid (GABA), serotonin, and norepinephrine also play a role in memory function (76). Neuromodulators, such as neuropeptides (e.g., opioids and vasopressin), are also involved in memory processes (77). The operation of memory systems is likely the result of the interaction of multiple neurochemicals. It is naive to believe that treatment directed at a single neurotransmitter can affect memory significantly. Thus, an innovative approach for improving memory function that should be attempted in the future would be to influence several neurotransmitter systems, especially systems that are less affected but nevertheless interact in memory processes.

Clinical Case Presentation

A.C. is a 49-year-old female with a history of migraine headaches who presented to the hospital with a complaint of the "worst headache of her life." While watching a movie, she suddenly developed a terrible headache and lost consciousness. On the way to the ER she vomited, and in the ER she had a generalized tonic-clonic seizure. An emergent CT of the head was performed, which showed that there was subarachnoid blood especially anteriorly. Initial examination noted that she was lethargic but had reactive pupils and moved all four extremities to noxious stimuli. On that day, the patient underwent an angiogram, which showed that the patient had a 9-millimeter aneurysm of the anterior communicating artery. On the following day, the patient underwent a left frontoparietal craniotomy and clipping of this aneurysm. The patient did extremely well after surgery and was quickly extubated from the respirator. The patient slowly improved in the acute care hospital, except for confusion and confabulation. For example, the patient stated the bandages on her head were because she had an amniocentesis rather than recent brain surgery. She was subsequently transferred to a rehabilitation hospital 10 days after surgery.

On exam in the neurorehabilitation unit, she was awake and alert but distracted by the other people in her room. Her affect appeared flat and she showed little insight into her condition, denying having any problems. She often confabulated. When asked why part of her hair was shaved, she stated it was merely due to a recent haircut. She did not acknowledge being in a hospital, insisting that it was the "Metropolitan Museum of Art." She claimed she was able to say the months forward but made errors and was very slow with perseveration when she counted backward and said the months backward. She was not oriented to the date or hospital. She could not recall the hospital she was transferred from. She did know her name and address, but had trouble recalling past information. She did not know the current president, vice president, or governor. She also did not know any details about current events, such as the Gulf War that had recently ended. However, she was accurate when answering questions about episodes early in her life such as her marriage and the birth of her children. She had marked difficulty learning new information and after a delayed recall could not retrieve even simple information such as the name of the hospital which was told to her several times. She had poor executive function. She could not generate any words in the category "animals" in 1 minute. Her only response was "carrot." When asked to state her three favorite fruits she responded with pizza, chicken, and cole slaw over 45 seconds. She had difficulty with a task that required shifting set and alternating sequences. Her speech and language were intact. She did not have buccofacial or limb apraxia. She exhibited a poor strategy when drawing a geometric design. Her cranial nerves were fully intact, including visual fields. She had full strength and sensation, but appeared akinetic. Her reflexes were symmetric and coordination was normal. She could walk relatively normally and with minimal assistance.

A CT of the head performed 1 month after her SAH showed resorption of the subarachnoid blood. However, she had bilateral infarctions of the medial portions of the frontal lobes, the septum of the basal forebrain, and head of the caudate of the basal ganglia (Figure 3.8). About the time of this scan, she showed significant improvement in her spontaneity, attentional abilities, and response time to questions. There was also improvement in executive function, but it was still impaired. For example, she could now generate 10 fruits and vegetables and 7 animals in 1 minute. However, she continued to confabulate when prompted and was significantly amnesic.

Bilateral Thalamic Infarction (Dementia Syndrome)

Clinical Profile

A stroke that simultaneously damages the medial portion of both thalami causes a distinctive neurobehavioral syndrome (Figure 3.9). Although this is an uncommon syndrome, it is an excellent example of lesions to subcortical structures, such as the thalamus or basal ganglia, causing cognitive and behavioral impairments that are as severe as those caused by cortical lesions. This unusual stroke occurs because some patients have an anomalous arterial supply of the thalamus where there is a single origin for both of the paramedian thalamic arteries that supply the medial parts of the thalamus. This creates the pos-

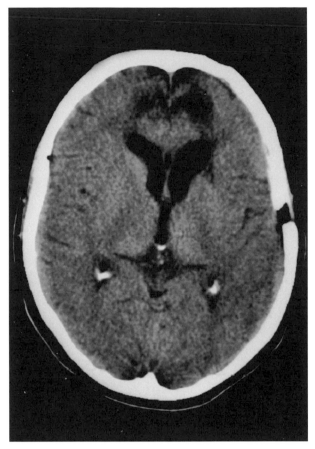

Figure 3.8 *CT scan from a patient with ACoA aneurysm rupture showing damage to medial frontal lobes, septum, and left caudate.*

sibility of a single embolus causing a blockage of flow to both the left and right thalamus simultaneously. The thalamus is a critical relay station and functional gateway for all information arriving from sensory receptors prior to projecting to the overlying cerebral cortex. The dorsomedial nucleus, one of several distinct thalamic nuclei, receives projection from the medial temporal lobes and projects forward to the dorsolateral frontal lobes. Thus, this thalamic nucleus is part of an important distributed network of brain regions that support memory and executive function. This strong interrelationship with these other brain regions accounts for the behavioral and cognitive deficits found on clinical examination.

Patients with bilateral thalamic infarcts present to the hospital with a depressed level of consciousness ranging from a drowsy state to a deep coma. Since acute strokes do not usually appear on initial neuroimaging studies, an emergent CT or MRI scan of the brain will not reveal the diagnosis. The initial workup of these patients often involves a search for metabolic and toxic etiologies of a hypoaroused patient.

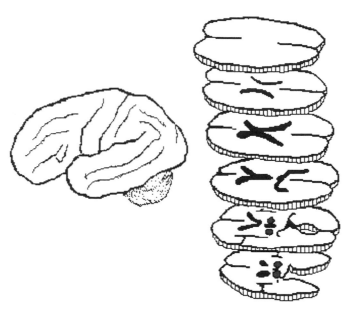

Figure 3.9 *Schematic drawing of the lesion site that causes the bilateral thalamic stroke syndrome.*

Patients will eventually awaken, and later neuroimaging will reveal small bilateral thalamic infarctions. The period of hypoarousal can last a few days or be prolonged for several weeks to months. There are even several reported patients that were hypersomnolent, remaining in bed most of the day, more than a year after their stroke (78). The early arousal deficits are probably due to damage of the ascending reticular activating system, projecting to the intralaminar nuclei of the thalamus.

Following this hypersomnolent state, patients can have significant cognitive impairments. Most noticeable is that despite regaining alertness, patients will demonstrate significant impairments in attention and mental control. Patients will respond very slowly when attempting to perform tasks to test these cognitive functions; simple observation of the patients will demonstrate their distractibility. Even after their attention improves, patients will exhibit deficits in executive function. Patients are initially disoriented, and memory testing will reveal impairments in both anterograde and retrograde memory. The pattern of memory deficit can be similar to the pattern found in other severe amnesic disorders such as Korsakoff's syndrome. Despite many significant cognitive deficits, there are several areas of preserved function; for example, language remains fluent with good naming, repetition, comprehension, reading, and writing.

Patients with this syndrome will also manifest several behavioral impairments, which are related to their executive and memory impairments. Patients have behaviors consistent with a frontal lobe syndrome; these include apathy, unconcern, and a lack of spontaneity and motivation. Patients will not typically engage in any spontaneous activity unless they are prompted. When patients do initiate responses, they are often perseverative. Confabulation can also be a prominent feature of the clinical picture.

In addition to the cognitive and behavioral abnormalities observed, other neurologic findings are present. Patients may have speech abnormalities that include dysarthria and hypophonia. Patients with lesions that extend into the midbrain may have deficits in eye movements such as limited upgaze and poor convergence. Incoordination such as limb and gait ataxia may also be present. Despite these findings on examination, motor and sensory deficits are uncommon.

In summary, patients with bilateral paramedian thalamic infarction have initial deficits in arousal, but eventually have normal wakefulness. Note that the critical factor for the presenting symptoms of this syndrome is that the lesions are bilateral, since a unilateral lesion will not cause an initial deficit in arousal (79). Behavioral and cognitive deficits are consistent with executive and memory dysfunction. Features of this syndrome are similar to other syndromes that damage frontal as well as septohippocampal systems (e.g., those previously described under ACoA syndrome). The clinical manifestations of bilateral thalamic stroke syndrome are outlined in Table 3.4.

Recovery and Prognosis

The outcome of patients with bilateral paramedian thalamic infarcts is poor. In one study, five (83%) of six patients with this syndrome showed no functional improvement (80). Of the patients with poor outcomes, one was institutionalized and the other patient was cared for at home but required constant supervision. The single patient that recovered functional independence in most of the activities of daily living

Table 3.4. Clinical Profile of
Bilateral Thalamic Stroke Syndrome

Cognitive impairment
- Transient coma followed by hypersomnolent state
- Impaired attention and mental control
- Anterograde and retrograde amnesia
- Slowness of thought and response

Behavioral impairment
- Apathetic, flat affect
- Lack of spontaneity and motivation
- Confabulation

Neurologic impairment
- Eye movement abnormalities are usually seen
- Motor and sensory deficits are uncommon

had a unilateral lesion. A conclusion that can be drawn from this study is that bilateral thalamic lesions will result in a poor functional outcome, whereas unilateral lesions may make a good recovery. However, since this condition is uncommon, there has not been a large enough study to substantiate this claim.

Therapeutic Remediation

Rehabilitation goals differ depending on what point in the course of recovery the patient is admitted to the rehabilitation unit. If the patient is admitted early in the course of recovery when still hypersomnolent, there is little to offer except supportive care while waiting for the patient to become more alert. Since the range of the recovery period is wide, it is possible that in some cases early admission to a rehabilitation unit is not rational. In some instances, patients can be admitted to a skilled nursing facility and transferred later when their level of arousal has improved. In many ways, the clinical state early in the course is analogous to patients with a closed head injury who are awakening from a vegetative state, and similar guidelines that have been outlined in earlier chapters should be followed.

After obtaining almost complete wakefulness, rehabilitation strategies may depend on whether the patient has bilateral lesions. Since bilateral lesions carry a poor outcome, goals should incorporate the assumption that patients will require some assistance with activities of daily living when discharged home, and efforts should be aimed at maximizing abilities necessary to regain as much of their independence as possible. Cognitive remediation therapies may be directed at the specific deficits identified in these patients, for example, memory impairment, which may be the most profound deficit. Strategies would be similar to those discussed for patients with ACoA rupture, since the nature of the memory deficit is similar. Unfortunately, since these patients often have deficits in several cognitive domains, effective cognitive rehabilitation is often difficult.

Clinical Case Presentation

S.J. is a 33-year-old female with a past medical history with hypothyroidism and borderline diabetes who presented to the hospital after being found by her husband unconscious on their bed. He did not observe tonic-clonic movements nor urinary incontinence. She was immediately brought to the ER, where it was determined that she had normal vital signs including an arterial blood gas. She could not be aroused but did withdraw to noxious stimuli; otherwise her neurologic exam was unremarkable. She did not respond to intravenous naloxone hydrochloride (Narcan) and glucose. Her stomach was ravaged but no pill fragments were noted. An emergent CT, lumbar puncture, and extensive blood work including a toxicology screen were all normal.

By the day following admission, she became arousable but was not following commands, and it was noted that her gaze was dysconjugate. Given the initially normal medical workup, the psychiatry service raised the possibility of a conversion disorder. Two days after her initial presentation, an MRI was performed which showed new bilateral thalamic infarcts. This prompted a workup for stroke occurring in young patients. She did not have evidence of vertebrobasilar atherosclerosis on transcranial dopplers; an echocardiogram was normal, ruling out a cardiac thrombus; and blood studies did not reveal any evidence for a hypercoaguable state. She was therefore started on aspirin for stroke prophylaxis. Over the first week, she began to wake up but exhibited long latencies for responses. her most profound difficulties were with attention and memory.

After 2 weeks in the hospital, she remained alert enough during the day to be transferred to a rehabilitation hospital. On examination, she was awake but not fully oriented. Her voice was dysarthric to a degree that most of her words were unintelligible. Her responses to most questions were slow. She had marked difficulty with tasks of mental control such as saying the months backward. She could not maintain set or sustain attention on a vigilance task. She had difficulty learning five new words, and after learning them she could not recall any of the items after a distracted delay. Her memory was just as impaired when she was asked to remember visual designs. Despite her impaired speech, her language was intact, including naming, repetition, and comprehension. She had no evidence of buccofacial or limb apraxia. She could copy geometric designs.

A follow-up MRI scan was performed approximately 1 month after her stroke, which again revealed bilateral medial thalamic infarcts (Figure 3.10). She continued to make steady gains in both attention and memory function, but as of 6 months post stroke, she still required assistance at home and could not take care of her children on her own.

CONCLUSION

Stroke is a common cause of neurologic disability and can result in many distinct syndromes. Four examples of specific stroke syndromes that cause a wide spectrum of cognitive, behavioral, and neurologic deficits have been presented in this chapter. This review should help the clinician abandon the notion that all strokes cause a homogeneous clinical profile. As stroke patients are encountered on neurorehabilitation units, a rational approach must be taken in their evaluation in order to develop appropriate rehabilitation goals. First, a careful mental

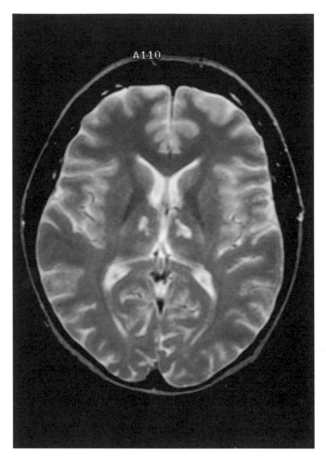

Figure 3.10   *MRI scan from a patient with bilateral medial thalamic strokes.*

status and neurologic exam must be performed. Such an examination, as outlined in the clinical case presentations, will properly characterize the cognitive and neurologic deficits caused by brain damage. These findings can then be correlated with the extent and location of the brain damage. Determining such clinicoanatomic relationships can allow the clinician to decide if the deficits found are consistent with the extent of brain damage. If there is mismatch between clinical findings and the lesion, it is possible that a coexisting pathology, such as anoxia or a metabolic encephalopathy, may be contributing to the clinical picture. Concurrent anoxia will markedly change the prognosis for most patients, whereas a coexisting metabolic derangement, such as hepatic encephalopathy, may be treated and lead to significant recovery. The nature of the deficits found on exam will help the clinician identify weaknesses that need to be addressed in therapy and possible strengths that can be used as anchor points for recovery.

Second, as a supplement to the examination, there is important clinical data that must be extracted from the medical records that are

Table 3.5: *Clinical Data to Gather from the Medical Records for Patients with Stroke or Subarachnoid Hemorrhage*

Stroke
- Early medical or neurologic complications
- Adequate stroke workup, including CT or MRI scan, carotid studies or angiogram, echocardiogram
- Initiation of aspirin or anticoagulation therapy
- Previous history of strokes or transient ischemic attacks
- Extent of lesion on CT or MRI scan

Subarachnoid hemorrhage
- Clinical grade on arrival at emergency room
- Evidence for vasospasm
- Exact site of aneurysm
- Complications during surgery
- Evidence for hydrocephalus
- Extent of lesion on CT or MRI scan

usually sent with the patient from the acute care hospital. No evaluation is complete without knowing the exact details of the care and workup that were previously provided. Depending on the type of vascular event that the patient suffered (e.g., stroke, subarachnoid hemorrhage), slightly different data will need to be determined. Table 3.5 highlights some of this important information. It is not uncommon for an additional workup to be necessary after the patient has arrived in the rehabilitation hospital.

Third, any neuroimaging studies such as CT or MRI scans must be reviewed. If these studies are not available on admission of the patient, every effort should be made to obtain them. A common theme throughout this chapter was that the location and extent of the lesion can predict recovery of function. Thus, review of the neuroimaging scans—not the dictated report—is essential for this determination. After these steps are taken on admission of a new patient to the neurorehabilitation service, a valuable and unique set of data will be obtained for each patient; there is no common formula that can be applied to all patients. This information can be used to plan directed and rational rehabilitation goals that will lead, one hopes, to a patient recovering with minimal neurologic dysfunction.

References

1. Feinberg T, Farah MJ. Behavioral Neurology and Neuropsychology. New York: McGraw-Hill, 1997.

2. Benson D. The neurology of thinking. New York: Oxford University Press, 1994.

3. Caplan L, Stein R. Stroke: a clinical approach. Boston: Butterworth, 1986.

4. McCormick W. Pathology and pathogenesis of intracranial saccular aneurysms. Semin Neurol 1984;4:291–303.

5. Hunt W, Hess R. Surgical risk as related to time of intervention in the repair of intracranial aneurysms. J Neurosurg 1968;28:14–20.

6. Alexander M, Fischette M, Fischer R. Crossed aphasias can be mirror image or anomalous. Case reports, review and hypothesis. Brain 1989;112:953–973.

7. Alexander M, Benson D. The aphasias and related disturbances. In: Joynt R, ed. Clinical neurology. vol. 1. Philadelphia: JB Lippincott Co., 1991:1–58.

8. Kertesz A. Recovery and treatment. In: Heilman K, Valenstein E, eds. Clinical neuropsychology. 3rd ed. New York: Oxford University Press, 1993.

9. Kertesz A, McCabe P. Recovery patterns and prognosis in aphasia. Brain 1977;100:1–18.

10. Lomas J, Kertesz A. Patterns of spontaneous recovery in aphasic groups: a study of adult stroke patients. Cortex 1978;5:388.

11. Naeser M, Helm-Estabrooks N, Haas G, et al. Relationship between lesion extent in Wernicke's area on computed tomographic scan and predicting recovery of comprehensions in Wernicke's aphasia. Arch Neurol 1987;44:73–82.

12. Hecaen H. Acquired aphasia in children and the ontogenesis of hemispheric functional specialization. Brain Lang 1976;3:114.

13. Kertesz A, Benson D. Neologistic jargon: a clinicopathologic study. Cortex 1970;6:362–387.

14. Helm-Estabrooks N, Albert M. Manual of aphasia therapy. Austin, TX: ProEd, 1991.

15. Jones L, Wepman J. Dimensions of language performance in aphasia. J Speech Hear Res 1961;4:220–232.

16. Naeser M, Haas G, Mazursky P, et al. Sentence level auditory comprehension treatment program for aphasic adults. Arch Phys Med Rehabil 1986;67:393.

17. Benson D. Aphasia rehabilitation. Arch Neruol 1979;36:187.

18. Heilman K, Valenstein E. Neglect and related disorders. In: Heilman K, Valenstein E, eds. Clinical neuropsychology. 3rd ed. New York: Oxford University Press, 1993.

19. Bisiach E, Luzzatti C. Unilateral neglect of representational space. Cortex 1978;14:129–133.

20. Coslett H, Bowers D, Fitzpatrick E, et al. Directional hypokinesia and hemispatial inattention in neglect. Brain 1990;113:475–486.

21. Daffner K, Ahern G, Weintraub S, Mesulam M. Dissociated neglect behavior following strokes in the right hemisphere. Ann Neurol 1990;28:97–101.

22. Denes G, Semenza C, Stoppa E, Lis A. Unilateral spatial neglect and recovery from hemiplegia: a follow-up study. Brain 1982;105:543–552.

23. Stone S, Halligan P, Greenwood R. The incidence of neglect phenomena and related disorders in patients with an acute right or left hemispheric stroke. Age Ageing 1993;22:46–52.

24. Cutting J. The study of anosognosia. J Neurol Neurosurg Psychiatry 1978;41:548–555.
25. Stone S, Patel P, Greenwood R, Halligan P. Measuring visual neglect in acute stroke and predicting its recovery: the visual neglect recovery index. J Neurol Neurosurg Psychiatry 1992;55:431–436.
26. Levine D, Warach D, Benowitz L, Calvanio R. Left spatial neglect: effects of lesion size and premorbid brain atrophy on severity and recovery following right cerebral infarction. Neurology 1986;1986: 362–366.
27. Weinberg J, Diller L, Gordon W, et al. Visual scanning training effect on reading-related tasks in acquired right brain damage. Arch Phys Med Rehabil 1977;58:479–486.
28. Weinberg J, Diller L, Gordon W, et al. Training sensory awareness and spatial organization in people with right brain damage. Arch Phys Med Rehabil 1979;60:491–496.
29. Robertson I, North N, Geggie C. Spatiomotor cueing in unilateral left neglect: three case studies of its therapeutic effects. J Neurol Neurosurg Psychiatry 1992;55:799–805.
30. Rossi P, Kheyfets S, Reding M. Fresnel prisms improve visual perception in stroke patients with homonymous hemianopia or unilateral visual neglect. Neurology 1990;40:1597–1599.
31. Gordon W, Hibbard M, Egelko S, et al. Perceptual remediation in patients with right brain damage: a comprehensive program. Arch Phys Med Rehabil 1985;66:353–359.
32. Butter C, Kirsch N, Reeves G. The effect of lateralized dynamic stimuli on unilateral spatial neglect following right hemispheric lesions. Restorative Neurol Neurosci 1990;2:39–46.
33. Butter C, Kirsch N. Combined and separate effects of eye patching and visual stimulation on unilateral neglect following stroke. Arch Phys Med Rehabil 1992;73:1133–1139.
34. Fleet W, Valenstein E, Watson R, Heilman K. Dopamine agonist therapy for neglect in humans. Neurology 1987;37:1765–1770.
35. DeLuca J, Diamond B. Aneurysm of the anterior communicating artery: a review of neuroanatomical and neuropsychological sequelae. J Clin Exp Neuropsych 1995;17:100–121.
36. Alexander M, Freedman M. Amnesia after anterior communicating artery aneurysm. Neurology 1984;34:752–757.
37. Irle E, Wowra B, Kunert H, et al. Memory disturbance following anterior communicating artery rupture. Ann Neurol 1992;31:473–480.
38. Gade A, Mortensen E. Temporal gradient in the remote memory impairment of amnesic patients with lesions in the basal forebrain. Neuropsychologia 1990;28:985–1001.
39. Carpenter M. Core text of neuroanatomy. 4th ed. Baltimore: Williams & Wilkins, 1991.
40. Shoqeirat M, Mayes A, MacDonald C, et al. Performance on tests sensitive to frontal lobe lesions by patients with organic amnesia: Leng & Parkin revisited. Br J Clin Psychol 1990;29:401–408.
41. Parkin A, Yeomans J, Bindschaedler C. Further characterization of the executive memory impairment following frontal lobe lesions. Brain Cogn 1994;26:23–42.
42. Damasio A, Anderson S. The frontal lobes. In: Heilman K, Valenstein E, eds. Clinical neuropsychology. New York: Oxford University Press, 1993:409–460.

43. Fischer R, Alexander M, D'Esposito M, Otto R. Neuropsychological and neuroanatomical correlates of confabulation. J Clin Exp Neuropsychol 1995;17:20–28.

44. Laiacona M, De Santis A, Barbarotto R, et al. Neuropsychological follow-up of patients operated for aneurysms of anterior communicating artery. Cortex 1989;25:261–273.

45. Stenhouse L, Knight R, Longmore B, Bishara S. Long-term cognitive deficits in patients after surgery on aneursyms of the anterior communicating artery. J Neurol Neurosurg Psychiatry 1991;54:909–914.

46. D'Esposito M, McGlinchey-Berroth R, Alexander M, et al. Cognitive recovery following anterior communicating artery aneurysm rupture. J Int Neuropsychol Soc 1995;1:364.

47. Prigatano G, Fordyce D, Zeiner H, et al. Neuropsychological rehabilitation after closed head injury in young adults. J Neurol Neurosurg Psychiatry 1984;47:505–513.

48. Godfrey H, Knight R. Cognitive rehabilitation of memory functioning in amnesic alcoholics. J Clin Exp Neuropsychol 1985;8:292–312.

49. Erickson R, Chase W. Acquisition of a memory skill. Science 1980;208:1181–1182.

50. O'Connor M, O'Connor CL, Cermak LS. Rehabilitation or organic memory disorders. In: Meier M, Benton AL, Diller L, eds. Neuropsychological rehabilitation. New York: Guilford Press, 1987.

51. Glisky E, Schacter D. Models and methods of memory rehabilitation. In: Boller F, Grafman J, eds. Handbook of neuropsychology. New York: Elsevier, 1991:233–246.

52. Wilson BA. Rehabilitation of memory disorders. In: Squire L, Butters N, eds. Neuropsychology of memory. 2nd ed. New York: Guilford Press, 1993.

53. Baddeley A. Amnesia: a minimal model and interpretation. In: Cermak L, ed. Human amnesia. Hillsdale: Lawrence Erlbaum, 1982:305–336.

54. Parkin A. Memory: phenomenon, experiment and theory. Oxford: Blackwell, 1993.

55. Harris J. External memory aids. In: Gruneberg M, Morris P, Sykes R, eds. Practical aspects of memory. vols. 172–179. London: Academic Press, 1978.

56. Sohlberg M, Sohlberg MC. Training use of compensatory memory books: a three stage behavioural approach. J Clin Exp Neuropsychol 1989;11:871–891.

57. Kapur N. The Wessex memory manual. 1989.

58. Beaulieu K, Knipe C, Selley S, Sunderland S. Burden memory group manual. 1990.

59. Evans J, Wilson B. A memory group for individuals with brain injury. Clin Rehabil 1992;6:75–81.

60. Glisky E, Schacter D, Tulving E. Learning and retention of computer-related vocabulary in memory-impaired patients: method of vanishing cues. J Clin Exp Neuropsychol 1986;3:292–312.

61. Glisky E, Schacter DL, Tulving E. Computer learning by memory impaired patients: acquisition and retention of complex knowledge. Neuropsychologia 1986;24:313–328.

62. Glisky E, Schacter DL. Long-term memory retention of computer learning by patients with memory disorders. Neuropsychologia 1988;26:173–178.

63. Glisky EL, Schacter DL. Extending the limits of complex learning in organic amnesia: computer training in a vocational domain. Neuropsychologia 1989;17:107–120.
64. Wilson B. A rehabilitation of memory. New York: Guilford Press, 1987.
65. Crow TJ, Grove-White IG, Ross DG. An analysis of the learning deficit following hyoscine administration in man. Br J Pharmacol 1973;49:322–327.
66. Crow TJ, Grove-White IG, Ross DG. The specificity of the action of hyoscine on human learning. Br J Clin Pharmacol 1975;2:367–368.
67. Drachman DA, Leavitt JL. Human memory and the cholinergic system: a relationship to aging? Arch Neurol 1974;30:113–121.
68. Drachman DA. Memory and cognitive function in man: does the cholinergic system have a specific role? Neurology 1977;27:783–790.
69. Thal L. Pharmacological treatment of memory disorders. In: Boller F, Grafman J, eds. Handbook of neuropsychology. New York: Elsevier, 1991:247–267.
70. Peters B, Levin H. Memory enhancement after physostigmine treatment in the amnesic syndrome. Arch Neurol 1977;34:215–219.
71. Goldberg E, Gerstman L, Mattis S, et al. Effects of cholinergic treatment on posttraumatic anterograde amnesia. Arch Neurol 1982;39:581.
72. Chatterjee A, Morris M, Bowers D, et al. Cholinergic treatment of an amnestic man with a basal forebrain lesion: theoretical implications. J Neurol Neurosurg Psychiatry 1993;56:1282–1289.
73. Brown R, Crane A, Goldman P. Regional distribution of monoamines in the cerebral cortex and subcortical structures of the rhesus monkey: concentrations and in vitro synthesis rates. Brain Res 1979;168:133–150.
74. Luciana M, Depue R, Arbisi P, Leon A. Facilitation of working memory in humans by a D2 dopamine receptor agonist. J Cogn Neurosci 1992;4:58–68.
75. Kimberg D, D'Esposito M, Farah M. The effects of bromocriptine, a D-2 receptor agonist, on the cognitive abilities of human subjects with different working memory capacities. Soc Neurosc Abstr 1994;20:1271.
76. Altman HJ, Normile HJ, Gershon S. Non-cholinergic pharmacology in human cognitive disorders. In: Stahl SM, Iverson SD, Goodman EC, eds. Cognitive neurochemistry. New York: Oxford University Press, 1987:346–371.
77. Zager EL, Black P. Neuropeptides in human memory and learning processes. Neurosurgery 1985;17:355–369.
78. Gentilini M, DeRenzi E, Girolamo C. Bilateral paramedian thalamic artery infarcts: report of eight cases. J Neurol Neurosurg Psychiatry 1987;50:900–909.
79. Castaigne P, Lhermitte F, Buge A, et al. Paramedian thalamic and midbrain infarcts: clinical and neuropathological study. Ann Neurol 1981;10:127–148.
80. Katz D, Alexander M, Mandell A. Dementia following strokes in the mesencephalon and diencephalon. Arch Neurol 1987;44:1127–1133.

Traumatic Brain Injury

Douglas I. Katz

Patients with traumatic brain injury (TBI) present many diagnostic and prognostic challenges for rehabilitation clinicians. First, injury to the brain produced by trauma may involve a number of different pathologic processes. This makes it difficult to attribute specific clinical problems to any single lesion. Second, many of the diffuse pathologic processes that occur as a result of injury cannot be directly detected by clinical examination or current neuroimaging techniques. Third, the most common impairments in these patients, such as those associated with enduring frontal systems dysfunction, are the most difficult to evaluate and quantify even with sophisticated neuropsychologic protocols. Nonetheless, there are some principled strategies that rehabilitation clinicians can use to arrive at meaningful diagnoses that guide thoughtful prognostication. To that end, this chapter presents a framework for determining the expected natural history of TBI. This framework strives to predict a functional outcome that can then be used to set realistic long-term goals and appropriate time frames in which they can be achieved.

EPIDEMIOLOGY

The incidence of TBI in the United States is 200 cases per 100,000 persons, or about 500,000 new cases per year, establishing it as the most commonly encountered serious brain disorder. Thus, the incidence of TBI now exceeds that of stroke and epilepsy (1). However, of that number only 20 percent are defined as moderate or severe injuries (2). Half of those patients with sustaining severe injuries die. The remainder of these patients as well as those with moderate injuries generally require extensive utilization of the health care system. Traumatic brain injury is largely a disorder affecting young men. As such, the peak incidence occurs between the ages of 15 and 24, with men outnumbering women by more than two to one. In this age group, motor vehicle accidents are the most common cause of TBI. Other common causes of TBI include falls, assaults, and sports injuries. The true prevalence of injury related to each of these causes is also dependent on such factors as age and geographic location. For example, assault and firearm injuries are the most common cause of TBI in high-density urban areas (2). On the other hand, falls are the primary cause of injury in the very young and the very old. Alcohol use contributes to about half of all injuries (3).

MECHANISM AND PATHOLOGY

Mechanical Force

The neuropathologic consequences of TBI are the result of primary damage from mechanical forces and a host of secondary, reactive processes. The mechanical forces fall into two categories: direct contact and acceleration/deceleration. As expected, *direct contact* forces involve an invariable interaction between the object producing the force, such as a club, the calvarium, and ultimately the central nervous system (CNS). It is this translation of the force to the CNS that causes damage to the underlying brain tissue, primarily producing *focal* injury.

Acceleration/deceleration forces are typically produced during motor vehicle accidents or falls of more than 6 feet. They cause damage by creating shear and tensile strains in the parenchyma and vascular supply of the brain, due to displacement of brain tissues. These dynamisms cause both focal and *diffuse* damage. Focal injuries occur because decelerational forces produce movement of the brain itself within the skull. The polar and inferior frontal and temporal cortical surfaces are particularly vulnerable to abrasion because of 1) the bony configuration of the anterior and middle fossas of the calvarium, and 2) the confinement of these brain areas to a small volume in the calvarium, allowing for a higher gradient of strain to be produced with deceleration forces. Cortical contusions such as these are the primary cause of focal pathology occurring as a result of closed TBIs. The primary diffuse pathology of TBI is diffuse axonal injury.

Table 4.1. Focal and Diffuse Injuries Associated with Trauma to the Brain

	Focal	**Diffuse**
Primary injury	Focal cortical contusion Deep cerebral hemorrhage Extracerebral hemorrhage*	Diffuse axonal injury Petechial white matter hemorrhage
Secondary injury	Delayed neuronal injury Microvascular injury Focal hypoxic-ischemic injury Herniation	Delayed neuronal injury Microvascular injury Diffuse hypoxic-ischemic injury

*Exerts effect on brain by way of secondary injury.

Understanding the neuropathology differentially associated with both diffuse and focal injuries is clinically important because each has a unique natural history and a particular pattern of recovery. A host of secondary processes are associated with either type of neuropathology and can lead to many patterns of delayed CNS injury (Table 4.1).

Diffuse Pathophysiology

Diffuse axonal injury (DAI) is caused when shear and tensile strains produce a deformation of neuronal axons, which sets off a cascade of destructive processes beginning with defective axonal transport, progressing to axonal swelling, and ending with separation of the proximal and distal axonal segments over 12 to 24 hours (Figure 4.1) (4). Diffuse axonal injury occurs throughout the cerebral hemispheres and brainstem; the amount and location are directly related to the magnitude of the accelerational forces involved. The overall severity of CNS injury is also directly related to the amount of DAI produced by these forces (5). The distribution of DAI seems to follow a gradient from the peripheral cerebral cortex to the central midbrain and concentrates in susceptible locations, such as the medial frontal lobes, the corpus callosum, and the superior cerebellar peduncles (Figure 4.2; see also Figure 4.15).

The complete picture of diffuse traumatic damage involves a number of associated secondary phenomena. In addition to axonal disruption, damage to the dendritic neuronal processes of the soma may also occur (6). Secondary neuronal injury may also be created by biochemical insults—such as surges of excitatory neurotransmitters, which produce toxicity by creating massive neuronal depolarization—and by forming free radicals, which cause membrane lipoperoxidation (7). Diffuse microvascular damage, contributing to edema, ischemia, or hemorrhage is another important source of secondary injury. It is produced by mechanical rupture of small blood vessels, loss of cerebrovascular

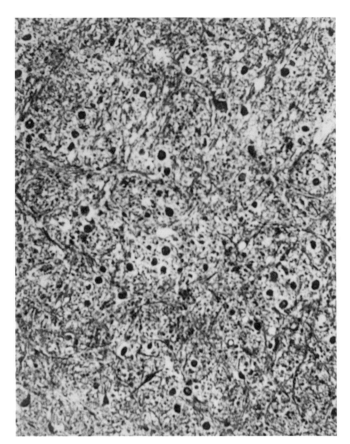

Figure 4.1   Microscopic picture of diffuse axonal injury (DAI) showing axonal swelling (or retraction balls), which are swollen separated portions of axons. (Reprinted from Esiri MM, Oppenheimer DR. Diagnostic neuropathology: a practical manual. Oxford: Blackwell Scientific, 1989:93.)

autoregulation, breakdown of the blood-brain barrier, and endothelial damage leading to delayed hemorrhages (8). These secondary insults compound the sequelae produced by primary CNS injuries and must be considered when attempting to predict outcome. Currently, they are the targets of early treatment interventions, for example, the induction of total body hypothermia, which is aimed at limiting the overall damage trauma creates within the CNS.

Focal Pathophysiology

Focal cortical contusions (FCC) are the main residua of localized trauma associated with closed brain injuries. These involve consolidated areas of tissue destruction, hemorrhage, and edema extending from the cor-

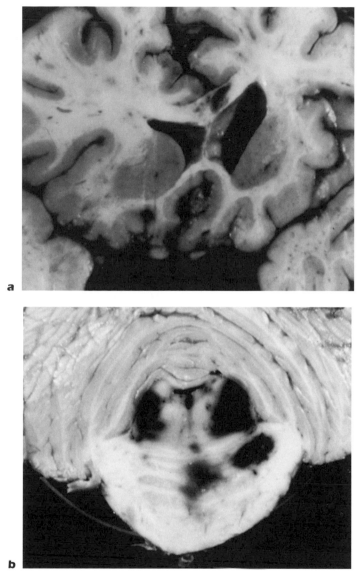

Figure 4.2   Hemorrhagic tears in corpus callosum (a) and superior cerebellar peduncles (b) associated with diffuse axonal injury. (Reprinted from Esiri MM, Oppenheimer DR. Diagnostic neuropathology: a practical manual. Oxford: Blackwell Scientific, 1989:93.)

tical surface into varying depths of the underlying white matter. As previously noted, the areas most susceptible to this type of damage are the anteroinferior and lateral regions of the frontal and temporal lobes (Figure 4.3). These focal lesions evolve as would be expected of any type of localized brain injury, leaving behind scarred (gliotic) parenchyma with retracted cavities that fill with cerebral spinal fluid

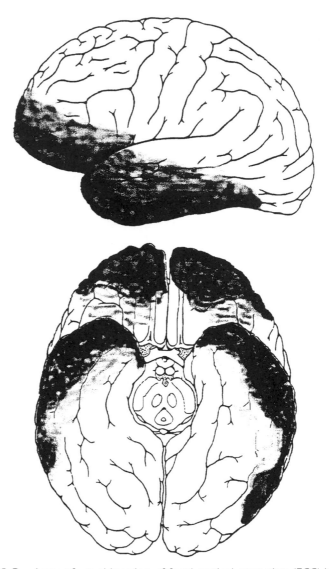

Figure 4.3 Areas of usual location of focal cortical contusion (FCC) in frontal and temporal lobes.

(CSF). The size of the residual lesion can be substantially smaller than the area of acute involvement apparent on clinical examination or visualized by neuroimaging studies (Figure 4.4). Occasionally, large focal hemorrhages, related to rupture of deep penetrating vessels, occur in subcortical structures such as the basal ganglia, unassociated with surface pathology (9).

Given the incompressibility of the brain and the limited capacity of the calvarium, focal hemorrhagic lesions can produce a number of remote effects. Some occur by compressing contiguous neural and vascular structures until infarction ensues. Others happen when pressure

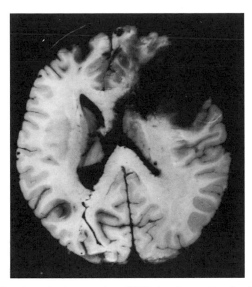

Figure 4.4   Focal cortical contusion (FCC): horizontal brain slice showing large frontal FCC with deep hemorrhagic extension. (Reprinted from Esiri MM, Oppenheimer DR. Diagnostic neuropathology: a practical manual. Oxford: Blackwell Scientific, 1989:90.)

gradients build to the point where portions of the brain are forced to shift out of their normal compartments (*herniate*) into other potential spaces. Common examples include the herniation of the medial temporal lobe into the posterior fossa, producing pressure against the brainstem and the medial frontal lobe under the midline dural membrane (falx), compromising its vascular supply (Figure 4.5).

Pupillary dilatation caused by the compression of the third cranial nerve may be the earliest clinical sign of temporal lobe herniation. Further compression of the brainstem causes a progression of clinical signs, and ultimately death, when vital centers such as those responsible for respiratory control are lost. Herniations can also produce stroke syndromes due to the compression of larger blood vessels; the most common occurs following entrapment of the posterior cerebral artery as the temporal lobe herniates under the tentorium (Figure 4.6).

Apart from the pressure effects noted above, focal lesions may be associated with the same array (albeit more circumscribed) of secondary neuronal and microvascular insults that occur following more widespread CNS injury (10).

Extracerebral hemorrhages such as epidural (EDH) and subdural (SDH) hematoma are other common focal lesions. EDHs typically occur following skull fractures that lacerate the closely associated meningeal arteries (Figure 4.7). SDHs usually result from accelerational forces that rupture the bridging veins in the subdural space. The immediate pathophysiologic consequences of these lesions occur as a result of their mass effects (see Table 4.1).

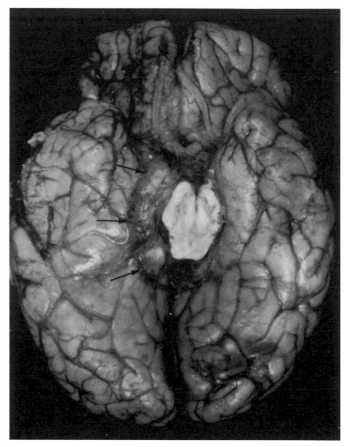

Figure 4.5 Herniation: shift of brain out of normal compartments. Base of cerebrum illustrating shift of medial temporal lobe distorting brainstem (arrows). (Reprinted from Esiri MM, Oppenheimer DR. Diagnostic neuropathology: a practical manual. Oxford: Blackwell Scientific, 1989:23.)

NATURAL HISTORY

Diffuse Injury

Patients with diffuse neuropathology caused by DAI and its secondary complications have a stereotypic pattern of recovery. This *pattern* is independent of injury severity and can be defined by three epochs of recovery. The first epoch is associated with immediate alteration of awareness or unconsciousness. The second is characterized by confusion and continuing anterograde amnesia (*post-traumatic amnesia* [PTA]). The third and final epoch begins with the restoration of continuous memory and ends with the individual recovering from or compensating for as many handicapping conditions as possible (Figure 4.8).

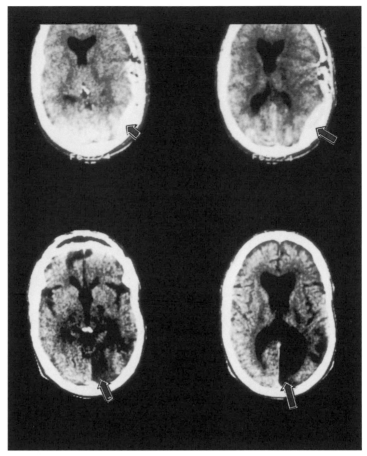

Figure 4.6   CT scan illustrating posterior cerebral artery (PCA) infarction
following herniation. A 33-year-old man suffered an acute left epidural
hematoma (EDH) and skull fracture in an assault. Top two CT scan slices were
from acute CT, showing acute EDH (arrows). Bottom two slices were from two-
month follow-up CT, showing L PCA infarct (arrows).

Table 4.2. Rancho Los
Amigos Levels of Cognitive Functioning

I.	No Response
II.	Generalized Responses
III.	Localized Responses
IV.	Confused—Agitated
V.	Confused—Inappropriate
VI.	Confused—Appropriate
VII.	Automatic—Appropriate
VIII.	Purposeful and Appropriate

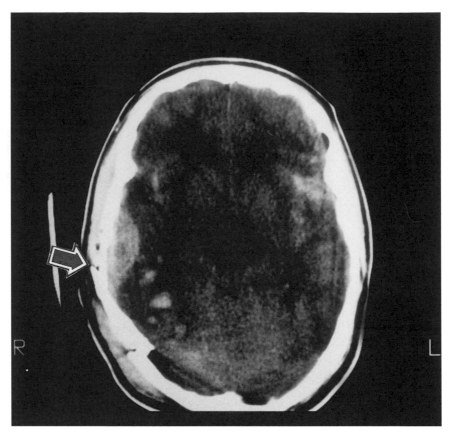

Figure 4.7 *CT scan illustrating an acute right epidural hematoma (lens-shaped high-density area). There is also an overlying skull fracture (arrow) and underlying focal cortical contusion.*

Recovery from diffuse TBI

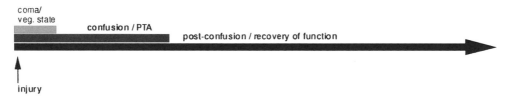

Figure 4.8 *Epochs of recovery following diffuse TBI (PTA = post-traumatic amnesia).*

The *duration* of these epochs is related to the severity of injury (Figure 4.9). It is the relationship between severity of the pathology and the expected rate of recovery that forms the basis for predicting the course and outcome in patients with diffuse injuries.

These epochs of recovery from injuries principally characterized by diffuse axonal injury have been further subdivided according to various descriptive schemas. The most well known is the Rancho Los

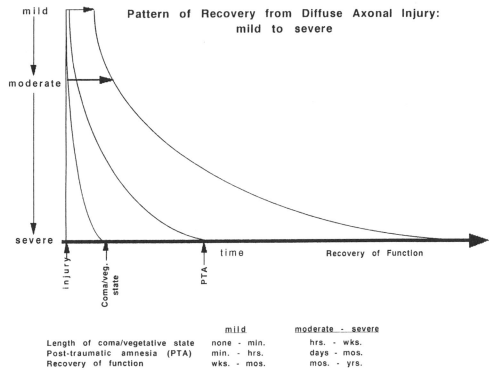

Figure 4.9   *Recovery time in relation to injury severity after diffuse TBI.*

Amigos (*Rancho*) levels of cognitive functioning (Table 4.2) (11). Another system, first introduced by Alexander in 1982 (12), and later modified by Mills and Katz, is similar but better follows neurologic nomenclature (13) (Table 4.3) (12,13). This schema is used throughout this chapter:

1. Coma: The first stage (corresponding to Rancho level I) is defined by unconsciousness without any spontaneous eye opening. The depth of coma in the first few hours following injury is an important early index of severity and is commonly measured by the Glasgow Coma Scale (GCS) (Table 4.4). Total GCS scores range from a low of 3 [(E = 1) + (V = 1) + (M = 1) = 3] to a high of 15 [(E = 4) + (M = 6) + (V = 5) = 15]. Patients with no eye opening (E + 1), no verbalizations (V = 1), and no motor response to noxious stimuli (M = 1) or those who demonstrate decerebrate (M = 2) (extension of all four extremities in response to pain) or decorticate (M = 3) (flexion of the upper extremities with extension of the lower extremities) posturing are in the worst prognostic category (GCS = 3 to 5).

Table 4.3. *Stages of Recovery from Diffuse Axonal Injury*

1. **Coma**
   Unresponsive
   Eyes closed
2. **Vegetative state**
   No cognitive responsiveness
   Gross wakefulness
   Sleep-wake cycles
3. **Minimally conscious state**
   Purposeful wakefulness
   Responds to some commands
   Often mute
4. **Confusional state**
   Recovered speech
   Amnesic (PTA)
   Severe attentional deficits
   Agitated
   Hypoaroused or labile behavior
5. **Postconfusional, evolving independence**
   Resolution PTA
   Cognitive improvement
   Achieving independence in daily self-care
   Improving social interaction
   Developing independence at home
6. **Social competence, community reentry**
   Recovering cognitive abilities
   Goal-directed behaviors, social skills, personality
   Developing independence in community
   Returning to academic or vocational pursuits

SOURCE: Adapted from Alexander MP, Traumatic brain injury (12) and Katz DI, Neuropathology and neurobehavioral recovery from closed head injury (13).

2. Vegetative state (corresponding to Rancho level II to III): Within 4 weeks, all survivors spontaneously open their eyes and develop sleep-wake cycles, but demonstrate no purposeful attention or cognitive responsiveness. Approximately 2 percent of these patients remain *permanently vegetative*, a term applied to patients with TBI who remain at this stage for 1 year or more (14).

3. Minimally conscious state (corresponding to Rancho level III): The vast majority of survivors progress to a state of directed, albeit at first erratic, purposeful responsiveness. Initially, they are mute or have sparse hypophonic speech. The earliest signs of this transition are visual fixation and tracking or purposeful movements toward stimuli. Often these purposeful responses are difficult to distinguish from generalized automatic or reflexive responses. The transition is confirmed

Table 4.4. Glasgow Coma Scale*

	Points
Eye Opening	
Spontaneous	4
To speech	3
To pain	2
None	1
Best Motor Response	
Obeys commands	6
Localized to pain stimuli	5
Withdraws from pain stimuli	4
Decorticate flexion	3
Decerebrate extension	2
None	1
Verbal Response	
Oriented	5
Confused conversation	4
Inappropriate words	3
Incomprehensible sounds	2
None	1

*Score for the scale ranges from 3 to 15 points.
SOURCE: Teasdale G, Jennett B. Assessment of coma and impaired consciousness: a practical scale. Lancet 1974;2:81–83.

when these individuals begin to follow verbal commands. Patients with very severe injuries may remain in this condition for an extended time or even permanently plateau at this stage.

4. Confusional state: As patients begin to speak and respond more reliably to commands, they transition to the confusional state, which is characterized by severe attentional disturbances and continuing dense, anterograde amnesia or PTA. This stage corresponds to Rancho levels IV, V, and part of VI. Patients at this stage have difficulty focusing or sustaining attention on cognitive tasks. They demonstrate little ability to control their behavioral responses, which can lead to impulsive and exaggerated reactions to even trivial events. In this context, both directed and nondirected aggression may be seen. Less frequently, patients in the confusional state remain hypokinetic and underaroused, exhibiting apathy, paucity of movement, and little speech. Although they are unable to learn new information or recall day-to-day experiences (*episodic memory*), patients at this stage of recovery can be taught motor tasks and routines associated with activities of daily living via *procedural* or *implicit learning*, even though they demonstrate no recall of the therapy itself (15). Although organized retrieval may be difficult, previously acquired knowledge (*semantic* or *crystallized memory*) and recall for events before the injury (*remote memory*) are relatively well preserved. There is typically loss of memory of the accident itself and, depending on injury severity, lack of awareness of events that occurred days, weeks, or months before the incident (*retrograde amnesia*). This lack of awareness improves with time and may resolve as recovery proceeds. Nonetheless, recovery of the anterograde gap in memory (PTA) never occurs. The resolution of the confusional state is marked by substantial improvement in attention and the return of continuous, episodic memory. This marks the end of PTA. The length of PTA serves as another standard index of injury severity. When improvement in one or another of these components lags, one should suspect that the underlying diffuse neuropathology has been exacerbated by the effects of focal lesions or secondary damage, which give rise to very different recovery curves. For instance, prefrontal contusions may contribute to prolonged behavioral disturbance or confabulation. Likewise, secondary complications that lead to severe hypoxic injury to the CNS produce extensive bilateral hippocampal damage that presents as unrelenting amnesia.

5. Postconfusional, evolving independence (corresponding to Rancho levels VI and VII): This stage is characterized by growing independence in the performance of basic activities of daily living. Cognitive problems are related to difficulties in higher level attention, speed of processing information, appropriate memory retrieval, and impaired executive functions. As global attentional disturbances wane, impairments in specific cognitive functions such as language become more noticeable, and meaningful evaluation is possible. Patients are usually ready for discharge from inpatient rehabilitation programs during this stage, although accompanying motor or orthopedic problems may prolong dependency and hospitalization. Severe behavioral disturbances usually resolve at this time, although disinhibition and poor social awareness may remain. Despite typically underestimating their impairments, patients usually exhibit a return of basic insight and safety awareness at this point in recovery. However, deficits in reasoning and judgment, especially when combined with impulsivity and forgetfulness, lead many to need continuing supervision to ensure safe reentry into the home.

6. Social competence, community reentry (corresponding to Rancho levels VII and VIII): This stage is somewhat arbitrarily marked by the resumption of household independence. Community independence and a return to previous societal roles are the major functional objectives of this stage. This final stage of recovery is better delineated by psychosocial criteria than by specific neurologic milestones. As such, the impact of the underlying neurology on recovery lessens and an individual's premorbid personality and social resources become increasingly important in predicting outcome. Premorbid developmental, medical or psychiatric disorders, and the support of the person's social network all play increasingly important roles in determining how fast and how far he or she will progress. If progression continues, higher level cognitive capacities such as divided attention, executive function, and complex memory improve. These improvements permit a return to previous social roles, for example, provider, automobile driver, or student. Accomplishing these goals paves the way for restoration of higher level self-awareness, which is the necessary foundation for the development of a new personal identity.

Timeline of Recovery for Diffuse Injuries

Several points about the natural history of diffuse injury deserve reemphasis. First, the duration of the epochs of recovery is proportional to injury severity. In those with the least severe injuries (*mild* or *minor brain injury*), the transition through all these stages is more rapid and often unwitnessed. However, in patients with more severe injuries, the rate of progression slows and may plateau at any stage along the continuum of recovery. Second, most patients, irrespective of injury severity, pass through these stages. Survivors rarely skip stages; for example, unconsciousness is always followed by a period of amnesia and confusion.

Injuries can be designated as *mild (minor)*, *moderate*, or *severe* depending on how quickly these stages resolve (see Figure 4.9). If rendered unconscious (coma and vegetative stages), patients with mild injuries remain so for only seconds to minutes. They are then amnestic and confused (minimally responsive and confusional stages) for minutes to an hour, and usually evolve through the later stages (evolving independence and social competence) in days to weeks. Patients with severe injuries are unconscious for days to weeks, remain confused and resolve PTA only after weeks or months, and progress through the later stages over months to years, leading to one of the most protracted recoveries seen in the practice of neurology. Each epoch is proportionally longer than its predecessor. This proportionality is useful in predicting the time course of recovery from diffuse injuries. For example, the relationship between duration of unconsciousness and duration of PTA was defined by the following regression model in a sample of patients with diffuse TBI (16):

$$\text{PTA in weeks} = \left[(0.4)(\text{length of coma in days})\right] + 3.6.$$

Therefore, a patient in coma for 2 weeks will be predicted to remain in PTA approximately 9 weeks [(0.4) × (14 days) = 5.6] + 3.6 = 9.2 weeks.

The impact of this predictability for treatment planning is immediately obvious. However, factors such as age (>40), compounding focal injuries (especially temporal), and secondary complications (such as hypoxemia) alter this relationship by increasing the duration of PTA for any given interval of unconsciousness (17).

Motor Problems

Besides cognitive problems, severe DAI frequently produces motor deficits. Clinical examination typically reveals a mixture of signs resulting from damage to a number of systems involved in the production or control of movement (e.g., pyramidal, extrapyramidal, cerebellar, and vestibular). Spastic paresis of the extremities, impairments in bulbar control (causing dysarthria and swallowing problems), and abnormalities in balance and posture are common problems. Hypokinesia may also occur due to lesions created by DAI in parasagittal frontal areas that initiate movement. Motor deficits caused by diffuse injury may take longer to recover than similar impairments produced by focal damage (18). However, most patients with spastic paresis recover arm function and independent ambulation within 2 to 4 months post injury (19). Nevertheless, motor deficits typically evolve more rapidly than impairments associated with cognitive or behavioral dysfunction (20).

Focal Injury

The evolution of focal lesions produced by trauma is similar to that of other antecedents that produce discrete CNS pathology, particularly brain hemorrhages. Maximal deficits occur immediately or develop within several hours after the insult, as edema and other secondary problems develop. These secondary effects may or may not cause acute impairments in consciousness, which mask the specific deficits associated with the focal lesion itself. When the global impairments wane, a subacute phase of recovery begins and continues for the next 1 to 2 months as transient physiologic abnormalities resolve and brain plasticity permits some reorganization of function. During this time, the particular localizing effects of the lesion become more apparent. Much of the expected recovery from focal lesions occurs within the first 3 months following injury. Nevertheless, some further improvement can occur during the residual phase, especially within the first 6 months.

As seen with other focal neuropathologic processes, the critical issues determining the clinical effects of traumatically induced lesions are their *location*, *size*, and *number* (see Chapter 1).

Table 4.5. Focal Lesions—Typical Locations and Consequences

Lesion	Location	Consequences
Focal cortical contusions	Frontal polar and orbital frontal	Alterations in affect and behavior (apathy or disinhibition)
		Higher level intellectual abilities (processing, executive functions, self-awareness)
	Anterior-inferior temporal	Alterations in affect and behavior
		Auditory association deficits (e.g., aphasia)
		Visual association deficits (e.g., agnosia)
Deep hemorrhages	Basal ganglia area	Hemiparesis
		Discoordination
		Hypertonia
		Movement disorders
		Aphasia (left)
		Neglect
		Visuospatial problems (right)
Focal hypoxic-ischemic artery infarct	Posterior cerebral	*Left side*
		Hemianopia
		Amnesia
		Aphasia (alexia and anomia)
		Right side
		Hemispatial neglect
		Topographic disorientation
		Prosopagnosia

Location: Brain lesions occurring in some locations are associated with predictable neurologic syndromes. This is particularly true in areas of the brain that subserve discrete functions (*idiotypic* or *unimodal cortex*); for example, lesions in the right, primary visual cortex will always produce left visual field deficits. In traumatic brain injury, the clinical presentation of underlying focal pathology is less predictable because it preferentially involves areas of brain that serve more broad functional purposes (*heteromodal cortex*). As previously noted, the typical neurologic syndromes of focal TBI are associated with contusional lesions in frontal and temporal heteromodal cortex and as such, broad, difficult to quantify problems occur in cognition, personality organization, and emotional control. Table 4.5 lists focal lesions of other sites that produce corresponding problems. Hemorrhages in the basal ganglia cause contralateral motor dysfunction and other signs depending on their distribution (e.g., neglect with right-sided lesions, aphasia with left-sided ones). Posterior extension of left temporal contusions will affect language function. Focal ischemic injuries produced by left posterior cerebral artery strokes cause amnesia and contralateral visual field loss, as well as other visual association problems (e.g., alexia).

Size: Size, but particularly *depth*, of the lesion is another critical factor influencing the outcome of focal lesions. Relatively large but superficial cortical lesions produce few long-term consequences, except for increasing the risk of post-traumatic epilepsy. On the other hand, smaller lesions that extend into and interrupt subcortical pathways produce lasting clinical effects. Even small differences in the location of a subcortical insult can significantly influence the nature of the presenting clinical syndrome. The deficits caused by focal lesions evolve with time; early effects are widespread, but tend to wane as the lesion consolidates. This can be seen with serial neuroimaging studies, which demonstrate significant diminution in size of acute lesions over the ensuing months following injury. As might be expected, the individual's lasting impairments correspond much more closely to the residual, rather than the acute lesion.

Number: The number of focal lesions is also important in predicting outcome. The effects of multiple lesions are not simply additive, and prognosis is far worse if they occur bilaterally, especially when involving homologous brain areas.

Natural History— Combined Focal and Diffuse Injury

The natural history of focal deficits after TBI is often difficult to discern because their clinical effects are often embedded in the aftermath of diffuse pathology. Particular localizing syndromes may be impossible to detect in early stages when arousal and attentional problems predominate and become demonstrable only after confusion clears. Furthermore, the usual cognitive and behavioral effects of focal pathology appear identical to those that occur in the later stages of diffuse pathology (e.g., frontal system dysfunction). Even the early effects of focal pathology may mimic the first stages of recovery from diffuse pathology because confusion can be caused by secondary effects. However, unconsciousness is not a direct result of focal pathology unless it occurs in critical mesencephalic or diencephalic structures or causes distortions of these areas by secondary mass effect.

When prognosticating, several principles help separate the contributions of focal and diffuse injury.

1. For patients with severe TBI, the recovery pattern is largely driven by the effects of diffuse injury.

2. The effects of focal lesions emerge a ＿＿＿＿＿＿＿＿＿＿＿ stages associated with diffuse injury and cause additional problems in a particular modality (e.g., aphasia with left perisylvian lesions) or the persistence of a problem in a specific functional domain while overall recovery continues (e.g., amnesia with hippocampal lesions or confabulation with frontal lesions).
3. Recovery from focal pathology will occur more rapidly and reach an earlier plateau, whereas recovery from diffuse pathology will have a longer, more steady progression (see Chapter 1).
4. Over time the clinical effects of small, superficial focal lesions are negligible.

RESIDUAL SYNDROMES

The life-long impairments associated with TBI result from the residual effects of both diffuse and focal CNS damage and are largely a function of the location and severity of these forms of neuropathology.

Diffuse Injury

Diffuse injury can produce a number of residual cognitive, behavioral, and motor problems. Cognitive problems involve deficits in attention, memory, and higher-level regulatory or executive processes. Even after the basic elements of attention resolve with the passage of the confusional stage, more complex attentional problems remain. Patients usually have a slowed rate of mental processing, increased susceptibility to distracting interference, and difficulty dividing attention among two or more tasks (21). The functional implications of these problems include slowed completion of more complex everyday activities (e.g., meal preparation) and difficulty concentrating on more than one thing at a time (e.g., talking and driving).

Although dense amnesia is not usually seen in uncomplicated injuries, memory problems remain. Patients are often forgetful, have trouble with "automatic," passive memory (22), and have less effective learning strategies (23). Even when tests of general intellectual function have normalized, higher cognitive processes such as those associated with the frontal systems remain dysfunctional. These so-called executive problems present during tasks that require flexible thinking, deviation from routine, and self-reflection. Due to such problems, planning an alternate route when encountering heavy traffic or efficiently organizing a number of errands may become overwhelming. Frontal system dysfunction also leads to the emotional and behavioral problems that are so common following brain injury. With the loss of orbital frontal supervisory control over emotions and appetitive drive states, impulsivity, disinhibition, and personality changes occur. However, when lateral frontal dysfunction predominates, patients are apathetic, unconcerned (*abulic*), and unmotivated.

As with other problems of diffuse injury, the amount of personality change relates to injury severity, and profound changes generally occur with the most severe injuries. Limbic disconnection syndromes produce mood disorders, irritability, and on occasion outright aggression. Families of survivors report that these behavioral disorders are far more stressful and produce much more long-term familial strife than any of the individual's residual physical impairments (24).

Motor problems have already been reviewed and do not necessarily correspond to the severity of cognitive deficits. Residual deficits are usually bilateral, asymmetric, and involve multiple components. The most common residual problems include balance and gait dysfunction, eye motility difficulties (vertical gaze, pursuits, and accommodations), and spastic paresis, although dysmetria, dysarthria, and swallowing problems also occur.

Minor Diffuse Brain Injury

In principle, the problems associated with minor brain injury are the same as those seen in more severe injuries, but of less severity and shorter duration. However, the residual syndrome of minor TBI, known as *persistent concussive disorder*, may take on a life of its own due to a number of unique issues that present in this patient population. One such issue is the incongruity between what the patient's medical evaluation reveals and how he or she feels. To the examining clinician, these patients usually look quite normal, have normal medical evaluations, and have unrevealing imaging or electrophysiologic studies. However, early on in the course of this disorder, most patients do not feel normal and are not able to function at their normal capacity. Nonetheless, they may be advised by others or choose on their own to resume normal roles before they have had adequate time to recover. This mismatching of expectations and abilities may lead to forms of psychologic distress that can prolong concussive symptoms beyond that which would be predicted by the natural history of the disorder (25). Other symptoms such as headache, dizziness, and neck pain may take on greater importance in more mild injuries and may interact to produce persistent cognitive and emotional problems. However, it must be emphasized that the vast majority of patients with MBI have resolution of their symptoms within a few weeks or months. Those with persistent concussive disorder likely retain these other features of the disorder as the precipitating neural injury resolves.

Focal Injury

As previously noted, the residual syndromes associated with focal injuries relate to the location and extent of the remaining lesions. The syndromes associated with contusional frontal lobe injuries reflect the regulatory role of the prefrontal areas. These problems are consistent with those seen resulting from diffuse injuries, but generally show less resolution with time. Poor initiation of behavior; impaired organization, sequencing, and planning; disinhibition; confabulation; shallow or rapidly changing mood; and failure to anticipate the consequences of behavior are recognized manifestations of these "frontal" problems.

Residual syndromes associated with temporal lesions devolve from the disconnection of limbic structures and their regulatory sensory associations. Emotional lability, delusional thinking, and perceptual distortions can result from this disassociation. Larger lesions that encroach on medial temporal structures may directly affect memory, while more posterior extension on the left side affects language, usually leading to anomic or transcortical sensory aphasia. Bilateral posterior temporal lesions may cause visual recognition problems. Focal posterior cerebral artery strokes are another common residual focal syndrome whose manifestations include hemianopia, alexia, agnosia, and anomia.

Table 4.6. *Elements of a Complete Diagnostic Profile*

1. Cause of injury
2. Loss of consciousness—immediate or delayed?
3. Depth of coma over the first few hours (Glasgow Coma Scale score [see Table 4.4])
4. Duration of unconsciousness—time to follow commands
5. Duration of confusion and PTA—time to full orientation and continuous day-to-day memory
6. Neuroimaging—acute and follow-up CT and MRI scans
7. Risk of secondary hypoxic-ischemic injury—sustained systemic hypotension (<80 mm Hg) or intracranial hypertension (>20 mm Hg)
8. Probability of herniation—mass lesion, unreactive pupil on same side
9. Delayed secondary problems—hydrocephalus, chronic subdural hematomas, and hygromas
10. Important non–brain injury factors—age, premorbid medical neurologic or psychiatric problems, other medical complications, associated injuries, learning disability, substance abuse, social/family network, education, occupation, habits, personality, hobbies

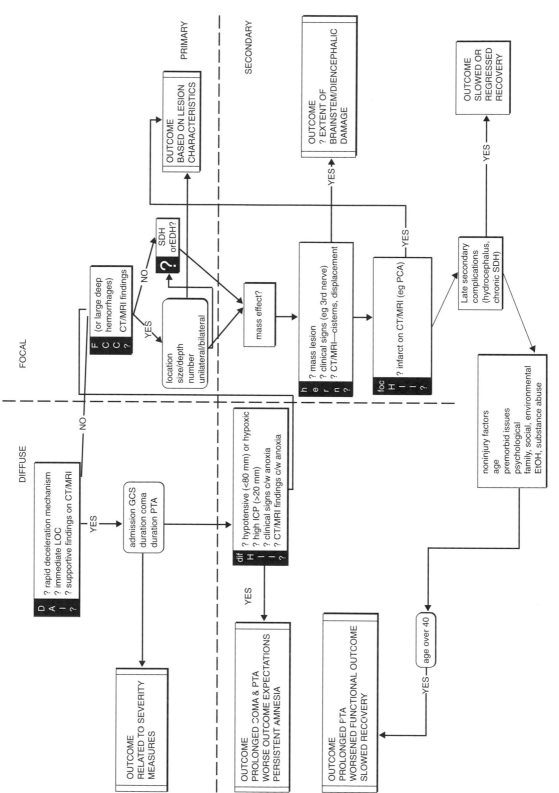

Figure 4.10 Algorithm for clinical diagnosis of pathologic type, severity, and associated factors in formulating prognosis.

PROGNOSIS

Predicting outcome after TBI using the neurologic model presented in this chapter requires the development of an organized clinical approach that separately considers the individual components of the injury. Several historical facts of the accident and its immediate consequences are necessary (Table 4.6), and most can be gleaned from the patient's acute medical records. The clinical algorithm presented in Figure 4.10 illustrates the decision tree used in formulating diagnosis and prognosis. The steps are as follows:

   1. Diffuse axonal injury: First, was there diffuse brain injury? If so, how severe was it? Due to the lack of direct measures, the diagnosis of diffuse injury relies on established clinical criteria which include a significant mechanism leading to acceleration and then deceleration (e.g., motor vehicle accident or fall of over 6 feet), immediate loss of consciousness (i.e., no lucid interval), and supportive neuroimaging

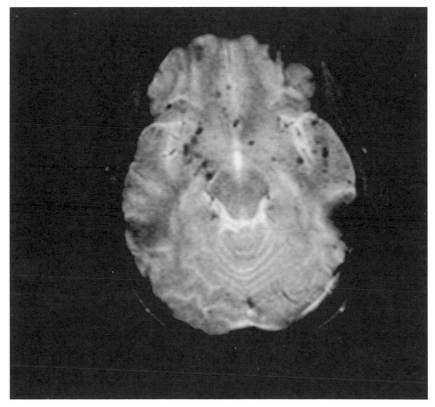

Figure 4.11   Petechial white matter hemorrhages associated with DAI (dark, low signal areas on gradient echo MRI scan).

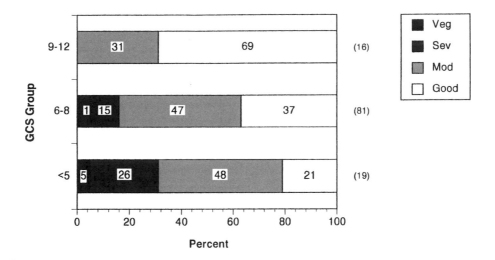

12 Month Outcome by GCS Class
(Patients with moderate to severe DAI, n=116)

Figure 4.12   *Probabilities of outcome at 1 year (Glasgow Outcome Scale scores) in series of survivors of TBI based on admission Glasgow Coma Scale (GCS) scores (Veg = vegetative state; Sev = severe disability; Mod = moderate disability; Good = good recovery).*

findings (petechial white matter hemorrhages [Figure 4.11] and small subarachnoid or intraventricular hemorrhages).

Severity of DAI is also best determined by clinical measures, such as the early Glasgow Coma Scale (GCS) score, duration of unconsciousness, and duration of PTA. From this one can construct probabilities of outcome guided by information from large TBI outcome studies (e.g., Figures 4.12, 4.13, and 4.14). The lowest postresuscitation GCS score in the first few hours has a strong relationship to outcome (26). The traumatic coma data bank study reported odds of a 16% good recovery or moderate disability in a cohort with GCS of less than 6, but up to 63% had good recovery or moderate disability in those with GCS ranging from 6 to 8 (27). In another series of cases evaluated at 1 year following injury, of those with initial GCS of less than 6 only 21% achieved good recovery, and 26% were left with severe disability. In those individuals with GCS ranging from 6 to 8, 37% reached good recovery and only 15% remained with severe disability (see Figure 4.12).

Extent of loss of consciousness (LOC) and PTA have even stronger relationships with outcome (16). For instance, in a rehabilitation sample, LOC between 1 day and 1 week predicted 49% good recovery at a year, whereas LOC over 3 weeks predicted no chance of good recovery and a 64% chance of severe disability or vegetative state (see

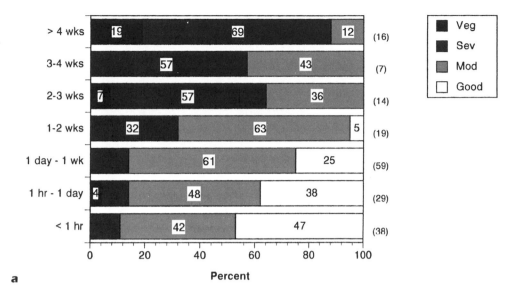

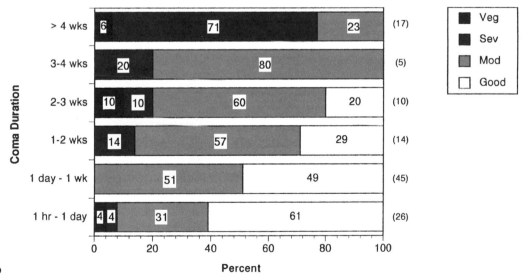

Figure 4.13 *Probabilities of outcome at (a) 6 months and (b) 1 year (Glasgow Outcome Scale scores) in series of survivors of TBI based on duration of unconsciousness (coma) (Veg = vegetative state; Sev = severe disability; Mod = moderate disability; Good = good recovery).*

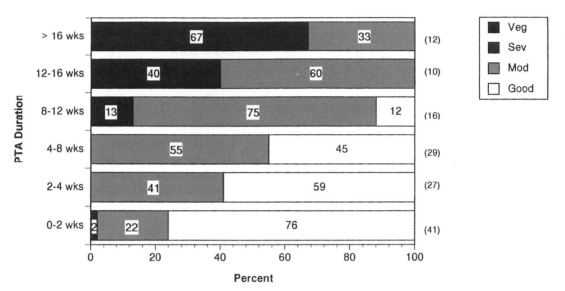

12 Month Outcome by PTA Class
(patients with DAI, n = 135)

Figure 4.14 *Probabilities of outcome at 1 year (Glasgow Outcome Scale scores) in series of survivors of TBI based on PTA duration (Veg = vegetative state; Sev = severe disability; Mod = moderate disability; Good = good recovery).*

Figure 4.13). Of those with PTA duration less than 2 weeks, nearly 75% achieve a good recovery by 1 year post injury, but PTA extending 8 to 12 weeks was associated with only a 12% chance of good recovery (see Figure 4.14).

2. Secondary diffuse hypoxic-ischemic injury (DHII): If DAI has occurred, then the next diagnostic question centers on determining how much secondary injury exists. This determination is also a challenge of clinical probability, since there are no extant tools that can directly measure these processes either. However, two routinely assessed parameters have been implicated in producing DHII: a critical drop in systemic blood pressure (i.e., systolic BP <80 mm Hg) or a sustained rise in intracranial pressure (i.e., >20 mm Hg) (28). Diffuse secondary injury predicts a longer confusional state and overall worse functional outcome than for uncomplicated DAI (17).

3. Focal pathology: The next major diagnostic question to be answered is if focal brain injury has occurred as focal cortical contusions (FCC), deep hemorrhages, or focal hypoxic-ischemic injury (FHII). In these circumstances, neuroimaging studies (brain CT or MRI) are diagnostic. Their specific clinical effects can be estimated by lesion characteristics, that is, location, size, depth, bilaterality, and the production of distal brain damage. Neuroimaging studies performed later in the patient's recovery (>2 months) are of greater salience in predicting the long-term prognosis associated with these types of injury than are earlier scans demonstrating its existence.

4. Extracranial hematomas (ECH): In addition to intracranial focal lesions, the existence of subdural and epidural hematomas is an important prognostic consideration. These pathologic processes exert their clinical effects by producing mass effects within the bony calvarium, which can lead to herniation syndromes—a significant cause of mortality and morbidity. Rapid neurosurgical evacuation of these hematomas, however, can mitigate such disastrous consequences.

5. Herniation and focal hypoxic-ischemic injury (FHII): If the mass effects produced by extra- or intracranial hemorrhages are excessive, localized ischemia and herniation may occur. Clinical signs of temporal lobe herniation include progressive signs of brainstem compression, usually initiated by an unreactive pupil and eventuating in death. Posterior cerebral artery strokes and their corresponding posterior brain syndromes are other possible consequences of herniation.

6. Late secondary complications: Delayed complications, if not emergently recognized and treated, impact prognostication by worsening outcome beyond which would have been expected based on primary pathology alone. *Hydrocephalus,* resulting from an obstruction in cerebrospinal fluid circulation or absorption is treated surgically by the placement of a ventriculoperitoneal shunt. Obstructive hydrocephalus must be distinguished from ventricular enlargement that occurs passively as a result of brain atrophy (*hydrocephalus ex vacuo*) which is not amenable to surgical treatment. Other potentially treatable late complications include chronic fluid collections, especially those occurring beneath the dura, that have the potential to exert direct pressure on the brain or lead to herniation syndromes. Late complications should be suspected whenever deviation from the patient's projected recovery curve occurs, as one cannot rely upon any specific early clinical signs to aid in their discovery. Besides neurosurgically remediable problems, medical complications may also occur. Some examples of the latter include seizures, deleterious CNS side effects of commonly prescribed medications, and adult respiratory distress syndrome.

7. Noninjury factors: Other factors being equal, advancing age, beginning as early as 40, is associated with slower recovery and worse outcome. In addition to age, premorbid personality characteristics and social functioning are other factors that dramatically affect outcome (16,27,29). In fact, changes in cognitive or functional capacity are meaningful only when understood in the context of an individual's previous functioning. Therefore, in order for a global outcome to assume personal relevance, it must be viewed in the setting of individual, familial, and societal expectations, which are often shaped by cultural forces more powerful and less malleable than medical insight. As such, this algorithm is at best a general guide for defining prognosis. Although there may never be a complete diagnostic model to precisely predict outcome for the individual, the paradigm proposed here has at least moved the endeavor beyond pure conjecture to a nascent science that will surely improve with diagnostic advances and increasingly sophisticated epidemiologic studies.

IMPLICATIONS FOR REHABILITATION AND GOAL SETTING

The central theme of this book is that natural history, predicated on accurate diagnosis, serves as the foundation of treatment planning for patients with neurologic disorders. For instance, severe deficits in declarative memory have vastly different implications for treatment planning if they persist long past the expected end of the confusional state. If they do, longer lasting memory impairments should be expected, and compensatory strategies must be identified far earlier in the treatment process. In the initial stages of recovery, biologic and environmental factors govern most functional improvement seen; however, if recovery continues, the influence of social forces directed toward retraining and learning increase the rate and quality of recovery. Thus, treatment planning and goal setting must recognize that ongoing functional improvements result from a complex calculus of biologic recovery and directed treatment, with the latter assuming greater importance as time progresses.

Particular features of the natural history of diffuse and focal injury, discussed below, define reasonable long-term goals for treatment and certain treatment help strategies for achieving them.

Diffuse Injury

For diffuse injuries, the main issues influencing treatment planning are the stage of recovery and the expected rate of progression through it. Within this context, the treatment plan should recognize the following.

First, certain cognitive problems define the parameters of therapy for each of the different stages of recovery: impaired arousal in the initial stages; defective basic attention and amnesia in the subsequent early stages; and higher level attention, memory, and executive functions in the later stages. Attempts to evaluate and treat cognitive deficits beyond these limitations are futile and improvident.

Second, advancement through the early stages of recovery—including coma, vegetative state, minimal consciousness, and confusion—largely occurs independent of treatment. As such, many early problems resolve on their own as recovery progresses and require nothing more than expectant medical care, vigilant nursing, and regulation of environmental stimulation.

Third, different learning and memory capabilities (e.g., procedural vs. declarative) are best exploited at phases of recovery where their efficient functioning can be relied on in therapy. For example, procedural learning permits relearning of some basic activities of daily living even when declarative memory is so severely impaired that acknowledgment of such learning cannot be verbalized.

Fourth, the expected rate of improvement through the stages of recovery should help guide the amount of time devoted to the treatment of specific deficits presenting within each phase, given their expected impact on the patient's final outcome.

A clinical example will help illustrate these four points.

Case 1

A 21-year-old man was in a motor vehicle accident. He was rendered immediately unconscious and had a postresuscitation GCS score of 6 (eyes closed [E = 1], nonverbal [V = 1], withdrew to pain [M = 4]). An emergent brain CT scan demonstrated diffuse swelling, no major focal lesions, but a few tiny white matter hemorrhages and a small amount of intraventricular and subarachnoid blood (Figure 4.15). There were no known secondary complications. He had a left tibial fracture requiring surgery for open reduction and internal fixation, following which he was not allowed to bear weight on this leg for several weeks. He was unconscious for 4 days, after which he began to follow commands, and after 10 days he was transferred to an acute rehabilitation hospital.

On admission to this hospital, he was restless, highly distractible, and rapidly escalated to the point of verbal aggression and physical combativeness whenever the staff attempted to touch him. He was disoriented and had no idea he had been in an accident. He continually called out for his brother and confabulated he was at work in a bottling factory.

Thus the neurologic diagnosis was severe diffuse axonal injury, and he had progressed to the *confusional stage* of recovery at the time he

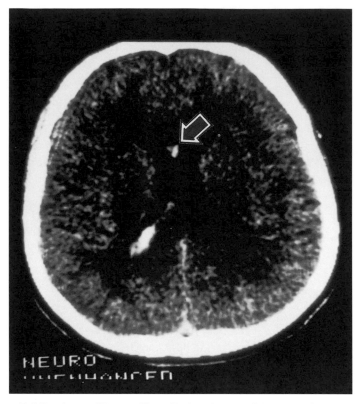

Figure 4.15 *Acute CT scan (Case 1) showing small intraventricular hemorrhage and a small corpus callosum hemorrhage (arrow). These findings are consistent with diffuse TBI. (see also Fig 4.2a).*

entered rehabilitation. He evolved through the earlier stages during his first few days in the acute care hospital without receiving any formal rehabilitation such as "coma stimulation," given that this improvement was driven by biologic factors. Much of the early "treatment" rendered at the rehabilitation hospital revolved around *management* of the patient's confusional state. Just as seen in the recovery of consciousness, there is no evidence that the duration of the confusional state can be modified by any sort of therapy. There may be alterable factors, such as sedating medications or delayed neurologic complications, that lengthen this state, but as yet no direct treatment can shorten it. Commonly used strategies such as "reality orientation groups" or "attention training" do not alter natural recovery at this point in the recovery process. Patients may learn to "proceduralize" responses to orientation questions before confusion clears, but this recitation is without meaning to them and is certainly not generalizable. Some of these treatments may appear to benefit the confused patient, but generally not for the presumed therapeutic reasons. Thus, frequent orientation may serve to improve behavior not because the individual comes to know where she or he is, but rather due to the reassuring human contact that is established during such an interaction. Similarly, staff-led group activities help provide containment of dysregulated behavior by permitting interpatient modeling, rather than by teaching control that can be generalized to the unstructured community.

Thus, the general goal of treatment is managing patients as safely and as comfortably as possible through their confusional state. Beneficial measures include reducing environmental stimulation to appropriate levels and, within reason, tolerating idiosyncratic behavior that does not jeopardize individual or group safety. The timing and duration of activities are also important. In this case, the patient became agitated when stimulated too much or too little. When overwhelmed by physical or cognitive demands in therapy, he became resistive, then combative; when left alone in his room restrained to a chair or in bed, he would yell out for help. However, he remained calm when engaged with staff in activities of appropriate complexity and length, especially when they incorporated his premorbid interests, such as soccer. Surrounding him with pictures and other items from home and on occasion having family members assist in the performance of therapeutic activities was also calming.

As with many confused patients, his sleep was disrupted and fatigue worsened his agitation. Keeping him awake and out of bed for much of the day, except for a structured nap after lunch, went a long way toward reducing daytime fatigue and its associated agitation. Other helpful measures were structuring his schedule with more demanding activities in the earlier, better part of his day, matching the duration of activities to his attention span, and building in breaks that refreshed him but did not lead to boredom.

Treatment of this patient recognized that inattention and amnesia were the defining problems at this stage of his recovery. It is of no value to perform elaborate cognitive evaluations at this level because attentional problems limit performance in all cognitive domains. Likewise, there is nothing to gain by setting short-term treatment goals aimed at advancing cognitive capabilities beyond those achievable while still confused. Attempting to incorporate declarative memory strategies in therapy tasks while the patient is still densely amnesic will not work and will not promote recovery. However, attempting to exploit procedural learning, which is likely preserved even during PTA, is often helpful. Thus, the patient learned to avoid weight-bearing on his left leg and ran through appropriate stand-pivot transfers on the right leg even without any explicit knowledge of the steps involved in completing the task or recall of having practiced it. He had used procedural (*implicit*) learning through oft-repeated practice, bypassing any declarative (*explicit*) capacities.

Providing for the safety of patients, families, and staff is another central management concern at this stage. Appropriate use of restraints may be necessary, especially if, as in this patient, balance problems and weight-bearing constraints preclude standing or walking. Medications should be used judiciously, as some commonly used sedatives may actually worsen confusion and prolong recovery. Once the therapeutic environment was modified for this patient, anxiolytic medications were no longer necessary. The treatment plan should be modified at regular intervals that vary based on the expected duration of confusion. In a patient with primarily diffuse injury, agitation should resolve as confusion clears. Expectations of a more prolonged agitated confusional state might influence longer-term treatment by incorporating the use of appropriate medications or more elaborate behavioral management strategies.

Calculating the expected length of confusion helped guide this patient's treatment planning. Knowing the duration of unconsciousness (4 days), having ruled out confounding factors such as focal injury or late secondary neurologic complications and observing his past rate of progress indicated that the total duration of his confusional stage should be about 5 weeks. This allowed planning for the management of his confusion to focus on short-term environmental strategies and predicted that his length of stay at the rehabilitation hospital would be about 1 month. As was seen with this patient, most survivors with uncomplicated, diffuse TBI can be discharged home shortly after their confusion clears. Those with more substantial motor problems or other factors that affect functional abilities require somewhat longer hospitalizations. Therefore, discharge goals were formulated early in the course of hospitalization and were implemented with the help of the family in a timely way. It was felt that once confusion cleared, he could be retaught to independently perform basic activities of daily living (ADLs) and ambulate safely with crutches. Furthermore, he would no longer require hospital containment, but would need continued supervision at home and close supervision outside of the home for at least another month. He was indeed discharged at that level, $4^1/_2$ weeks after admission. It was also projected that he had a better than 50% chance of returning to nearly normal functioning by 1 year post injury.

Outpatient therapies centered on reproceduralizing the tasks of everyday life. The patient had to relearn the contingencies of carrying out activities of increasing complexity. At this time, both declarative and procedural memory strategies could be incorporated into the learning process. Initial emphasis was placed on promoting safety awareness and judgment necessary to permit decreasing supervision while at home. Of course, retraining of instrumental ADLs such as appropriate telephone etiquette and cold-meal preparation was essential. Ambulation became an important goal once he was allowed to begin weight bearing on his left leg. Setting up a specific schedule, writing out "do's and don'ts" for allowable activities, and listing steps for more difficult tasks were important strategies employed to compensate for impaired executive functions during the later stages of recovery.

During the second month in outpatient treatment, the focus gradually shifted from the consolidation of home skills to the development of community competence. At $4^1/_2$ months post injury, he began a post-acute rehabilitation day program, set in the community, using a group-based treatment model. This program focused on the final steps to community independence: the refinement of social skills and vocational reentry. These goals are best accomplished in real-life settings using functionally based activities that model the accomplishments needed for independence. Finishing this program, the patient began part-time work at $7^1/_2$ months post injury.

Focal Injury

The main therapeutic issues confronting patients and clinicians following focal injuries occur as a result of the specific deficits produced by the residual lesion. The treatment plan should account for this in the following ways: First, therapists should understand the nature of the impairments related to the focal damage and prognosis to devise treatment strategies aimed at direct remediation (better prognosis) or compensation (worse prognosis) thereafter. Second, detailed evaluation of specific cognitive deficits and their treatment should wait until after the patient's confusion clears. Third, earlier intervention is indicated for problems related to focal damage since they tend to plateau earlier than their counterparts resulting from diffuse damage. Fourth, as suggested above, goal setting and treatment during the later phases of recovery should be directed toward teaching compensatory strategies, since in some cases the problem will not spontaneously resolve and direct treatment is to no avail.

The following case examples illustrate some of these points.

Case 2

A 19-year-old man was admitted to a rehabilitation unit 1 week after an assault. There was no loss of consciousness, but he became obtunded in the emergency room. A brain CT scan demonstrated a left temporal skull fracture, a small left-sided subdural hematoma, and a left temporal focal cortical contusion. Neurosurgery was not indicated for the removal of the small subdural. His confusion cleared in 2 days, but he was left with significant language problems. At the time of rehabilitation admission, his language output was fluent but highly paraphasic, as he often incorrectly substituted whole words and parts of words for those that he wished to communicate. His comprehension was severely limited, repetition broke down past a phrase of a few words, and reading and writing were severely impaired. This language profile was consistent with a *fluent aphasia*

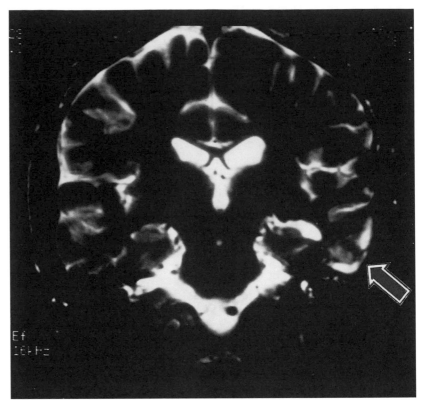

Figure 4.16   Follow-up MRI scan (3 weeks post injury) (Case 2) showing shallow left inferior-posterior temporal focal cortical contusion (FCC) (arrow). The patient had a rapidly improving fluent aphasia and a chronic mild anomia.

(Wernicke's aphasia). There were no motor problems beyond slight imbalance.

A follow-up brain MRI scan obtained at 3 weeks (Figure 4.16) revealed complete resolution of the subdural hematoma and significant, but not complete, resolution of the temporal contusion. The residual lesion affected the posteroinferior left temporal lobe, but did not extend much beneath the cortical surface. The patient's clinical progress and lesion characteristics suggested a favorable prognosis for language recovery, although some residual anomia was expected.

The language treatment plan included various semantic retrieval and circumlocution strategies. Other goals were designed to facilitate his awareness of the problem. His environment was modified by instructing the staff and his family to use contextual cues when communicating with him and by asking them to avoid lengthy and complex conversation. Given the favorable prognosis, the overall plan involved employing direct treatment strategies aimed at improving retrieval and the implementation of compensatory tactics until his condition improved.

When evaluated 3 months after the injury, the patient's language was much improved, but, as expected, he had difficulty retrieving names and less familiar words during conversation. Although his reading comprehension returned to its baseline, he reported that his reading rate was significantly slower. His language was functional for everyday activities, but it was clear that he was too compromised to return to the level of academic performance expected by his college. Therefore, the next goals of therapy centered on treatment strategies that would make such a reentry possible. Once he learned some compensatory techniques (e.g., tape recording lectures) and some environmental modifications were permitted by the college (e.g., allowing him more time to complete tests), this goal was accomplished.

Case 3

A 59-year-old man was struck by a car, causing a closed head injury. He was rendered briefly unconscious, but began talking again at the scene of the accident. He was lethargic and confused when initially evaluated in the emergency room, but rapidly became comatose. A brain CT scan showed bilateral skull fractures, a right epidural hematoma, and bilateral temporal cortical contusions. The patient's condition worsened, and clinical signs of herniation became evident. Emergency neurosurgery was performed to remove the expanding epidural and debride the temporal contusions. A stormy postoperative course ensued over the next 9 weeks; however at that point, the patient regained consciousness and his confusion cleared. The patient claimed he could not see, although on evaluation his basic vision (acuity, visual fields, color perception) was intact. He could not identify objects placed in front of him or describe their function, but on occasion was able to use them properly. Initially, he could not recognize his family, but after interacting with them and hearing their voices, he was able to identify them by name.

A subsequent brain MRI demonstrated bilateral temporal lesions, extending into the posteroinferior temporal-occipital junction (Figure 4.17). The patient's problem was *visual agnosia*. Diagnosis of this syndrome allowed a more focused treatment plan and avoided unnecessary evaluations of vision or inappropriate therapies directed at remediating anomia or apraxia. There are no direct treatments for this syndrome, thus compensatory strategies included promoting tactile exploration of objects and verbal interaction with people to aid their identification, teaching him to probe for distinctive features of people and objects, and making verbal identifications of salient objects for him during functional activities. The problem evolved over the next month such that *everyday objects became easily identifiable*. The patient still could not make complex discriminations involving facial recognition

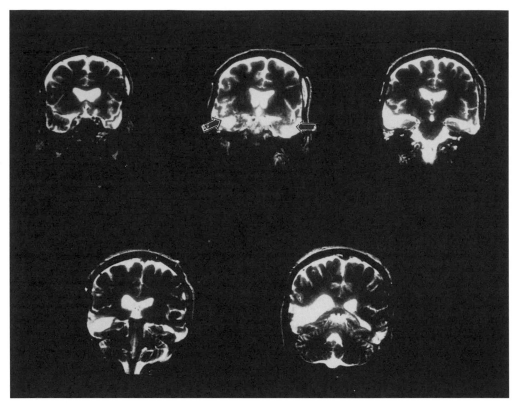

Figure 4.17   Follow-up MRI scan (Case 3) showing bilateral inferior temporal and temporal-occipital focal cortical contusions. This patient had visual agnosia and later prosopagnosia.

(*prosopagnosia*) or identify a particular member of a set of items, such as his comb amongst many.

Case 4

A 49-year-old man was an unrestrained driver in a motor vehicle accident. He was rendered immediately unconscious at the scene, but began following commands the next day. However, he remained very confused for the next $3^1/_2$ weeks. His brain CT scan at 6 weeks showed large bilateral orbitofrontal contusions (Figure 4.18). Disinhibition and confabulation were distinct features of his confusion; however, these behaviors remained despite improvement in his mental status. He was frequently agitated and made unwanted sexual advances toward women staff members. Given the diagnosis of focal frontal pathology, his behavioral prognosis was poor. The treatment plan therefore called for early behavioral interventions, including consistent contingencies designed to reduce the frequency of his inappropriate behavior. Direct treatment of confabulation was not possible since these beliefs are resis-

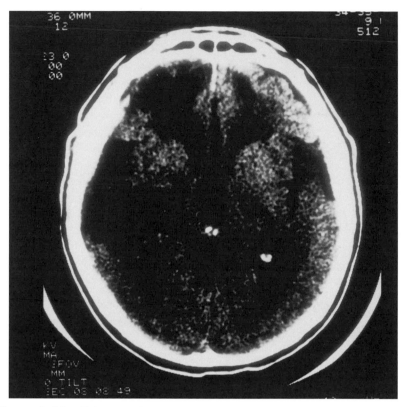

Figure 4.18   Follow-up CT scan (Case 4) showing bilateral orbital frontal (right > left) and right anterior temporal focal cortical contusions. This patient had chronic behavior problems.

tant to any environmental intervention. Gentle redirection and medication were the best strategies to manage this problem area.

The patient's behavioral program resulted in a dramatic decrease of inappropriate behavior while the patient was hospitalized. Unfortunately, the improvement did not generalize after discharge, and his inappropriate behavior led his partner to abruptly conclude their relationship and his landlord to evict him from his apartment because of directed, physical aggression. Attempts at behavior modification in a day program were of modest success, but ultimately failed when the patient refused to continue treatment.

CONCLUSION

In summary, treatment planning evolves from making an accurate diagnosis and knowing the natural history of the disorder diagnosed.

This process should elaborate the particular impairments attributable to the specific stage of recovery following diffuse injury or the clinical syndrome expected because of more localized, focal injury. Prognosis informs treatment by establishing achievable goals within expected time frames. It also prevents the indiscriminate delivery of costly and often useless treatment while guiding the deployment of appropriate interventions when indicated. Finally, treatment planning should be relevant to the individual whose life it is directed to restore. As such, it must account for premorbid strengths and weaknesses, the constraints imposed by the person's social resources, and perhaps most important, an outcome that will be ecologically viable to that singular human being.

References

1. Kurtzke JF, Kurland LT. The epidemiology of neurologic disease. In: Baker AB, Joynt RJ, eds. Clinical neurology. Philadelphia: Harper & Row, 1987:1–143.
2. Kraus JF. Epidemiology of head injury. In: Cooper PR, ed. Head injury. 2nd ed. Baltimore: Williams & Wilkins, 1987:1–25.
3. Corrigan JD. Substance abuse as a mediating factor in outcome from traumatic brain injury. Arch Phys Med Rehabil 1995;76:300–309.
4. Povlishock JT. Traumatically induced axonal injury: pathogenesis and pathobiological implications. Brain Pathol 1992;2:1–12.
5. Gennarelli TA, Thibault LE, Adams JH, et al. Diffuse axonal injury and traumatic coma in the primate. Ann Neurol 1982;12:564–574.
6. Gallyas F, Zoltay G, Balas I. An immediate light microscope response of neuronal somata, dendrites and axons to non-concussive contusing head injury in the rat. Acta Neuropathol 1992;83:386–393.
7. Hayes RL, Jenkins LW, Lyeth BG. Neurochemical aspects of head injury: role of excitatory neurotransmission. J Head Trauma Rehab 1992;7:16–28.
8. Maxwell WL, Irvine A, Adams JH, et al. Response of cerebral microvasculature to brain injury. J Pathol 1988;155:327–335.
9. Katz DI, Alexander MP, Seliger GM, Bellas DN. Traumatic basal ganglia hemorrhage: clinicopathologic features and outcome. Neurology 1989;39:897–904.
10. Cortez SC, McIntosh TK, Noble LJ. Experimental fluid percussion brain injury: vascular disruption and neuronal and glial alterations. Brain Res 1989;482:271–282.
11. Hagen C, Malkmus D, Durham P. Levels of cognitive functioning. Downey, CA: Ranchos Los Amigos Hospital, 1972.
12. Alexander MP. Traumatic brain injury. In: Benson DF, Blumer D, eds. Psychiatric aspects of neurologic disease. New York: McGraw-Hill, 1982:251–278.

13. Katz DI. Neuropathology and neurobehavioral recovery from closed head injury. J Head Trauma Rehab 1992;7:1–15.
14. MultiSociety Task Force on PVS. Medical aspects of the persistent vegetative state (1 & 2). N Engl J Med 1994;330:1499–1508, 1572–1579.
15. Ewart J, Levin HS, Watson MG, Kalisky Z. Procedural memory during post-traumatic amnesia in survivors of closed head injury: implications for rehabilitation. Arch Neurol 1989;46:911–916.
16. Katz DI, Alexander MP. Predicting outcome and course of recovery in patients admitted to rehabilitation. Arch Neurol 1994;51:661–670.
17. Katz DI, Alexander MP, Roberts MB. Functional outcome after closed head injury: the effects of multiple neuropathologies. Arch Phys Med Rehabil 1993;74:661–662.
18. Katz DI, Klein RB, Roberts MB, Alexander MP. Recovery of ambulation after traumatic brain injury. J Neurol Rehab 1995;9:134.
19. Klein RB, Katz DI, Roberts MB, Alexander MP. Recovery of arm function after traumatic brain injury. Neurology 1995;45(suppl 4):330.
20. McLean A, Dikmen SS, Temkin NR. Psychosocial recovery after head injury. Arch Phys Med Rehab 1993;74:1041–1046.
21. Stuss DT, Stethem LL, Hagenholtz H, et al. Reaction time after traumatic brain injury. Fatigue, divided and focused attention and consistency of performance. J Neurol Neurosurg Psychiatry 1989;52:742–748.
22. Levin HS, Goldsstein FC, High WM, Eisenberg HM. Disproportionately severe memory deficit in relation to normal intellectual functioning after closed head injury. J Neurol Neurosurg Psychiatry 1988;51:1294–1301.
23. Levin HS. Memory deficit after closed head injury. J Clin Exp Neuropsychol 1989;12:129–153.
24. Oddy M, Humphrey M, Uttley D. Stresses upon the relatives of head injured patients. Br J Psychiatry 1978;133:507–513.
25. Alexander MP. Mild traumatic brain injury: pathophysiology, natural history and treatment. Neurology 1995;45:1253–1260.
26. Levin HS, Gary HE, Eisenberg HM. Neurobehavioral outcome one year after severe head injury: experience of the traumatic coma databank. J Neurosurg 1990;73:699–709.
27. Marshall LF, Gautille T, Klauber MR, et al. The outcome of severe closed head injury. Neurosurgery 1991;75(suppl):28–36.
28. Marmarou A, Anderson RL, Ward JD, et al. Impact of ICP instability and hypotension on outcome in patients with severe head trauma. J Neurosurg 1991;75(suppl):59–66.
29. Ruff RM, Marshall LF, Crouch J, et al. Predictors of outcome following severe head trauma: follow-up data from the Traumatic Coma Data Bank. Brain Injury 1993;7:101–111.

Anoxic-Hypotensive Brain Injury and Encephalitis

David Bachman and Douglas I. Katz

Although stroke and traumatic brain injury are the most common disorders for which patients receive inpatient neurologic rehabilitation, hosts of other diagnoses are encountered in working with patients admitted to rehabilitation. In this and the following chapter, three other disorders are discussed that present a variety of cognitive, behavioral, and physical problems. The two disorders reviewed in this chapter, anoxic-hypotensive brain injury and acute viral encephalitis, have several similarities. First, they both are associated with a variety of diffuse or focal clinical presentations. Second, they frequently present with profound, but isolated memory impairments. Along with traumatic brain injury, herpes simplex encephalitis is one of the few neurologic disorders with a particular predilection for limbic-related structures.

ANOXIC-HYPOTENSIVE BRAIN INJURY

Overview

The growing number of successful resuscitations following cardiopulmonary arrest has led to a corresponding increase in the number of referrals of patients with anoxic-hypotensive brain injury to rehabilitation (1). Nevertheless, patients with anoxic-hypotensive brain injury

145

still make up a relatively small proportion of those admitted to neurologic rehabilitation services. Anoxic-hypotensive brain injury accounted for about 3% of patients evaluated on a neurologic rehabilitation service in the United Kingdom over a 16-year period and about 1% of admissions to a brain injury rehabilitation unit in the United States over a 1-year period (2).

It appears that relatively smaller proportions of patients with anoxic-hypotensive brain injury than patients with traumatic brain injury are referred for rehabilitation. One reason for this discrepancy is a more dichotomous distribution of outcome for anoxic-hypotensive brain injury than for traumatic brain injury. Outcomes for patients with anoxic-hypotensive brain injury tend to have a bimodal distribution at the extremes of the spectrum of outcome, either relatively intact or neurologically devastated. This is in contradistinction to those with traumatic brain injury whose outcomes tend to be more evenly distributed throughout the outcome continuum. There is rapid recovery in most patients with mild anoxic-hypotensive brain injury and usually dismal outcome for patients with more severe anoxic-hypotensive brain injury, such as those who are admitted to the acute hospital in coma. Further, following coma of similar duration, the prognosis for patients after anoxic-hypotensive brain injury is much worse than for patients following traumatic brain injury. Since most mildly impaired patients return directly home, and most patients in a persistent vegetative state would likely be sent to a nursing service rather than a rehabilitation program, there are few studies that address rehabilitative outcomes in large series of patients with anoxic-hypotensive brain injury. Much of the published literature consists of case reports. Despite this paucity of information, anoxic-hypotensive brain injury survivors represent an important patient population with a variety of residual cognitive, motor, and behavioral problems. This chapter will focus on those patients whose recovery is sufficiently advanced to justify intensive rehabilitation efforts.

Neuropathology

Cerebral hypoxia refers to the relative deprivation of oxygen to the brain. *Cerebral hypotension*, as used in this chapter, refers to the inadequacy of cerebral perfusion pressure or blood flow necessary to sustain brain oxygenation. Cerebral hypoxia is usually associated with some degree of hypotension. Most types of trauma sufficient to produce significant cerebral hypoxia almost invariably result in circulatory collapse (i.e., shock) or cardiac arrest. For this reason, most cases of cerebral hypoxia demonstrate a mixed picture of anoxic and hypotensive cerebral damage.

Barcroft divided anoxic-hypotensive brain injury into four types that provide a useful etiologic and pathologic classification (3):

- *Anoxic anoxia* (due to an inadequate oxygen supply)
- *Anemic anoxia* (due to inadequate oxygen carrying capacity of the blood)
- *Stagnant hypoxia* (due to a critical reduction of cerebral blood flow or pressure)
- *Toxic anoxia* (due to toxins or metabolites that may interfere with oxygen utilization)

Examples of these types of anoxic-hypotensive brain injury are given in Table 5.1. Of 100 consecutive, unconscious patients due to nontraumatic etiology evaluated by Szabon and colleagues, 34 had cardiorespiratory disease and 15 suffered an anesthesia accident. Of 25 children with severe anoxic/hypotensive brain injury, 11 were drowning victims, 7 were suffocations, and 3 were cardiac arrests; other causes included near sudden infant death syndrome, electrocution, and strangulation (4).

In humans, the critical threshold for the minimal oxygen level necessary to result in brain damage is not known. Normal partial pressure of oxygen in cerebral venous blood is about 4.5 kPa (34 mm Hg). It is estimated that a brief episode of hypoxia to oxygen levels as low as 0.13 kPa (1.0 mm Hg) may occur without permanent brain injury (5). In humans, cerebral blood flow remains constant between mean arterial blood pressures of 65 to 140 mm Hg because of cerebral autoregulation.

Table 5.1. Some Causes of Anoxic-Hypotensive Brain Injury

Anoxic anoxia
    Asphyxiation
    Drowning
    Crush chest injury
    Respiratory arrest from any cause
    Natural gas asphyxiation
    Anesthesia accident
    Status epilepticus
Anemic anoxia
    Massive blood loss
    Severe nutritional anemias
    Carbon monoxide poisoning
Stagnant hypoxia
    Cardiac arrest
    Shock
    Prolonged cardiac arrhythmia
    Strangulation
    Massive myocardial infarction
Toxic anoxia
    Cyanide poisoning
    Hypoglycemia

Below 65 mm Hg, the degree and pattern of brain injury will depend on the rapidity of pressure loss, the age of the patient, the health of the cerebral blood vessels, and the intracranial pressure. The adult brain accounts for 15% of cardiac output although it constitutes less than 3% of total body weight.

If circulatory arrest starts and stops fairly abruptly, lasting for more than 3 to 4 minutes, brain damage will be fairly generalized throughout the cerebral and cerebellar cortex and will also involve the basal ganglia (6). However, certain areas of the brain are particularly susceptible to anoxic-hypotensive injury and demonstrate "selective vulnerability." Although any area of the cerebral cortex may be affected, the occipital/parietal cortex and Purkinje's cells of the cerebellum are especially vulnerable to injury. The neurons of the primary motor and sensory regions are less vulnerable. The hippocampus is highly susceptible to ischemic damage, especially the portion referred to as Sommer's sector (CA 1). Ischemic damage may also involve the basolateral nuclei of the amygdala, caudate nucleus and putamen, globus pallidus, and anterior and dorsomedial nuclei of the thalamus. Occasional damage is also seen in the subthalamic nuclei and hypothalamus. The brainstem is relatively spared, although damage to the reticular zone of the substantia nigra, inferior colliculi, and inferior olives may be seen.

If a circulatory arrest of less than 3 to 4 minutes' duration is preceded or followed by a prolonged period of relative hypotension, then the arterial border zones, being at the most distant extreme of vascular flow, will be especially susceptible to ischemic injury (6). The most commonly affected border zone is that between posterior cerebral and middle cerebral arteries (see Figures 2.2a and 2.2c).

The penetrating arterioles of the basal ganglia and white matter of the centrum semiovale are also susceptible to anoxic-hypotensive injury. Damage to these structures may be evident in carbon monoxide poisoning with bilateral focal necrosis of the inner segment of the globus pallidus and diffuse or patchy demyelination of cerebral white matter (Figure 5.1). Occasionally, patchy demyelination of the corpus callosum, internal and external capsules, and optic tracts has been described.

Although persistent vegetative state following anoxic brain injury is usually attributed to severe, diffuse, cortical injury, that assumption was recently called into question. In the well-known case of Karen Ann Quinlan, a patient who remained permanently vegetative after anoxic-hypotensive brain injury, autopsy revealed extensive thalamic damage instead of prominent cortical damage; there was also limited damage to occipital pole, parasagittal parieto-occipital regions, and bilateral cerebellum and basal ganglia (7). These authors suggest that in some cases of anoxic-hypotensive brain injury, thalamic sparing may play a more important role in recovery of consciousness than was previously appreciated.

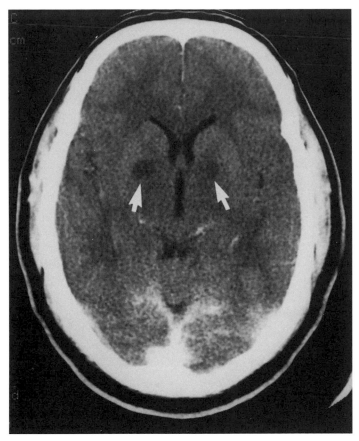

Figure 5.1   *Horizontal section of CT scan at level of basal ganglia. Arrows indicate low-density lesions bilaterally in the globus pallidus.*

Natural History

In 1969, Richardson and colleagues nicely summarized the hypothetical anoxic-hypotensive brain injury recovery time line (8).

The clinical sequence of recovery in those patients who survived without relapse, although of variable rate, is similar in all cases and may be arrested at any stage. An early deep coma, or state of unresponsiveness, gives way to a decerebrate condition of stupor and delirium and then a decorticate state with confusion and automatism, before recovery of the highest cerebral functions. Superimposed on this general pattern of recovery there occur an immense variety of focal symptoms, psychotic reactions, spatial disorientation, and motor disorders, such as hemiparesis, athetosis, or Parkinsonism. Frequently in the later stages of mild confusion or automatism, one can demonstrate agnosias, constructional apraxia, or dysphasia.

Bertini and colleagues performed follow-up evaluations on 113 patients resuscitated from out-of-hospital cardiac arrest and compared them to a control group with myocardial infarction without cardiac arrest (9). The mean follow-up interval was 29.5 months. There was no difference between the two groups, even for the subgroup that underwent extensive neuropsychologic testing. These findings are consistent with those of other investigators given that most patients that survive hospitalization (and are not unconscious for more than a brief period of time) make a nearly complete recovery. However, for patients with carbon monoxide poisoning, Smith and Brandon reported subtle cognitive or behavioral deficits that did not lead them to seek medical attention (10).

The only prospective study of neuropsychologic recovery following out-of-hospital cardiac arrest is that of Roine and colleagues, who followed 155 cardiac arrest survivors (11). The mean level of performance on most tests of intellectual function and memory were normal at 3 and 12 months post arrest for the group as a whole. The only exception was the delayed recall subtest of the Wechsler Memory Scale. Delayed recall scores were abnormal at all follow-up visits, but demonstrated gradual improvement from 3 months to 12 months post arrest. Despite the good performance for the group as a whole, 30% to 33% of patients demonstrated moderate to severe memory impairment, dyscalculia, or visuoconstructive impairment at 12 months. Improvement from 3 to 12 months was demonstrated in some spheres. At 3 months, 35% had symptoms of depression, 37% had motivational problems, and 60% had some neuropsychologic deficits compared to standardized norms. By 12 months, 31% had symptoms of depression, 20% had motivational problems, and 48% had some neuropsychologic deficits. These findings suggest that although there is a rapid period of improvement during the first 3 months following the arrest, some neuropsychologic and behavioral improvement can be demonstrated throughout the first year of injury. According to these investigators, speech, reading, writing, and visual perceptual functions were the least likely neuropsychologic parameters to be impaired. Memory, visuoconstructive function, programming of activities, and arithmetic were most likely to be affected. Patients who present without coma or in coma lasting up to 12 hours make a rapid and complete recovery over several days or weeks. However, inexplicably, a small percentage may have a prolonged postexposure confusional state or a permanent amnestic syndrome (9,12).

When coma extends past 12 hours to about 2 weeks, outcome is much poorer. Under these circumstances, coma is often associated with marked motor impairment, with decorticate or decerebrate posturing, and/or rigidity. Almost all survivors develop intermittent spontaneous eye opening by 4 weeks, even if they remain cognitively unresponsive (unconscious). This clinical condition is termed *vegetative state* (see Table 4.3). Patients may plateau at this stage and become classified as being in a *permanent vegetative* state at 3 months following arrest.

Patients who recover from coma enter a stage where they begin to demonstrate some awareness of the environment (consciousness). Often they are confused and agitated or mute and stuporous. Some patients with severe anoxic-hypotensive brain injury have a more prolonged period of inconsistent, low-level responsiveness (*minimally responsive*) associated with generalized convulsions, multifocal myoclonus, and tremor. Focal deficits including hemiparesis, visual field cut, or aphasia become apparent during this stage. EEG recordings during this phase of recovery demonstrate diffuse slowing in the delta range. Neuroimaging studies will appear normal or demonstrate generalized cerebral edema.

As the confusional state resolves in the weeks to several months following coma, specific cognitive deficits are more easily demonstrated. Common neuropsychologic deficits include amnestic syndrome, visual spatial impairment, deficits of executive functioning, and behavioral problems. Motor syndromes of parkinsonism, chorea, or dystonia may emerge. These deficits may improve during the first 3 to 6 months; however, after this time they are generally fixed.

The EEG shows that normal background activity may be restored, although some mixed slow frequencies are usually seen. Focal slowing may correspond to structural lesions, such as at the areas of border-zone arterial territory infarction. Interictal discharges (e.g., spikes or spike/slow wave complexes) are occasionally seen. CT or MRI scans demonstrate some degree of ventricular enlargement. Generalized cortical atrophy may also be seen. Focal areas of infarction, again, usually in an arterial border-zone distribution, are also seen.

Patients with coma duration greater than 2 weeks rarely survive their hospitalization. If they do survive, they remain in a vegetative state or regain consciousness, but with little hope of meaningful recovery. Patients who remain in a vegetative state for 3 months or more after anoxic-hypotensive brain injury are considered permanently vegetative with no expectation of regaining consciousness (13). However, as expected, there are rare exceptions.

Common Residual Deficits

Patients with residual deficits who recover beyond a vegetative or minimally responsive state have a variety of cognitive impairments, predominantly in the areas of attention, memory, and executive functions. The memory disorder may take several forms. The most common is an anterograde memory disorder similar to Korsakoff's syndrome, most likely caused by anoxic/ischemic damage to the hippocampus (14–16). These patients have difficulty with new learning, especially free recall, but demonstrate relatively preserved remote memory, except for a retrograde amnesia of weeks to months prior to the anoxic-hypotensive event. Verbal and nonverbal memories are equally impaired.

Smith and Brandon prospectively identified and followed all cases of carbon monoxide poisoning in Newcastle upon Tyne over a 3-year period (12). One hundred and forty-seven cases were identified. Most had attempted or completed suicide. Of the 135 survivors, only 5 were reported to have permanent neurologic deficits on initial examination. However, in a follow-up evaluation of these same cases after 3 years, the authors found that 21 (33.3%) survivors had experienced postexposure personality changes and 27 (43%) had complaints of memory impairment (10). The authors suggest that mild neurologic and psychiatric impairment frequently may be overlooked in this population.

Two studies suggest that the neuropathology and thus the neuropsychologic profile of memory loss following anoxic-hypotensive brain injury may vary from patient to patient. De Renzi and Lucchelli describe a 26-year-old man who suffered an episode of anoxic-hypotensive brain injury following a tractor accident (17). This patient had great difficulty recalling remote, autobiographical information, although new learning and intellectual function were relatively intact. Zola-Morgan and colleagues presented a case of a 52-year-old man who suffered an episode of hypotension following cardiac surgery (15). On recovery, he experienced a profound, persistent deficit in new learning, intact general intellectual functioning, and very little retrograde amnesia. At autopsy, cerebral pathology was limited to the CA 1 field of the hippocampus.

With severe hypotension, patients may experience cerebral infarction (stroke), especially in a border-zone arterial distribution, as described earlier in the neuropathology section of this chapter (Figure 5.2). However, in patients with pre-existing stenosis in major cerebral vessels, stroke may follow the distribution of this vessel. In such cases, the neuropsychologic deficits are consistent with those seen following classic stroke syndromes (see Chapter 3). The prognosis and clinical course of these deficits is similar to that for a thrombotic or embolic stroke.

Certain clinical syndromes are commonly identified after border-zone ischemia (18,19). Bilateral parieto-occipital ischemic damage, the most common border-zone injury pattern, results in partial or complete Balint's syndrome: difficulty with voluntary directed eye movements (optic apraxia), difficulty with visually guided upper extremity movements (optic ataxia), and difficulty appreciating the gestalt or overall perspective of a complex visual scene, although details of the stimulus may be correctly identified (simultanagnosia). Some patients may experience visual distortions or illusions and/or visual field defects. A patient who had survived a respiratory arrest secondary to an asthma attack often had difficulty locating objects in visual space. For instance, when asked to point to the clock in her room, she looked up at the wall

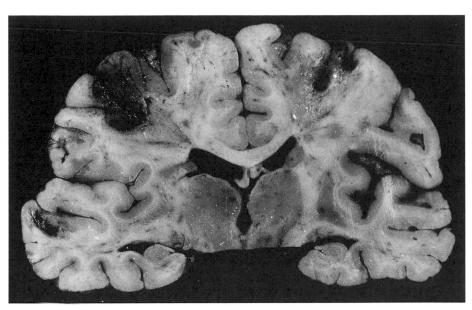

Figure 5.2   Border-zone ("watershed") infarcts in a 47-year-old woman with aortic valve disease leading to heart failure, who experienced confusion and coma for 1 month before death. There is hemorrhagic softening in the border zones of the middle and anterior cerebral arteries on both sides, and of the middle and posterior cerebral arteries on the left side. There were similar softenings in the border zones of the superior and inferior cerebellar arteries on both sides. (Reprinted from Esiri MM, Oppenheimer DR. Diagnostic neuropathology: a practical manual. Oxford: Blackwell Scientific, 1989:116.)

and said, "I know if I watch the wall and wait, the clock will move into view" (Bachman, personal communication). Cortical blindness has also been described, especially in cases of carbon monoxide poisoning. Additionally, transcortical sensory aphasia (fluent speech, intact repetition, and poor auditory comprehension) and isolation of speech area (sparse spontaneous speech, intact repetition, and poor auditory comprehension) have been reported (20). Varying degrees of dyslexia, dysgraphia, and anomia have also been noted.

Particularly intriguing is the pattern of motor and neuropsychologic dysfunction seen after anoxic-hypotensive damage to the basal ganglia. Any pattern of abnormal movement including parkinsonism, chorea, tics, athetosis, various forms of dystonia, and myoclonus has been reported (21). Parkinsonism includes features of akinesia, rigidity, tremor, dysarthria, and postural instability. Often, motor symptoms of parkinsonism are combined with other motor signs such as spasticity or cerebellar ataxia. Neuropsychologic deficits associated with basal ganglia damage produce frontal system dysfunction, including apathy, inertia, impaired insight, impulsivity, and poor problem solving/abstraction (22). Memory and other spheres of intellectual function are often relatively intact. LaPlane and colleagues demonstrated frontal lobe hypometabolism by positron emission tomography

(PET) scan in seven patients with this syndrome (22). These authors speculate that the frontal lobe dysfunction is secondary to the inability of neostriatal structures to activate prefrontal cortex rather than to direct damage to the frontal cortex per se. Damasceno reported the case of a 27-year-old woman who recovered from an episode of suspected anoxic-hypotensive brain injury with decerebrate rigidity but relatively preserved intellectual function (23).

Voluntary tremor may occur secondary to anoxic damage to Purkinje's cells in the cerebellum. A characteristic pattern of motor dysfunction following anoxic-hypotensive injury is bibrachial weakness (19). Patients exhibit bilateral arm-hand weakness with relative sparing of the face and legs. Bilateral border-zone ischemia in the anterior cerebral/middle cerebral artery territories, damaging the arm/hand component of the motor strip in the precentral gyrus, is thought to cause this type of motor dysfunction. Ischemic injury limited to the spinal cord has been described (24).

Neuropsychiatric symptoms may occur in isolation or in association with other neuropsychologic or motor deficits. Roine and colleagues report that almost one third of patients surviving out-of-hospital cardiac arrest suffered from depression (11). Smith and Brandon reported that personality change was common in patients surviving carbon monoxide poisoning, even among those without a premorbid history of psychiatric illness (10). Personality changes included moodiness, irritability, and aggressiveness. Obsessive compulsive disorder has been described in some patients, particularly in those with basal ganglia damage (22). Klüver-Bucy syndrome has occasionally been reported after anoxic-hypotensive brain injury and may include any or all of the following: apathy, impaired memory, visual agnosia, oral exploration of objects, dyssexuality, aggressivity, hyperphagia, hoarding behavior, and persistent touching and picking behavior (hypermetamorphosis) (25,26).

Prognosis and Treatment

There is very little data available to guide the clinician in assessing patients' prognosis for recovery once they have recovered from coma. Diagnostic studies such as brain CT scans or EEGs are of limited help during the acute phase of illness in predicting recovery. Much of the literature has focused on predicting recovery from coma. Factors that seem to predict a good outcome from coma depend on the neurologic examination and include spontaneous roving horizontal eye movements at 12 to 24 hours; purposeful movements of face, arms, or legs; and intact speech and comprehension within 48 hours of the event (27). Poor prognostic signs include absent brainstem reflexes at 12 and 24 hours (pupillary response, corneal reflex, doll's eyes, or calorics), absent deep tendon reflexes, and decorticate or decerebrate posturing after 24 hours (24). The Brain Resuscitation Clinical Trials I Study Group evaluated neurologic scores and signs to predict outcome after cardiac arrest (27). At 24 hours after arrest, the predictors of poor outcome were no eye opening to pain, no motor response to pain, and absent pupillary light reflex.

Most clinicians agree that *duration of coma* is an important predictor of outcome. Bell and Hodgson found that few patients in coma for more than 3 days even survived their hospitalization (28). Almost all patients with persistent neurologic sequelae from cardiac arrest or carbon monoxide poisoning are comatose at least 24 hours or longer. In general, the longer a patient is comatose, the worse the prognosis. Levy and colleagues determined that outcome after hypoxic-ischemic coma was highly related to the duration of unconsciousness and abnormal brainstem signs (e.g., pupillary abnormalities, decorticate/decerebrate posturing) early in the course of recovery (29). Patients with abnormal brainstem signs who were comatose more than 24–48 hours, or those without brainstem abnormalities comatose over 1 week, had virtually no chance of recovery better than vegetative state or severe disability.

Outcome for patients with anoxic-hypotensive brain injury in prolonged coma is markedly inferior to those with traumatic brain injury with similar coma durations (1) (see Chapter 4). At 1 month, more than 85% of adults in a coma immediately after nontraumatic brain injury are either dead or in a vegetative state. Of those in a vegetative state 1 month after anoxic-hypotensive brain injury, only 11% recover consciousness by 3 months and 15% by 1 year. In contrast, of patients with traumatic brain injury who are vegetative for 1 month, 33% regain consciousness by 3 months and 52% by 1 year (13).

Table 5.2 summarizes relevant clinical data that imply a worse prognosis for a patient recovering from anoxic-hypotensive brain injury.

Table 5.2. *Factors Predicting a Worse Outcome after Anoxic-Hypotensive Brain Injury*

Older age

Longer duration of coma

Anoxia associated with significant hypotension

Associated medical factors (e.g., heart failure)

Abnormalities of neurologic examination during and immediately after coma (see text)

Premorbid psychiatric illness (e.g., depression)

Presence of a relapsing course after anoxic injury

Borderline or low intellectual function prior to injury

Prolonged vegetative state prior to recovery

Delayed emergence of motor symptoms

Evidence of extensive infarction on CT/MRI scan

Significant cortical atrophy and/or ventricular enlargement on follow-up CT/MRI scan

---

For children with anoxic-hypotensive brain injury, the prognosis is similar to that for adults. Twenty-five children remaining comatose 24 or more hours after anoxic-hypotensive brain injury were reevaluated at more than 1 year by Kriel et al (30). Of the original 25, five had died, six were in a persistent vegetative state, and only one was cognitively normal. This group also reported that for children with very severe anoxic-hypotensive brain injury (unconscious for 90 days or longer), no child regained functional cognitive or motor skills (31).

Late Complications

One of the late complications of anoxic-hypotensive brain injury is delayed decline in functioning. This syndrome is often observed following carbon monoxide poisoning, but may be seen after any cause of anoxic injury. The pathologic correlate of this delayed deterioration is extensive demyelination of deep cerebral white matter. The clinical course of these patients has been summarized by Plum and colleagues in 1962 (32).

Anoxia is usually severe; most patients are in deep coma when found but awaken within 24 hours. Nearly all patients resume full activity in 4 or 5 days. A clear and seemingly normal interval follows which may last for weeks but usually lasts for 2 to 10 days. Then, abruptly, patients become irritable, apathetic, and confused. Some are agitated or manic. Motor control is clumsy, walking changes to a halting shuffle and diffuse skeletal muscle spasticity or rigidity develops, which occasionally suggests Parkinsonism. Neurologic deterioration either may progress to coma and death or may become arrested at any point. Some patients have a second recovery period that leads to full health.

Another delayed complication of anoxic-hypotensive brain injury is the emergence of *movement disorders*. Although parkinsonism, rigidity, or spasticity may be seen soon after the acute injury, other abnormal movements including rigidity, tremor, dystonia, chorea, and tics may not evolve for weeks or months. In adults, an akinetic-rigid syndrome emerges at 3 months. Many of these patients also develop dystonia some months later. Children and young adults tended to develop a pure dystonic syndrome with a mean onset of 10 months after injury. Dystonia was generalized and often progressed. Although the specific clinical syndrome seen was primarily determined by the age of the patient, the akinetic-rigid syndrome was more often seen after globus pallidus lesions and the dystonic syndrome with putamenal lesions.

Action myoclonus may be another delayed onset symptom. First described by Lance and Adams, these rapid, involuntary jerks may involve a single limb, multiple limbs, or the entire body (33). They may evolve from what appear to be generalized or more complex convulsions during the coma and immediate post-coma period or may begin with subtle jerks that worsen over days or weeks. Myoclonus may improve over time or persist as a significant disability. Sensory stimuli or attempts at movement often exacerbate the jerks. One patient, with significant global intellectual dysfunction following cardiac arrest, experienced myoclonus so severe as to require him to be strapped into a chair and to wear a helmet for protection. Without these safeguards, he was in danger of being thrown to the floor (Bachman, personal communication).

Treatment

There is no literature to indicate whether patients with anoxic-hypotensive brain injury respond to therapy any differently than patients with other types of brain injury. Only scattered case reports address the issue of rehabilitation in this specific population. It has been our experience that the amnestic syndrome seen after anoxic-hypotensive brain injury does not substantially improve beyond the first few months. However, some *compensatory strategies* can be taught. It has also been our experience that linguistic disorders in this population are resistant to traditional aphasia therapy strategies. These patients suffer from more extensive cognitive deficits than is seen in more classic aphasia syndromes following a focal stroke. Behavioral deficits, especially those resembling the frontal systems syndrome, are difficult to treat; however, behavioral strategies and pharmacotherapy may be helpful.

Because of the limited information available on this patient population, most therapists resort to assessments and therapeutic efforts based on experience with other types of brain injury, particularly traumatic brain injury (Chapter 4) or stroke (Chapter 3).

On transfer to a rehabilitation program, patients may vary considerably in their clinical condition. Many patients will be in the midst of a marked confusional state that may be associated with significant motor deficits. At this time, therapy should be directed at addressing the patient's general nutritional status, skin integrity, mobility, physical endurance, and independence in basic activities of daily living. To reduce agitation, the environment should be regulated to avoid excessive stimulation. Patients who are easily overstimulated should be treated in quiet treatment areas. At this time, it is inappropriate to perform extensive neuropsychologic or language testing. However, behavioral analysis can lead to treatment interventions to help regulate behavior while natural recovery continues. Once the confusional state begins to resolve, more specific neuropsychologic deficits often may be identified. Some patients may have marked, generalized cognitive impairment, others may exhibit the specific neurobehavioral syndromes described earlier.

Given that anterograde memory deficits often persist even as the patient's attention improves, providing orientation with the use of simple time and place cues can be useful in this initial period of recovery. Some patients may benefit from the use of more sophisticated compensatory memory strategies, such as organizational and memory aids. Attentional deficits and problems with new learning may make teaching compensatory strategies a protracted process that requires substantial repetition. A number of investigators have demonstrated that amnestic patients with brain injury (some with anoxic-hypotensive brain injury) can proceduralize use of compensatory strategies (memory books, cueing systems) even with persistent dense anterograde memory deficits (34,35).

If and when confusion has sufficiently improved, a formal neuropsychologic evaluation should be performed. Particular spheres of neuropsychologic function that should be addressed include attention, new learning for verbal and nonverbal material, frontal system functioning, and visuoperceptual and visuomotor function. In addition, language should be assessed, especially if aphasia is suspected. Behavioral problems may be sufficiently severe as to limit the assessment and treatment of cognitive deficits. Based on this initial assessment, a treatment plan can be implemented.

In general, by 3 months post injury, the confusional state has largely resolved, and the clinical picture is dominated by more stable deficits. Memory, executive functioning, and visuoperceptual problems are often the most significant deficits. Specific treatment plans shoule focus on the patient's handicapping conditions and are appropriately modeled after those used with the traumatic brain injury population (see Chapter 4).

Behavioral deficits, particularly apathy and denial of illness, become problematic because patients with these deficits make little effort in therapy. Some patients may be irritable and even aggressive. Pharmacotherapy, which may be helpful in some of these situations, is fully discussed in Chapter 11. Clinicians must also be sensitive to the presence of depression, which may also warrant treatment. When possible, care should be taken to avoid medications that may impair arousal, attention, and memory.

Follow-up assessment at 1 year is appropriate to monitor the patient's condition. A neurologic evaluation will identify any late neurologic complications. If there are areas of unexpected decline, one must suspect a late medical, neurologic, or psychiatric complication. Certainly at this time, but generally sooner, spontaneous improvement has plateaued. At this stage of recovery, therapy should focus on the patient's reacclimation to home and when possible, to work. A final neuropsychologic assessment can define the patient's cognitive strengths and weaknesses that delimit community and vocational reentry. For lower functioning patients, physical therapy and occupational therapy might reassess issues of self-care, mobility, tone and positioning, environment, and equipment needs. Higher functioning patients may be appropriate for community reentry programs or vocational services. Efforts at memory and cognitive deficit compensation should focus on practical solutions related to teaching skills required to adequately function in home and vocational environments with reduced supervision.

If behavior is a problem, referral to a professional with expertise in this area should be made. Practical behavioral strategies to be used in the home should be provided to caregivers by the treatment team. The behavior plan will need to be periodically monitored and updated. When behavior is severely disruptive or potentially harmful, an inpatient admission or residential placement may be necessary. Again, pharmacologic treatments may be useful in some cases.

Case Report

A 35-year-old man with a history of closed head injury and seizures was in good health until December 31, 1992. He had made a good recovery from his head injury and his seizures were well controlled. One morning, after spending the night at a friend's house, he was found slumped in a chair unconscious. When the emergency services arrived, he was incontinent and unconscious with "clenched teeth." He was breathing spontaneously, although on 100% oxygen his arterial partial pressure of oxygen (Po_2) was only 63. Other metabolic abnormalities included metabolic acidosis, hyperkalemia, and mild renal failure. A brain CT scan demonstrated symmetric, low-density lesions in the globus pallidus bilaterally (see Figure 5.1). Because of a fever, he was treated for possible sepsis, but antibiotics were eventually discontinued when no source of infection was identified. Two weeks later, he was much improved and although his mentation was described as "a little slow," he seemed nearly back to his baseline and returned home to live with his wife.

Comment: The etiology of this hypoxic episode was never identified with certainty. He may have fallen asleep near a gas heater, but this was never confirmed. Alternatively, he may have had an unobserved seizure and been found in a postictal state. Drug ingestion was also possible. Benzodiazepines and barbiturates were found on a urine drug screen, but he was prescribed these drugs for therapeutic reasons. In any event, he appeared to make a full recovery. Unfortunately, detailed memory testing was not available at the time of discharge from the hospital.

He was readmitted to the hospital 4 weeks after his original illness. He had been doing well until approximately 5 days before his readmission when he became increasingly withdrawn, lethargic, and ataxic. On the day of readmission, he had been found on the floor at home. It was unclear whether he had had a seizure. In the emergency department, his behavior was described as bizarre, and he had difficulty following commands. His neurologic examination was otherwise unremarkable.

During the next 4 to 5 days, his condition continued to deteriorate and became unresponsive. Muscle tone was extremely rigid, and at times he developed decerebrate and decorticate posturing. He was markedly febrile with a temperature up to 107°F and ultimately was placed on a ventilator and transferred to the intensive care unit. An EEG demonstrated slowing but no epileptiform activity; other diagnostic studies were unrevealing. During the next month, the patient improved and was weaned from the respirator.

Comment: This patient almost certainly suffered a delayed neurologic deterioration secondary to an anoxic brain injury.

A few weeks later he had sufficiently improved so that physical therapy and occupational therapy evaluated him. Strength appeared to be intact though there was a mild increase in flexor tone in both lower extremities. Seated balance was good, but he required minimum assistance of two when standing. There was moderately spastic tone in both upper extremities as well as mild ataxia, left greater than right. He was completely dependent in all activities of daily living. He was disheveled with near constant motion of his legs.

Cognitively, he was oriented to person and inconsistently oriented to place and time. His attention span was approximately 2 minutes in a quiet room, but he was easily distracted by visual and auditory stimuli. The patient was able to recall three out of three items immediately and one out of three after a 10-minute delay. Because of his distractibility, he had difficulty following directions. A few weeks later, he continued to be highly distractible but was able to participate in tasks for up to 10 minutes. He was alert and responded correctly to orientation questions about 50% of the time. New learning was clearly impaired. He was not significantly dysarthric and produced syntactically well-formed sentences though with occasional word-order errors. Frequent errors in confrontational naming were probably secondary to visual misperception and diminished attention. Responses to open-ended questions resulted in irrelevant and occasionally confabulatory responses.

Comment: During this time, the patient was recovering from a marked confusional state. Language appeared to be relatively intact aside from confusional responses and nonaphasic misnaming. Higher cognitive function, including memory, was difficult to assess at this time but appeared impaired. Physically, his strength appeared to be relatively good, but there was increased muscle tone, somewhat greater in the arms than in the legs. This pattern of deficit was consistent with border-zone ischemia with bibrachial involvement. The ataxia may have been secondary to anoxic injury to the cerebellum.

This patient's therapy was directed at minimizing confusion and agitation while focusing on practical short-term goals. Physical therapy concentrated on improving physical endurance as well as balance and safety for transfers and ambulation. Occupational therapy was directed at helping the patient regain independence in basic activities of daily living (ADLs). Motor function and task performance improved, and some new learning was proceduralized despite continuing anterograde amnesia.

The patient was discharged from the hospital after 8 weeks and was transferred to a nursing home where he remained for another month before returning home. He received no further rehabilitation in the nursing facility. Ten months after onset of his illness, he had a neuropsychologic evaluation. His behavior was characterized as apathetic, irritable, and impulsive with diminished social graces. He would impulsively call telephone numbers he had seen displayed in television advertisements in order to place orders. His personal hygiene was poor. He demonstrated some decline from his estimated premorbid level of function with a Verbal IQ score of 79, Performance IQ score of 65, and Full Scale IQ of 72. Immediate and short-term verbal and nonverbal memories were quite impaired. His immediate recall of verbal passages was poor (18% level); however, he was able to retain some of what little he had learned (13% level). He demonstrated mild difficulty on constructional tasks with no visual inattention or neglect. He demonstrated marked difficulties on tasks requiring flexibility of thinking, such as Trail Making Test B. Throughout his evaluation he demonstrated significant deficits in his ability to reason, plan his behavior, or negotiate novel situations. The patient had an unsuccessful trial on both valproic acid and thiothixene in order to reduce his anger and irritability.

In July of 1995 ($2\frac{1}{2}$ years post onset), the patient underwent a neurobehavioral evaluation. By this time, the patient's wife was in the process of divorcing him, and he was living with his mother. The behavioral difficulties described by the neuropsychologist 2 years earlier were virtually unchanged; irritable, angry outbursts were common. The patient would repetitively telephone people all hours of the day or night. Once he made the call, he would say very little and then hang up. He would then proceed to place another call. No other ritualistic behavior was present. The patient would sometimes expose himself and masturbate at inappropriate times. On neurologic examination, he demonstrated a mild dysarthria. His speech was soft and often delivered with such rapidity that it affected his intelligibility. There was a reduction in facial expression but no true akinesia. Muscle tone was slightly increased, left greater than right, and there was mild dysmetria on finger-to-nose examination. Otherwise, his neurologic examination, including gait and posture, was normal.

The patient had no insight into the nature of his deficits and was completely unconcerned. When asked why he was not working, he replied, "No one will hire me." On the Mini-Mental State Examination, he scored 26 of 30 possible points. He would have had a perfect score except that his responses were extremely rapid and impulsive, resulting in some errors. Naming, repetition, and auditory comprehension were excellent. Writing was micrographic. On a five-word supraspan, he recalled $^4/_5$, $^4/_5$, and $^5/_5$ objects on sequential presentations. After a 5-minute filled delay, he recalled four of five objects with one intrusion. Proverb interpretation varied from the abstract to the concrete.

Comment: After resolution of the confusional state, the patient began to exhibit behavioral and cognitive deficits similar to those seen in patients with frontal systems dysfunction. These findings, combined with the mild extrapyramidal motor findings are similar to those described by LaPlane with bilateral basal ganglia lesions (22). This patient did not have a distinct amnestic syndrome associated with anoxic-hypotensive brain injury, but in fact gradually improved such that he was oriented and able to make new memories. Shallow, ineffectual learning limited immediate memory but retention was reasonably good.

Therapy at this time was directed at minimizing the burden on his family. His mother was instructed how to approach him during periods of increased irritability and anger. She was taught to structure his time by providing him with a regular, daily schedule, including time for exercise and household chores. Suggestions were given for providing substitute activities, including the possibility of computer programs, to reduce his telephoning. Finally, she was encouraged to continue to work with a community reentry program and vocational rehabilitation counselor to see if sheltered work could be found for him. However, because of the severity of his behavioral problems, it was unclear if he would ever be capable of competitive employment.

ENCEPHALITIS

Infectious disorders are another cause of diffuse brain damage in patients admitted for neurorehabilitation. Infectious agents may involve the meninges (*meningitis*), the brain parenchyma (*encephalitis*), or both (*meningoencephalitis*). Abscesses (usually bacterial) may occur in the brain parenchyma or the meninges. Bacteria, fungi, and parasites can all affect the central nervous system, but the most common cause of brain infection is viral. In the United States alone, 20,000 cases of acute viral encephalitis occur each year (36).

Many viruses cause encephalitis. The clinical patterns produced by these pathogens are divided into the following four categories (37):

- Acute viral encephalitis
- Postinfectious encephalomyelitis (probably of autoimmune etiology)
- Slow viral infections
- Chronic degenerative diseases of viral origin.

Most of the discussion in this chapter will be limited to acute viral encephalitis.

Herpes simplex is the most common cause of sporadic acute viral encephalitis (Figure 5.3). It occurs sporadically throughout the year, in all age groups and in all parts of the world. In the United States. 5% to 10% of acute encephalitis cases are attributable to herpes simplex virus (36). Outside of North America, the most common cause of epidemic encephalitis is *Japanese B encephalitis* (38). Epidemic and seasonal encephalitis is usually caused by arthropod-borne viruses (arboviruses). Mosquitoes transmit these viruses from infected vertebrate carriers (e.g., horses, birds, and rodents) to humans or other hosts. These infections occur during the peak mosquito seasons, summer and early fall. Certain viruses also have a predilection for various geographic regions. Examples in the United States include *Eastern Equine*, *Western Equine*, *California Virus*, and *St. Louis Virus*. Eastern equine

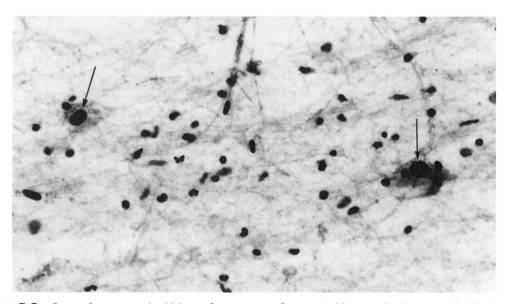

Figure 5.3   *Smear from a cerebral biopsy from a case of suspected herpes simplex encephalitis. A positive reaction in the nuclei of the two neurons (arrowed) was obtained with a rabbit antiserum to herpes simplex type I virus. Normal rabbit serum gave a negative reaction on a second smear. Immunoperoxidase with hematoxylin counterstain. x220.* (Reprinted from Esiri MM, Oppenheimer DR. Diagnostic neuropathology: a practical manual. Oxford: Blackwell Scientific, 1989:83.)

encephalitis is the most devastating form of arboviral encephalitis in the United States.

In addition to the acute forms of encephalitis, several forms of sub-acute or chronic viral encephalitides also occur. Recently, the most important type has been *HIV* encephalitis, sometimes referred to as *AIDS dementia complex*. The cause of this disorder is believed to be due to direct infection of the brain with HIV.

Neuropathology

Except for encephalitis caused by herpes simplex virus, the pathologic effects of acute viral encephalitis are nonspecific. There may be widespread destruction of neurons in one or more areas of the cerebral hemispheres, or damage may be limited to small, microscopic foci. The presence of mononuclear inflammatory cells, particularly around blood vessels and in the meninges, is characteristic of these disorders.

The pathologic picture of herpes simplex virus is distinctive. The hallmark is hemorrhagic necrosis of the inferior and medial temporal lobes, and basal and orbital portions of the frontal lobes (Figures 5.4 and 5.5). Sometimes the lesions extend laterally into the temporal lobes or medially in the frontal lobes up to the cingulate gyrus. The insular cortex, deep to the Sylvian fissure is frequently involved (see Figure 5.4). The distribution of the infection is thought to be related to the virus activating from a latent state in the trigeminal ganglion and spreading along fibers that innervate the meninges in the anterior and middle cranial fossas. This localization accounts for the typical clinical effects of herpes simplex virus encephalitis.

Clinical Features, Natural History, and Residual Syndromes

The clinical course of acute viral encephalitis may be considered in the acute, subacute, and chronic phases of recovery. In the acute phase (days after onset), all types of encephalitis present as an acute febrile illness with evidence of meningeal involvement. The patient may go on to have seizures, confusion, delirium, decreased arousal, or coma. Some particular signs may occur early, such as aphasia, mutism, hemiparesis, involuntary movements, ataxia, myoclonus, nystagmus, ocular palsies, and facial weakness. However, patients with less severe infections present with fewer and less severe symptoms and make a more rapid recovery.

In the subacute phase, beginning after the first week or two post onset, patients who survive begin to regain consciousness, and some

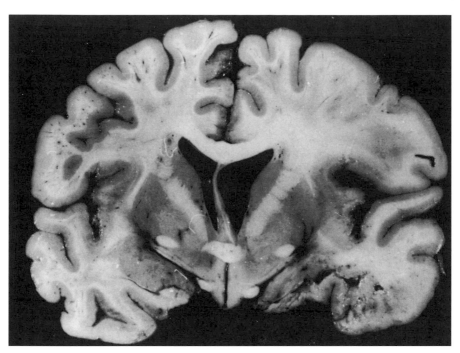

Figure 5.4 *Coronal slice through the temporal and frontal lobes of the brain from a patient with acute herpes simplex encephalitis. There is softening and necrosis of medial and inferior parts of the temporal lobes, more extensive on the right. The insula is also affected on both sides. The right cerebral hemisphere is swollen, causing a shift of midline structures to the left, and a downthrust of diencephalic structures. The slight dilatation of the right lateral ventricle has resulted from compression of the third ventricle and foramen of Munro. (Reprinted from Esiri MM, Oppenheimer DR. Diagnostic neuropathology: a practical manual. Oxford: Blackwell Scientific, 1989:140.)*

specific neurologic impairment may become evident. As with any acute neurologic disturbance, the evolving clinical profile is difficult to characterize until early arousal and basic attentional disturbances abate. Most forms of encephalitis do not have a distinct clinical profile. Generally, global cognitive and behavioral problems occur, and a variety of motor impairments such as hemiparesis, ataxia, or movement disorders is evident. Seizures may continue at this phase of recovery. Patients with herpes simplex virus often have a more characteristic clinical profile due to its predilection for limbic structures, cortical structures associated with the limbic system, and nearby neocortical structures in the temporal and frontal lobes. Other viral agents may also cause areas of focal damage, but none has the same predictable distribution as herpes simplex virus.

The persistence of clinical problems in the chronic phase of recovery depends on a host of factors relating to the type of virus causing the infection and the severity of the initial inflammatory reaction. These factors help predict the distribution and amount of residual brain

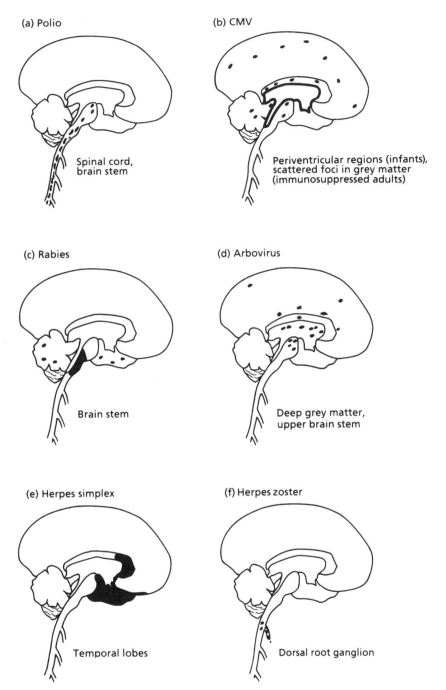

(a) Polio

Spinal cord,
brain stem

(b) CMV

Periventricular regions (infants),
scattered foci in grey matter
(immunosuppressed adults)

(c) Rabies

Brain stem

(d) Arbovirus

Deep grey matter,
upper brain stem

(e) Herpes simplex

Temporal lobes

(f) Herpes zoster

Dorsal root ganglion

Figure 5.5 Variations in topographic sites of maximal damage to the nervous system in some cases of viral encephalitis. (Reprinted from Esiri MM, Oppenheimer DR. Diagnostic neuropathology: a practical manual. Oxford: Blackwell Scientific, 1989:144.)

injury. Patients may fully recover or be left with a decline in neurologic function either of a more generalized nature or in a specific localizing pattern. As with any focal or multifocal brain disorder, patients with herpes simplex virus display one or more clinical syndromes largely depending on how the lesions disrupt various overlapping functional neural networks. If the lesion affects medial temporal limbic structures including the hippocampus, anterograde episodic memory and new learning deficits will be prominent. If the lesion extends into the anterior temporal higher-order association areas and the insular area, as in the case described by Damasio and colleagues in 1991, the patient also may have prominent retrograde, episodic memory loss (38). Involvement of the basal forebrain may produce confabulation, executive function impairments, as well as memory encoding and retrieval deficits. (For discussion of the basal forebrain syndrome, see the section on anterior communicating aneurysm rupture in Chapter 3.) If the lesion involves more lateral, temporal structures on the left side, the patient may also have semantic language and memory deficits (39). Patients with herpes simplex virus encephalitis sometimes report olfactory or gustatory hallucinations, presumably from involvement of olfactory pathways in the basal forebrain and anterior medial temporal areas (prepiriform and entorhinal cortex). Mood and personality changes such as euphoria, mania, aggressiveness, irritability, and depression are also common, affecting up to 65% of patients with herpes simplex virus (40). Disruption of limbic structures and closely related cortical areas in the orbital frontal and anteromedial temporal areas accounts for these signs. Finally, a frontal opercular syndrome with anarthria and dysphagia resulting from bilateral frontal opercular involvement (Broca's area and the right hemisphere analogue) has been described in young patients with herpes simplex virus (41).

The variety and heterogeneity of the cognitive and memory deficits associated with herpes simplex virus and other types of viral encephalitis were characterized in a consecutive series of patients with acute viral encephalitis by Hokkanen in 1996 (43). An important observation from this series of patients was that severe localizing impairments such as amnesia (characteristic of herpes simplex virus) was observed in patients with nonherpetic encephalitis. In general, however, patients with herpes simplex virus were more likely to have disruption of verbal memory and verbal semantic functions. Overall, patients with herpes simplex virus encephalitis were two to four times more likely to have significant cognitive deficits than patients with non–herpes simplex virus encephalitis. The amnesic deficit observed in patients without herpes simplex virus was heterogeneous. Three patterns of memory involvement were described: one pattern involved prominent semantic memory loss, another was characterized by abnormal executive functions, and the last by rapid forgetting. These patterns generally correspond to the syndromic relationships described above for lateral temporal, basal frontal, and medial temporal syndromes, respectively. Lesion analysis supported these relationships for some of the patients described.

Formulating Prognosis

Outcome from viral encephalitis is highly variable. Studies providing a systematic analysis of recovery and outcome are lacking. Some broad guidelines are available, but the most important predictor is *viral etiology* (Table 5.3). Some viruses, such as herpes simplex virus or eastern equine encephalitis are associated with significant mortality. Without antiviral therapy, death from herpes simplex virus encephalitis may exceed 70%, and only 2.5% infected with this virus regain normal function (37). Antiviral agents, such as acyclovir, have substantially reduced mortality (28%) and lessened morbidity (38% normal or mild impairment) (37). Mortality from eastern equine encephalitis has ranged from 31% to 68%; more than half of the survivors had no or only mild sequelae (42).

The effects of most other viruses is less serious; for example, mortality of western equine encephalitis ranges from 5% to 15%. Survivors have a low incidence of long-term sequelae. With St. Louis encephalitis, mortality runs from 2% to 20%, and 20% of the affected group have long-term sequelae.

In reviewing a series of 77 patients with encephalitis caused by herpes simplex or other viruses, Hokkanen and colleagues observed full recovery at postacute follow-up (average 28 days) in 44% of patients with non–herpes simplex virus encephalitis but only 12% of those with herpes simplex virus encephalitis, despite treatment with acyclovir (43). Longer term follow-up of a subgroup of the patients with herpes simplex virus encephalitis reported by the same group of

Table 5.3.   *Factors Predicting a Worse Outcome After Viral Encephalitis*

Viral etiologies with high mortality and morbidity (e.g., herpes simplex, eastern equine)

Lack of early treatment with antiviral agents

Coma and low Glasgow Coma Scale score during acute phase of recovery

Bilateral distribution of neuropathology

Focal signs on neurologic examination or neuroimaging

More rapid onset, shorter prodrome

Signs of brainstem dysfunction (e.g., abnormal oculocephalic responses)

High intracranial pressures

Decreased regional cerebral blood flow on subacute SPECT study

Younger age (?)

investigators revealed that 75% of the patients had significant memory problems, but by 1 year 50% of these survivors had restoration of normal memory (40). Persistent global amnesia was observed in 12.5% of this group. This report of the prognosis for herpes simplex virus is somewhat better than that seen in other studies, where 60% had persistent amnesia (44). The likelihood of returning to work is worse for patients with herpes simplex virus than other forms of encephalitis. Hokkanen and colleagues found 46% of surviving patients with herpes simplex virus returned to work, whereas patients with non–herpes simplex virus encephalitis returned to work at nearly twice that rate (89%) (43).

To reiterate, viral etiology is an important determinant of outcome. As noted above, herpes simplex virus and eastern equine arborvirus carry a worse prognosis. However, the use of antiviral agents such as acyclovir has improved the outlook for those contracting herpes simplex virus.

Another factor predicting recovery is the *presence and depth of coma* during the acute phase of the illness. Although duration of coma has not been well studied, the absence of coma was seen as a good prognostic sign in a group of patients with eastern equine encephalitis (42). A low Glasgow Coma Scale score (see Table 4.4) was a sign of poor outcome in a group of patients with a number of common encephalitides (45). In a study of children with encephalitis, the Glasgow Coma Scale score was a predictor of outcome only if it was profoundly depressed (i.e., <6) (46).

The *distribution of neuropathology* is a recognized factor in recovery (see Figure 5.5). The presence of focal signs on examination or imaging studies were the main factors predicting poor outcome in children with encephalitis (46). As it is for most neurologic disorders, the extent of bilateral involvement is an important variable in predicting outcome (see Chapter 1). In herpes simplex encephalitis, patients with unilateral involvement have substantially better recoveries than those with bilateral presentation (43,47,48). Antiviral agents may play a role in preventing unilateral lesions from progressing to involve both hemispheres.

The effect of *age* on recovery from encephalitides has been discussed in several reports. Paradoxically, older age was found an advantage in two of them. An investigation of patients with eastern equine encephalitis concluded that those over 40 had a better outcome than those under 40 (42). In evaluating a group of children and adults with various types of encephalitis, Kennedy and colleagues found that younger age was associated with poorer outcome (45). However, another report looking at children with encephalitis concluded that young children (<1 year) did not have a worse prognosis (46). Thus, at this point in time, the effect of age on recovery after encephalitis is inconclusive. The possible advantage of older age raises the question of a protective factor, perhaps related to immune function or genetic predisposition.

Other factors proposed as negative prognosticators include more rapid onset or shorter prodrome; abnormal oculocephalic responses, indicators of brainstem or vestibular dysfunction; and very high intracranial pressures (42,45,49). Pressures over 29 mm Hg were associated with high mortality, but low Glasgow Coma Scale scores did not correlate as well with mortality as intracranial pressure.

Outcome after viral encephalitis in children was predicted by serial evaluation of regional blood flow by single-photon emission CT (SPECT) (50). The acute SPECT studies showed increased regional cerebral blood flow in almost all patients. If the subacute SPECT was normal, rather than showing a decrease in regional cerebral activity, a good outcome was predicted by 1 year. Although SPECT may prove to be a good prognostic tool for encephalitis, more study is required before this test becomes an accepted guide clinically.

Rehabilitation Planning

The principles that guide rehabilitation planning are similar to those described above for anoxic-hypotensive brain injury. During the acute rehabilitation period, specific impairments, particularly those related to focal brain damage, will not be fully apparent and cannot be adequately evaluated until early arousal and basic attentional deficits resolve. At that point, more elaborate evaluations can be performed and used to develop management strategies for specific impairments. Most patients present with cognitive and behavioral disabilities, but motor disorders of various types, such as imbalance or hemiparesis may occur. For patients with herpes simplex encephalitis, memory will be the most frequent management problem. The memory disorder should be characterized by its various components, such as anterograde vs. retrograde, episodic vs. semantic vs. procedural, verbal vs. nonverbal, encoding vs. retrieval. Related behavioral problems are understood best in relation to disorders of executive dysfunction, inattention, or language disorders.

The treatment plan should emphasize compensation strategies consistent with a patient's anticipated real-world needs and prognosis for recovery. During the subacute phase of recovery, treatment centers on cognitive therapy aimed at establishing household safety awareness and compensation strategies for recall and follow-through of everyday activities. At the chronic phases of recovery, treatment focuses on returning to full household and community independence and, if possible, return to work or school. The extent of residual impairments (especially memory) at 3 to 6 months post infection will determine the feasibility of these more ambitious goals.

Case Studies

Case 1

A 63-year-old man, who owned a retail grocery store, was admitted to the hospital with mental status changes and new onset seizures. Two days before admission, he began experiencing strange metallic odors. The next day he developed slurred speech, confused language, and vomiting. On the day of admission, he had a generalized seizure. When examined at the hospital, he had a temperature of 103°F and was lethargic. The acute brain CT scan demonstrated a vague low-density area in the left insula and inferomedial temporal lobe. Spinal fluid analysis was positive for a mildly elevated protein, but normal for glucose levels; white blood cell count was elevated—a picture consistent with viral meningoencephalitis. Specific viral studies of this and a subsequent spinal fluid sample demonstrated a high cerebral spinal fluid (CSF) to serum antibody ratio, supporting a diagnosis of herpes simplex virus encephalitis. The patient had been started on both antibiotics and an antiviral agent (acyclovir).

Over the first 3 days of hospitalization, he became comatose, responding only to painful stimulation. By the second week of hospitalization, he began regaining consciousness and when fully responsive was confused, perseverative, and his language was filled with semantic paraphasias. There were no motor abnormalities other than mild unsteadiness when standing. A repeat brain CT scan at this time demonstrated bilateral lesions and swelling in the inferior temporal lobes, insula, and basal frontal areas, significantly worse on the left than right side.

By the third week he was afebrile and more attentive and appropriate in his responses; he was transferred to an acute rehabilitation hospital. On initial rehabilitation evaluation, he was alert, distractible, oriented only to person, and unable to demonstrate any awareness of his illness or hospitalization. He gave vague and inaccurate responses to biographical questions, even about his family, residence, and occupation. It was not always clear that he recognized family members. His speech was at time hesitant and empty, and he appeared somewhat anomic. He was ambulatory with contact guarding and needed continual cueing to follow through on basic ADLs.

Over the next week, his attention and language output considerably improved. He remained mildly anomic, but his responses to most basic biographical questions were accurate and he had no problems recognizing family. He was, however, still disoriented and densely amnestic for any day-to-day experiences. He was unable to learn new information after even a brief delay, and he was amnestic for personal and historic events going back several years. It was clear that he had evolved out of a confusional state, but was left with a profound amnestic syndrome.

By 6 weeks following onset of the illness, he was safely ambulating, could follow through on ADLs with a minimum of setup, yet he remained densely amnestic. He now knew he was in the hospital and could state that he had some kind of problem with his head. With personal warning signs positioned on the walls and frequent cueing, he learned to stay within the bounds of the unit (procedural learning), although he could not explicitly recount these limits when asked. Use of a memory and schedule book was attempted, but he needed cues to remind him of the purpose of the book, vitiating its usefulness.

The rehabilitation goal at this point was to set up a safe discharge plan. He went home on a day pass to evaluate his safety. Although safe moving about the house, he repeatedly attempted to begin various household chores such as mowing the lawn and perseverated about driving his car. He was discharged home after 4 weeks of inpatient rehabilitation with a recommendation for 24-hour distant supervision in the house. Various recommendations were instituted to assure safety, such as hiding the car keys and parking the car out of view, and placing a sign and a buzzer on the front door to keep him from wandering out unnoticed.

By 12 weeks after onset, he was showing ability to remember some day-to-day experiences, but his ability to learn new information was still impaired. He had developed regular day-to-day routines and was fully independent in basic ADLs. In outpatient rehabilitation therapies, he started to routinize the use of a memory book, but only occasionally generalizing its use at home. His wife was anxious to be able to leave him home alone and resume her place in the family grocery business.

The patient began a postacute cognitive rehabilitation day program. The main goal was to help him achieve household independence so he could be left safely alone for an extended period of time. A system of memory aids was set up, including an improved memory book to follow his daily schedule, appointments, and essential information; lists of important phone numbers, highlighting an emergency number list; a reminder system for taking medications; and a system for recording phone messages. Varieties of meal preparation tasks were proceduralized, including safe use of the stove. A number of household tasks and leisure activities were explored to fill the time he was home alone and improve the quality of his life. After 8 weeks in the program, he was able to safely stay home alone for the better part of the work day. Over subsequent weeks in the program, a variety of work tasks were explored so that he could participate in his family grocery business.

By 9 months post onset, he had returned to working at least 20 hours a week in the store. Although not as densely amnesic, he still had severe anterograde memory and new learning problems. However, he had much better insight into his problems and began to set his own limits in activities. He still needed supervision in community activities and could not manage finances, but had returned to a number of premorbid routines at home and work.

Case 2

A 57-year-old woman presented to the emergency department of a hospital with a 3-day history of flulike symptoms culminating in confusion, lethargy, high fever, and headache. She was somnolent and confused. The initial brain CT scan was negative, but her spinal fluid indicated abnormalities consistent with viral inflammation. She was started on acyclovir. For the next 2 days, she was difficult to arouse and may have been having brief seizures associated with lapses in responsiveness. She resumed full wakefulness over the next few days. An MRI scan revealed an abnormal area in the right orbital frontal and anterior temporal areas. Viral CSF studies were suggestive of herpes simplex encephalitis.

She was admitted to a rehabilitation hospital 2 weeks post onset. At that time, she was still confused, highly confabulative, and disinhibited. She was occasionally restless and agitated. Much of the early rehabilitative effort centered on managing her confusion by reducing stimulation and providing calming reassurance during ADL and other interactions.

The patient improved substantially over the next 2 weeks to the point that she was fully attentive, but she was still highly confabulative and at times behaviorally disinhibited. On tests of verbal memory, she had only mild retrieval problems that improved considerably with cueing. Visual memory was a little worse than verbal memory. She had great difficulty with even simple decision-making and problem-solving tasks. Consistent with neuroimaging, the clinical diagnosis was a basal frontal syndrome associated with primarily right-sided frontal and anterior temporal damage from herpes simplex encephalitis. The discharge plan included a behavioral program involving her family to help manage inappropriate behavior and a structured schedule to compensate for disordered executive functioning.

Over subsequent weeks, while in outpatient rehabilitation, the patient improved to the point that she could manage at home independently. Confabulation resolved, social behavior and personality returned to their baselines, but she still had difficulty with the structured home schedule designed to manage her disordered executive functioning. The remainder of outpatient rehabilitative efforts were directed toward independence in community activities and managing household finances. Over the next 3 months, she returned to a relatively normal level of functioning.

References

1. Grosswasser Z, Cohen M, Costeff H. Rehabilitation outcome after anoxic brain damage. Arch Phys Med Rehabil 1989;70:186–188.
2. Wilson BA. Cognitive functioning of adult survivors of cerebral hypoxia. Brain Injury 1996;10:863–874.
3. Barcroft J. Anoxemia. Lancet 1920;2:485–489.
4. Sazbon L, Zagreba F, Ronen J, et al. Course and outcome of patients in vegetative state of nontraumatic aetiology. J Neurol Neurosurg Psychiatry 1993;56:407–409.
5. Lubbers DW. The oxygen pressure field of the brain and its significance for the normal and critical oxygen supply of the brain. In: Lubbers DW, Luft VC, Thews G, Witzleb E, eds. Oxygen transport in blood and tissue. Stuttgart: Thieme, 1966:124–139.
6. Bierley JB, Graham DI. Hypoxia and vascular disorders of the central nervous system. In: Adams JH, Corsellis JAN, Duchen LW, eds. Greenfield's Neuropathology. 4th ed. New York: John Wiley & Sons, 1984:125–207.
7. Kinney HC, Korein J, Panigrahy A, et al. Neuropathological findings in the brain of Karen Ann Quinlan: the role of the thalamus in the persistent vegetative state. New Engl J Med 1994;330:1469–1475.
8. Richardson JC, Chambers RA, Heywood PM. Encephalopathies of anoxia and hypoglycemia. Arch Neurol 1959;1:70–82.
9. Bertini G, Giglioli C, Giovannini F, et al. Neuropsychological outcome of survivors of out-of-hospital cardiac arrest. J Emerg Med 1990;8:407–412.
10. Smith JS, Brandon S. Morbidity from acute carbon monoxide poisoning at three-year follow-up. Br Med J 1973;1:318–321.
11. Roine R, Kajaste S, Kaste M. Neuropsychological sequelae of cardiac arrest. JAMA 1993;269:237–242.
12. Smith JS, Brandon S. Acute carbon monoxide poisoning—3 years experience in a defined population. Postgrad Med J 1970;46:65–70.
13. The Multi-Society Task Force on PVS. Medical aspects of the persistent vegetative state (part 2). New Engl J Med 1994;330:1572–1579.
14. Cummings JL, Tomiyasu U, Read S, Benson FD. Amnesia with hippocampal lesions after cardiopulmonary arrest. Neurology 1984;34:679–681.
15. Zola-Morgan S, Squire LR, Amaral DG. Human amnesia and the medial temporal region: enduring memory impairment following a bilateral lesion limited to field CA1 of the hippocampus. J Neurosci 1986;6:2950–2967.
16. Kuwert T, Homberg V, Steinmetz H, et al. Posthypoxic amnesia: regional cerebral glucose consumption measured by positron emission tomography. J Neurol Sci 1993;118:10–16.
17. De Renzi E, Lucchelli F. Dense retrograde amnesia, intact learning capability and abnormal forgetting rate: a consolidation defect? Cortex 1993;29:449–466.
18. Howard R, Trend P, Russell RWR. Clinical features of ischemia in cerebral arterial border zones after periods of reduced cerebral blood flow. Arch Neurol 1987;44:934–940.
19. Mohr J. Neurological complications of cardiac valvular disease and cardiac surgery including systemic hypotension. In: Vinken PJ, Bruyn

GW, eds. Handbook of clinical neurology. Amsterdam: Elsevier Science 1977;38:143–171.

20. Geschwind N, Quadfasel FA, Segarra J. Isolation of the speech area. Neuropsychologia 1968;6:327–340.
21. Hawker K, Lang AE. Hypoxic-ischemic damage of the basal ganglia. Mov Disord 1990;5:219–224.
22. LaPlane D, Levasseur M, Pillon B, et al. Obsessive-compulsive and other behavioral changes with bilateral basal ganglia lesions. Brain 1989;112:699–725.
23. Damasceno BP. Decerebrate rigidity with preserved cognition and gait: a possible role of anoxic-ischemic brain damage. Int J Neurosci 1991;58:283–287.
24. Caronna JJ, Finklestein S. Neurological syndromes after cardiac arrest. Stroke 1978;9:517–520.
25. Tonsgard JH, Harwicke N, Levine SC. Kluver-Bucy syndrome in children. Pediatr Neurol 1987;3:162–165.
26. Lilly R, Cummings JR, Benson F, Frankel M. The human Kluver-Bucy syndrome. Neurology 1983;33:1141–1145.
27. Edgren E, Hedstrand U, Kelsey S, et al. Assessment of neurological prognosis in comatose survivors of cardiac arrest. Lancet 1994;343:1055–1059.
28. Bell JA, Hodgson HJF. Coma after cardiac arrest. Brain 1974;97:361–372.
29. Levy DE, Caronna JJ, Singer BH, et al. Predicting outcome for hypoxic-ischemic coma. JAMA 1985;253:1420–1426.
30. Kriel RL, Krach LE, Luxenberg MG, et al. Outcome of severe anoxic ischemic brain injury in children. Pediatr Neurol 1994;10:207–212.
31. Kriel RL, Krach LE, Jones-Saete C. Outcome of children with prolonged unconsciousness and vegetative states. Pediatr Neurol 1993;9:362–368.
32. Plum F, Posner JB, Hain RF. Delayed neurological deterioration after anoxia. Arch Int Med 1962;110:18–25.
33. Lance JW, Adams RD. The syndrome of intention or action myoclonus as a sequel to hypoxic encephalopathy. Brain 1963;86:111–134.
34. Kime SK, Lamb DG, Wilson BA. Use of a comprehensive programme of external cueing to enhance procedural memory in a patient with dense amnesia. Brain Injury 1996;10:17–26.
35. Glisky EL, Schacter DL, Tulving E. Computer learning by memory-impaired patient: acquisition and retention of complex knowledge. Neuropsychologia 1986;24:313–328.
36. Hanley DF, Johnson RT, Whitley RJ. Yes, brain biopsy should be a prerequisite for herpes simplex encephalitis treatment. Arch Neurol 1987;44:1289–1290.
37. Whitley RJ. Viral encephalitis. N Engl J Med 1990;323:242–249.
38. Damasio AR, Tranel D, Damasio H. Amnesia caused by herpes simplex encephalitis, infarctions in basal forebrain, Alzheimer's disease and anoxia/ischemia. In: Boller F, Grafman J, eds. Handbook of neuropsychology. Vol. 3. Amsterdam: Elsevier, 1989:149–166.
39. Pietrini V, Nertempi P, Vaglia A, et al. Recovery from herpes simplex encephalitis: selective impairment of specific semantic categories with neuroradiological correlation. J Neurol Neurosurg Psychiatry 1988;51:1284–1293.
40. Hokkanen L, Salonen O, Launes J. Amnesia in acute herpetic and nonherpetic encephalitis. Arch Neurol 1996;53:972–978.

41. Van der Poel JC, Haenggeli CA, Overweg-Plandsoen WC. Opercular syndrome: unusual feature of herpes simplex encephalitis. Pediatr Neurol 1995;12:246–249.
42. Przelomski MM, O'Rourke E, Grady GF, et al. Eastern equine encephalitis in Massachusetts: a report of 16 cases, 1970–1984. Neurology 1988;38:736–739.
43. Hokkanen L, Poutiainen E, Valanne L, et al. Cognitive impairment after acute encephalitis: comparison of herpes simplex and other aetiologies. J Neurol Neurosurg Psychiatry 1996;61:478–484.
44. Kapur N, Barker S, Burrows EH, et al. Herpes simplex encephalitis: long term magnetic resonance imaging and neuropsychological study of 9 cases. Rev Neurol (Paris) 1990;146:671–681.
45. Kennedy CR, Duffy SW, Smith R, Robinson RO. Clinical predictors of outcome in encephalitis. Arch Dis Child 1987;62:1156–1162.
46. Klein SK, Horn DL, Anderson MR, et al. Predictive factors of short-term neurologic outcome in children with encephalitis. Pediatr Neurol 1994;11:308–312.
47. Laurent B, Allegri RF, Michel D, et al. Primarily unilateral herpes encephalitis: long-term neuropsychological study of 9 cases. Rev Neurol (Paris) 1990;146:671–681.
48. Eslinger PJ, Damasio H, Damasio AR, Butters N. Nonverbal amnesia and asymmetric cerebral lesions following encephalitis. Brain Cogn 1993;21:140–152.
49. Barnett GH, Ropper AH, Romeo J. Intracranial pressure and outcome in adult encephalitis. J Neurosurg 1988;68:585–588.
50. Kao CH, Wang SJ, Mak SC, et al. Viral encephalitis in children: detection with technetium-99 m HMPAO brain single-photon emission CT and its value in prediction of outcome. Am J Neuroradiol 1994;15:1369–1373.

Multiple Sclerosis

Susan Pierson

OVERVIEW OF THE DISEASE PROCESS

Multiple sclerosis (MS) presents one of the most challenging neurologic diseases to predict patient progress, define rehabilitation goals, and anticipate outcome. Precise prognostication depends on a sound knowledge of the patient's disease type and progression within the natural history of the disease process. In addition, few other illnesses demand as much flexibility in readapting treatment plans as the course of the MS waxes or wanes. Although each case of MS must be considered individually because of the wide variety of clinical presentations, the syndrome itself is categorized into four major disease types. Multiple sclerosis is different from other diagnoses commonly treated by rehabilitation professionals in that it does not present with a defined catastrophic event or a solitary disabling episode, as is the case for traumatic brain injury, spinal cord injury, and stroke. As such, it is viewed as a difficult disease entity to include in rehabilitation programs because it is considered a progressive neurologic disorder without expected recovery. Thus, MS is often generically managed as one of a number of various disease processes grouped together for treatment on a "general rehabilitation unit."

177

Epidemiology

The current estimate of the incidence of MS in the United States is 250,000 cases (1). It is a disease predominantly affecting young women. The majority of patients are diagnosed between the ages of 18 to 40, and females outnumber males 2 to 1. Caucasians are primarily affected, and epidemiologic data support a greater incidence of MS in persons who have lived their lives prior to adolescence in the northern latitudes.

Genetics

Although the genetics of MS is not yet established, there is a familial tendency to acquire the disease. Genetic analysis of families with multiple cases of MS in siblings have not disclosed a fully penetrant (single gene) Mendelian pattern of inheritance (2). The familial rate for multiple sclerosis in the Vancouver, British Columbia, MS clinic approaches 20%, if the rates are combined for first-, second-, and third-degree relatives. Compared to the risk for the population at large (0.2% lifetime risk), the risk for a female sibling is 25 times greater (5% lifetime risk) (3). Twin studies reveal a concordance rate significantly higher for monozygotic twins than dizygotic twins. In fact, the concordance rate for dizygotic twins and siblings are similar. It appears, then, that the differences in concordance for monozygotic and dizygotic twins is genetically based (4).

Etiology

Older theories on the development of MS tried to identify an offending agent or infectious source in the environment, but current thinking suggests an interaction between a genetic predisposition to the disease and an inciting environmental antigen. This interaction produces an autoimmune, demyelinating response in a susceptible host. The pathophysiology of this autoimmune response may be explained by one of two possible theories (5). In the first, the organ becomes infected by a virus or other agent. Then the immune system targets the infectious agent and begins a series of immunologic events that lead to organ-specific autoimmune disease. The second hypothesis posits that autoimmune cells infiltrate the organ system (i.e., neuronal myelin) and recognize specific proteins presented by antigen-presenting cells that are associated with a major histocompatability complex (MHC) class II molecule labeled DR2, DRw1 (6).

Over the years, many infectious agents have been implicated, but no specific virus has ever been identified as the single causative agent in MS. It is more likely that the development of MS requires one of a variety of antigens, which may be found either in the environment or produced experimentally. Myelin basic protein (MBP) is the experimental antigen which induces the animal model of MS, experimental allergic encephalomyelitis (EAE). In MS, the environmental antigen activates an autoreactive T cell. This T cell recognizes the antigen in the context of an antigen-presenting cell that is encoded by the major histocompatibility complex (7). Then recruitment of effector T cells occurs and produces an inflammatory response within the central nervous system (CNS). Cytokines released by activated T cells (including interleukins and tumor necrosis factor) can then alter the integrity of the CNS epithelial cells and break down the blood-brain barrier.

NEUROPATHOLOGY

Microscopic Pathology

Central neuronal myelin is the target organ of the immune-mediated inflammatory response. Myelin at several sites, including the gray-white matter junction, the central white matter, and the root entry zones of the spinal and cranial nerves can be a potential target for MS lesions. The inflammatory lesion, called a *plaque*, has sharply delineated borders whose size can vary from less than a millimeter to several centimeters in diameter. Lesion location is typical. Plaques occur in proximity to the lateral ventricles where the subependymal veins line those structures. Other frequent lesion sites are the optic nerves and chiasm (but not the tracts), and randomly throughout the white matter of the brainstem, cerebellar peduncles, and spinal cord (Figures 6.1 and 6.2).

Microscopically, lesions occur in perivenular locations and are formed by the coalescence of multiple small foci of demyelination. The axon cylinder is spared, and, in acute lesions, macrophages infiltrate the lesions and an astrocytic reaction is seen. Older plaques show relatively acellular, fibroglial tissue with rare inflammatory cells. The lesions of MS are highly variable with respect to size, location, and evolution of lesion over time. Recurrent MS lesions develop with multiple demyelinating and remyelinating episodes. The end result is a chronic "burnt out" placque. From a clinical standpoint, the disease progresses on the basis of multiple lesion sites that are temporally dispersed in cycles of active demyelination. The myelin repair is incomplete, and, in the end stage, grossly visible plaques develop (Figure 6.3). Interestingly, incidental solitary plaques can be found by magnetic resonance imaging (MRI) in patients without neurologic symptoms, supporting the notion that the major factor in disease expression is the cumulative lesion load. In addition, there is a poor correlation

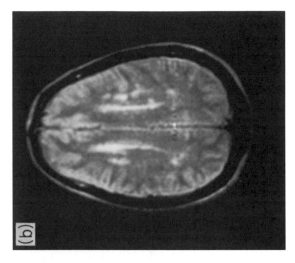

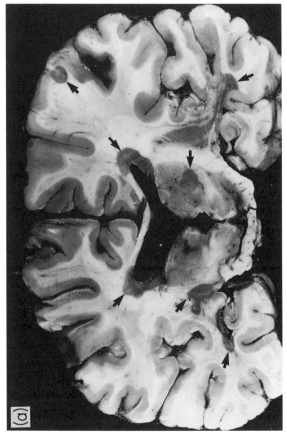

Figure 6.1 (a) Coronal slice through the cerebrum from a patient with severe MS. There are many sharply defined areas of gray demyelination in gray and white matter, including the lateral margins of the lateral ventricles, particlarly their inferior horns (arrowed). (b) NMR imaging of MS plaques during life; spin echo sequence, showing high signal intensity (bright) areas in the periventricular regions. (Courtesy NMR Unit, Hammersmith Hospital, London. Reprinted from Esiri MM, Oppenheimer DR. Diagnostic neuropathology: a practical manual. Oxford: Blackwell Scientific, 1989:227.)

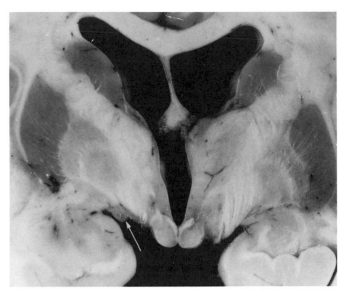

Figure 6.2 *Coronal section of the cerebrum at the level of the mamillary bodies from a patient with MS. The optic tracts (left one indicated by arrow) are shrunken and discolored as a consequence of severe, long-standing demyelination in the optic nerves. (Reprinted from Esiri MM, Oppenheimer DR. Diagnostic neuropathology: a practical manual. Oxford: Blackwell Scientific, 1989:229.)*

between the MRI location of a lesion and the patient's clinical symptomatology.

Immunopathology

Activated T cells are found within the perivascular spaces in the active disease state. These cells recognize the antigen via the interaction of the T-cell receptor and the MHC molecules presenting the antigen. The two types of T cells involved in neuroimmune disease are the CD4 (helper) and the CD8 (cytotoxic) cells. They are defined by one of two mutually exclusive antigens found on their cell surface. These antigens help regulate the interaction between T cells and the major histocompatibility complex. CD4 T cells are restricted to Class II MHC molecules, and CD8 are restricted to Class I. CD4 cells are helper T cells and produce cytokines. CD8 cells are cytotoxic. Suppressor T cells are not well defined and can be either CD4 or CD8. B cells are also activated in the neuroimmune process and are responsible for antibody production. They possess immunoglobulins on their cell surface. The type of immunoglobulin expressed (IgG, IgA, etc.) is a function of the B-cell interaction with the activated T cell.

Since all of the immune system cells arise from the bone marrow, they must actively cross the blood-brain barrier to enter the CNS. Activated CD4 T cells cross into the perivascular space when they recog-

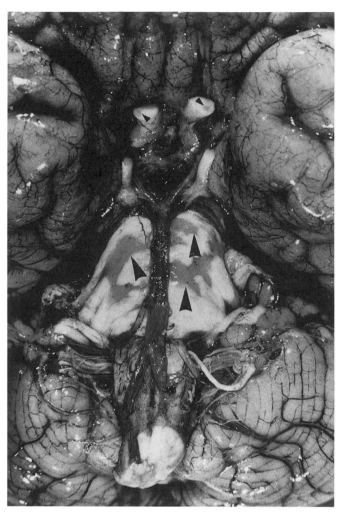

Figure 6.3   Surface of the pons from a patient with MS. There are irregular gray patches (large arrowheads) contrasting with the normal white appearance. Small plaques can also be seen in both optic nerves (small arrowheads). (Reprinted from Esiri MM, Oppenheimer DR. Diagnostic neuropathology: a practical manual. Oxford: Blackwell Scientific, 1989:225.)

nize neural antigen presented by the class II MHC molecule that is expressed by the capillary endothelial cells. An alternate hypothesis is that the T cells cross into the perivascular space when adhesion molecules are present on the blood-brain barrier endothelial cells. These adhesion molecules are produced by activated T cells within the periphery and facilitate interaction between the endothelial cells and the T cells, allowing the T cells to pass into the CNS (8). This process is one target for newer immunomodulating therapies designed to limit disease progression.

The cellular infiltrate in active plaques contain CD4 and CD8 cells and macrophages. The microglial cells and macrophages serve mostly as scavenger cells and intensify the inflammatory demyelination of axons. Macrophages may also have some role in the presentation of antigens to T cells. The role of astrocytes is not well understood, but they may cause further inflammation by producing tumor necrosis factor (TNF).

Magnetic resonance imaging has greatly advanced the understanding of the neuropathology of MS. It has demonstrated that dysfunction of neurons may arise out of inflammation and not only from demyelination. The lesions seen with the gadolinium-enhanced MRI have been pathologically correlated and found to represent areas of perivascular inflammation (9). These enhancing lesions may represent the initial phases of plaque development rather than demyelination. Therefore, demyelination appears to begin with oligodendrocyte damage and is associated with "dying back" of the myelin. Direct attack of myelin membranes may be mediated by antibody and complement, but the damage to oligodendrocytes and the dying-back phenomenon is induced by cytopathic cytokines (e.g., TNF). Pathophysiologically, inflammation, edema, and frank demyelination all translate into interrupted or inefficient nerve transmission.

Natural History

Rationale

The natural history of MS is a significant consideration in every diagnostic and treatment decision pertaining to the disease. The diagnosis of MS is clinically based. "Possible" and "probable" diagnoses of MS are still a part of the diagnostic continuum, especially when the laboratory and neuroimaging studies are negative. The natural course of the disease affects the decision to treat with immunomodulating therapies and for what period of time. It is also essential in the consideration of entry criteria for any well-designed clinical trial and in the prediction of rehabilitation outcomes. Stabilization of MS symptoms is the gold standard in judging the efficacy of any immunomodulating treatment, while improvement in physical incapacity is the goal in rehabilitation trials.

Disease Types

Multiple sclerosis has been traditionally categorized into four major disease types: relapsing remitting, chronic progressive, benign, and fulminant (Table 6.1). The most common subtype is relapsing-remitting (RR) disease. This comprises the onset of multiple sclerosis in approximately 60% to 70% of the MS population. These patients experience

Table 6.1. *Stages of Multiple Sclerosis*

Disease Type	Percentage of MS Patients at Onset
Relapsing remitting	20%–30%
Relapsing remitting progressive (secondarily progressive)	40%
Chronic progressive (primary progressive)	15%
Benign	15%–20%
Fulminant	<5%

episodes of rapid, abrupt deterioration with variable degrees of recovery over time. Those relapsing patients who accumulate residual disability move into the relapsing-remitting but progressive (RR-P) category (also known as "secondarily progressive"). A few unfortunate patients (approximately 15%), are diagnosed at onset with primary progressive (PP) or chronic progressive (CP) disease. These patients tend to be male in a female-dominated disease. The two final categories are "benign" multiple sclerosis (15% to 20%), wherein the patients remain fully functional even 15 years after the diagnosis, and the "fulminant" type whose course is rapidly progressive and leads to early, severe disability and death (10). These remain useful delineations, but it is important to recognize that any disease type is not a static phenomenon, and that MS may change course and character over time within the same patient.

Symptom clusters also can exist, and patients can have significant disability, including patients whose primary impairment is cognitive with relatively preserved sensory and motor function. Another subset of symptom clusters is predominant cerebellar ataxia, severe vibratory and kinesthetic loss, and brainstem signs. Patients with these symptoms and mobility dysfunction benefit the least of any group from a restorative rehabilitation program, but often benefit from a compensatory program. For the purposes of rehabilitation, there also exists another subset of patients who have primarily spinal cord disease without cognitive limitations and who still have viable employment options despite a long duration of disease.

Clinical Ratings

Clinical rating scales provide yet another scheme by which to classify patient groups. These scales can show, via serial measurements in the same patient, a temporal course to the disease according to physical, cognitive, and social markers. Some of the scales are insensitive to certain aspects of the disease, such as cognitive or psychosocial factors. They may also be heavily weighted toward lower-limb motor abilities (ambulation). Nonetheless, scales such as the Kurtzke Disability Status Scale and the Functional Improvement Measure are useful for scoring the progress of an individual's disease over time with treatment interventions (11,12). These provide some level of universal classification as well, which is important to critical interpretation of the medical literature and to the conduct of multicenter trials. There are, however, several difficulties inherent in defining the natural history of multiple sclerosis. It is not a uniform, homogeneous disease and demonstrates tremendous variability among individuals and over time. In addition, there are dwindling numbers of patients who have gone without any intervention during the course of their disease. Finally, there is a patient selection bias for the clinical trials on which natural history studies are based. These group studies exclude the extremes of the patient population who are either severely or mildly affected.

Similar Demyelination Diseases

There are other diseases of central demyelination that are also most likely due to an autoimmune process triggered by an environmental agent, such as a virus. Included in this group are solitary, optic neuritis, transverse myelitis, Devic's disease (neuromyelitis optica), acute disseminated encephalomyelitis (ADEM), and hemorrhagic disseminated encephalomyelitis (Weston Hurst syndrome). The incidence of multiple sclerosis following an episode of optic neuritis has been variably estimated between 15% and 90% (13). For patients presenting with acute transverse myelitis, the risk of developing subsequent MS has been cited as 7%, but a much higher rate (50%) appears to accompany those patients with partial myelitis syndromes (14). Whether these solitary demyelinating episodes represent a partially arrested form of multiple sclerosis is not clear.

Disease Modifiers

Factors that may worsen the disease course temporarily are reported in the epidemiologic literature, but the pathophysiologic basis is not well understood. These include concurrent systemic illness, prolonged bed rest, excessive fatigue or exhaustion, heat exposure, pregnancy, and the puerperium (15). Emotional stress has been implicated in several studies and reports, but these are contradictory and inconclusive (16–18).

Other elements that may have a longer-lasting impact on the disease course may include gender, genetics, personality, and climate. There is no clear consensus on the effect of gender, with results equally divided between worse outcomes in men and no effect of gender on disease progression. Patients living in warmer climates tend to do worse, but questions about how genetics and the various MHC molecules determine outcome remain unresolved. Outcomes between familial and sporadic MS do not differ significantly (19).

Survival is not significantly shorter in patients with mild disease when compared to the general population, but the risk of death is 4 times greater than expected in patients with severe disease (20). In general, the indicators of poorest outcome include the following (21):

- Older age at onset
- Primary progressive disease
- Pyramidal or cerebellar involvement at onset
- Frequent and prolonged exacerbations with incomplete recovery between attacks.

Kurtzke reported on the accumulation of disability in veterans and concluded that disability status at 5 years was predictive of disability at 10 and 15 years (22). As an aggregate, two thirds of patients with known MS remain ambulatory and functional 20 years after the onset of their illness (23). Unfortunately, only 30% of patients remain competitively employed after the same amount of time. Spasticity and incoordination were the main limiting factors in a study by Bauer (24). Another study noted that 49% of the variance in employment status could be attributed to walking ability, age, memory, and verbal fluency (25). Interestingly, very few patients (3.5%) reside in nursing homes (26), but the reasons for this may have more to do with the patients' ability to access this type of care financially and logistically than with their physical needs or incapacity (27).

RESIDUAL DEFICITS AND SURFACE CLINICAL MANIFESTATIONS

The clinical manifestations of multiple sclerosis are extremely variable and depend on the disease type, severity, and lesion location. Symptoms range from cognitive impairments to myelopathic findings (Table 6.2). Sensory complaints are among the most frequent presenting symptoms in multiple sclerosis and occur as patchy parasthesias or areas of numbness that do not correspond to dermatomal segments. Early physical signs include monoparesis, vestibular dysfunction, oculomotor palsy, and optic neuritis (Table 6.3).

Studies employing serial MRI have shown that lesion load by MRI exceeds that which would be clinically expected, and that poor correlation exists between clinical signs and site of lesion on MRI (28,29).

Table 6.2. Symptoms Present in a Series of Patients with Established MS

Motor impairment	94.2%
Sensory deficit	78.2%
Optic neuritis	63.9%
Sphincter and sexual disturbances	71.4%
Impaired facial sensation	23.5%
Diplopia	37.9%
Ataxia of limbs	71.6%
Intention tremor	23.5%

SOURCE: Adapted with permission from Francis GS, Antel JP, Duquette P. Inflammatory demyelinating diseases of the central nervous system. In: Bradley WG, Daroff RB, Fenichel GM, Marsden CD, eds. Neurology in clinical practise. Boston: Butterworth-Heinemann, 1991:1138.

Table 6.3. Initial Symptoms in Multiple Sclerosis

Symptom	
Motor	26.6%
Sensory	25.3%
Optic	21.4%
Cerebellar ataxia	14.2%
Sphincter disturbances	14.2%
Lhermitte or pain	3.2%
Brainstem	1.9%
Cerebral	1.4%
Blurred vision	0.8%
Transverse myelitis	0.6%
Gait problems	0.4%

SOURCE: Adapted with permission from Francis GS, Antel JP, Duquette P. Inflammatory demyelinating diseases of the central nervous system. In: Bradley WG, Daroff RB, Fenichel GM, Marsden CD, eds. Neurology in clinical practise. Boston: Butterworth-Heinemann, 1991:1138.

Cognitive Impairment

Cognitive profiles in MS are fairly predictable and reproducible among patients. Cognitive impairment in MS has previously been underestimated. More recent work indicates a much higher rate (54% to 65%) of cognitive dysfunction when determined by neuropsychologic testing.

Prior estimates of 5% to 10% were based on neurologic and mini-mental status exams (30). Rao suggests that the pattern of cognitive decline is similar to that seen with other diseases involving the subcortical structures, such as Huntington's and Parkinson's disease (31). In all of these entities, personality and mood alterations, impaired problem solving and abstraction, depressed visuospatial skills, poor executive and sustained attention skills, and slowed speed of cognitive processing are components of the cognitive deterioration. Modality-specific impairments such as aphasia, apraxia, and alexia seen with cortical injuries or stroke are *not* part of the dementia of multiple sclerosis.

Modest declines in verbal IQ are seen in multiple sclerosis patients in comparison to controls. More severe impairment in performance IQ is also seen, but is not unexpected given this group's motor impairments. These deficits are seen early in the course of the disease and do not deteriorate further. Both visual and auditory attention measures are consistently impaired in MS, especially in tasks that require vigilance or attention divided between simultaneous stimuli. Cognitive processing speed as tested by digit-span processing and recall is also slowed.

Patients with MS frequently complain of having a poor memory. Amnesia per se is rarely encountered in MS, but deficits in attention, visual and verbal learning, and memory retrieval all factor into this patient complaint. Immediate memory, registration, and storage, as measured by digit span, appear relatively intact in MS, but impairments in recent memory are evident. Both nonverbal and verbal information beyond immediate recall are poorly learned and recalled. However, patients tend to do better on recognition tasks when multiple choice cues are given to enhance retrieval. Remote memory is a relative strength in MS, and patients do reasonably well in recalling detail of current events, past presidents, and autobiographical data. The memory deficit in MS appears to be a result of inefficient encoding and retrieval mechanisms similar to that seen in other forms of subcortical dementia.

Patients with MS tend to perseverate with unsuccessful problem-solving strategies during nonverbal tasks such as the Wisconsin Card Sort and the Raven's Matrices. The performance is similar to that seen with frontal lobe lesions. Verbal abstraction skill (measured by similarities testing) is consistently deficient. Visuospatial and language skills are relatively preserved in MS, even in cases of advanced disease.

Cranial Nerve Impairment

Cranial nerve involvement is a clinical and pathologic hallmark of MS. Optic neuritis is the most common manifestation of visual pathway injury and presents with sudden visual loss, pain with extraocular movement, central scotomas, and an afferent pupillary defect (Marcus Gunn pupil). The optic disc appears normal on fundoscopy since the plaque is usually retrobulbar. In the later stages, the disc may appear pale. Optic neuritis may occur in a patient with established MS, or be an isolated finding that later proves to be the earliest sign of the disease. If optic neuritis is associated with abnormal white-matter lesions on MRI, the risk of subsequent MS is far higher than in the case of optic neuritis with a nomal brain MRI (32). Vision improves over weeks to months, but some residual scotoma or acuity loss usually persists. Optic neuritis may occur bilaterally and, even with resolution, symptoms can worsen temporarily with heating (Uhtoff's phenomenon).

Oculomotor abnormalities are also seen early in the course of MS. Patients can present with vertical or horizontal diplopia depending on the extraocular muscle involved. Generally, cranial nerves III and IV are more often affected than cranial nerve VI. Commonly, visuovestibular and brainstem intranuclear connections are disrupted by plaque. The patients then demonstrate spontaneous and/or gaze-evoked nystagmus or an intranuclear ophthalmoplegia (INO) due to the interruption of the medial longitudinal fasciculus (MLF) within the pons.

Trigeminal neuralgia in a young adult should be considered a manifestation of multiple sclerosis until proven otherwise. Taste is rarely affected, but central facial weakness is common. Subclinical dysphagia is more common than suspected and is more likely in the presence of dysarthria (33). Clinical measures of disease severity are better predictors of dysphagia than are patient complaints. Videofluoroscopy most often reveals an abnormal oral phase of swallowing characterized by a delayed pharyngeal phase initiation. Pharyngeal residue and transient or persistent entry of barium into the larynx also occur in a smaller number of patients (34). Vertigo is not usual, but hearing loss is. The dysequilibrium seen in MS is due in part to vestibular pathway involvement. It is manifested by impaired postural reactions and a widened base of support and is made worse by cerebellar ataxia and proprioceptive loss.

Sensory-Motor Dysfunction

Sensory complaints can be attributed to posterior column, spinothalamic, or dorsal root entry lesions. Radicular signs are caused by plaque at the dorsal root entry zone. Motor involvement in MS appears as weakness and spasticity. Initially, the weakness is generally more pronounced in the lower extremities—the result of disordered nerve conduction along demyelinated motor pathways throughout the subcortical white matter, brainstem, and spinal cord. Weakness may be worsened by disuse atrophy and by medications such as baclofen or klonopin.

Spasticity can be present in any distribution and may be tonic with extensor rigidity in the legs and flexor posturing in the arms. Alternately, patients may be troubled by phasic tone problems in the form of flexor or extensor spasms of the legs, which are mediated by spinal reflex mechanisms. The spasms and the tonic increase in tone can be useful if extensor spasticity is used for transfers and ambulation. It can also be painful or even throw patients out of their wheelchairs if the flexor or extensor spasms are powerful enough. The decision to treat spasticity is guided by the observations of the patient, therapist, and caregiver.

Cerebellar pathway lesions impart limb and truncal ataxia, gait ataxia, and scanning or explosive speech. Ataxia is frequently mixed with pyramidal signs and kinesthetic loss and is resistant to restorative therapeutic interventions.

Urinary Incontinence

Bladder dysfunction is another early sign in multiple sclerosis. The bladder is rarely spared as the course of the disease progresses, and 80% to 90% of patients report urinary symptoms at some point in their disease (35). The most common urologic findings are detrusor areflexia, detrusor hyperreflexia, and detrusor hyperreflexia with detrusor-sphincter dyssynergia (DSD). The common clinical complaints are frequency and urgency. However, clinical complaints are notoriously poor indicators of the specific type of bladder dysfunction. Disorders of storage and emptying result with any disruption between the pontine micturition centers and the sacral spinal cord. With interruption of the ascending afferent impulses from the detrusor muscle to the pons, the inhibition of the parasympathetic fibers to the detrusor muscle are lost during bladder filling, and the detrusor contracts inappropriately as the bladder volume increases (failure to store). Detrusor-sphincter dyssynergia occurs as a result of abnormal coordination of the external sphincter muscle as the detrusor muscle contracts to empty the bladder. This results in obstruction to voiding by an inappropriately contracting external sphincter and poor urine flow with incomplete bladder emptying (failure to empty). It appears that the lesion causing most of the bladder problems in MS is located in the spinal cord. There is a strong correlation between bladder dysfunction and pyramidal involvement, and the trend is toward worsening bladder function as pyramidal function worsens (36).

Sexual Dysfunction

Sexual lives change in 91% of males and 72% of females with severe disability from multiple sclerosis (37). Of those with more mild disability, there is still some degree of sexual dysfunction in 71% to 74% of patients (38). Sexual dysfunction in females with MS may be multifactorial, including perineal sensory loss, weakness of the pelvic floor musculature, adductor spasticity, hyperreflexic bladder contractions during intercourse, depression, and loss of self-esteem. In males, erectile dysfunction occurs and is manifest by rapid loss of the erection upon attempted intercourse, rather than loss of ejaculation. Other common problems in male sexuality include weak erection, generalized weakness, spasticity, frigidity of the spouse, and periodic loss of erection. It seems that the more important factor in impotence is the location of the plaque within the lumbar cord rather than the duration of the MS (39).

Heat Sensitivity and Fatigue

Heat sensitivity is marked by exacerbation of prior symptoms when nerve conduction along previously damaged pathways is slowed. This may identify a subset of patients because they seem to respond more dramatically to the potassium channel blocker, 4-aminopyridine (40). The fatigue of MS is unique in its character and proportions. It is described as a sense of exhaustion that is not necessarily related to the amount of physical exertion. The severity of the symptom is also not correlated with the extent of physical disability. It is relieved, to some degree, by rest periods and medication. The fatigue may be worsened by other components such as sleep disorder, depression, energy-consuming gait and mobility deviations, medication side effects, deconditioning, nutritional impairment, and neuromuscular fatigue. *Neuromuscular fatigue* is described as an increased muscle fatigue that develops as physical work is performed. Its physiologic basis is not well understood, but may include elements such as increased but inefficient energy consumption by demyelinated nerve fibers, changes in potassium conductance at the axonal membrane, and heating due to physical exercise (41). Pulmonary dysfunction occurs in patients with severe paraparesis and is marked by expiratory weakness. Expiratory weakness progresses as the upper extremities become increasingly involved and trunk control diminishes (42).

Psychiatric Disorders

Psychiatric disorders are more common in patients with MS than in the general population. The entire range of psychiatric symptoms can be seen, but irritability, anger, and somatic complaints are more common than apathy and withdrawal. Unipolar and bipolar depression are more common in MS than in general and probably comprise the bulk of psychiatric symptoms. Estimates of their incidence vary widely between 18% and 55% (43,44). The incidence of major depression is 3 times that of the general population, and bipolar depression is 13 times more common (45). Bipolar and unipolar depression are also more common in MS than in other chronic diseases. Whether the depression of MS is related to demyelination of the subcortical limbic structures or is a reaction to disability is unclear. It is probably a combination of both. Patients with the predominantly cerebral form of MS are more likely to be depressed than those with the spinal form of the disease (46). Euphoria ("la belle indifference") is not as common as is classically described. It is associated with subcortically medicated dementia.

Ritvo's study of patients with MS showed that they score below the mean of normals on the Mental Health Inventory (MHI). The best predictive factors for mental health in MS are the fatigue impact score, perceived social supports, and disease duration (47). Other factors found to impact mental health in MS include stressful life events, degree of chronic pain, self-perceived cognitive deficits, and clinically assessed cognitive deficits. No greater incidence of schizophrenia is seen in the MS population compared to controls, but the suicide rate is significantly higher. It is approximately 14 times greater than in the general population (48). The same factors that contribute to depression contribute to suicide. In a study by Berman, patients contemplating suicide tended to be male, and had advanced, chronic progressive disease. They were also unemployed and experiencing financial distress. These patients were more severely disabled physically and displayed signs of unendurable psychic pain (45).

PREDICTING OUTCOME IN MULTIPLE SCLEROSIS

The most important piece of information that permits an accurate prediction of outcome is a thorough understanding of the natural history of each individual's disease. By investigating the history of the current illness, one can specify those precipitants that have created the exacerbation or contributed to the progression of the disease (Table 6.4).

When a patient with MS initially encounters the rehabilitation system, assessment of the degree of disease activity is the first step in defining the rehabilitation goals and expectations. Patients with deteriorating physical function due to an active, demyelinating process are unlikely to have that process directly impacted or reversed by physical rehabilitation measures alone. Rather, immunosuppression or immunomodulating therapies, such as methylprednisolone or

Table 6.4. Clinical Data
Collection in MS Rehabilitation

Age and gender

Age at disease onset

Duration of disease

Symptoms at onset

Number and frequency of relapses

Recovery pattern from prior relapses

History of disease pattern, treatment, and patient
response
Immunosuppressive treatment?
Immunomodulating treatment?

Current symptoms and level of disability (adm.
EDSS)

Level of disability prior to admission (pre-adm.
EDSS)

Factors precipitating current admission

Potential medication problems

Presence of cognitive and affective disorders

Social supports

Employment status

EDSS = Expanded Disability Status Scale.

betaseron, are indicated. Where physical incapacitation worsens without actively progressive or exacerbating disease, precipitating factors need to be identified. Their impact and the feasibility of reversing them must be addressed. For example, a patient with progressive dysequilibrium due to accumulating plaques within the brainstem vestibular apparatus can not halt their progressive disability with a vestibular rehabilitation program. However, a 3- to 5-day course of intravenous methylprednisolone may make their symptoms more quiescent.

Alternately, deterioration in functional status due to concurrent medical illness or deconditioning will generally respond well to physical interventions as long as the MS itself is not active. Other factors that temporarily worsen neurologic function (such as heat-induced symptoms, excessive fatigue, poor nutrition particularly as it relates to skin healing and constipation, intervening surgical procedures, and cardiopulmonary deconditioning) have a good prognosis for resolving. Medication side effects should also be considered when looking for reversable causes of deterioration, regardless of any associated medical or surgical illness. Careful evaluation of recent medication changes or potential drug interactions, which can create new problems such as depression, weakness, or urinary incontinence, should be done. A favorable statement can be made regarding return to previous level of functioning if it is determined that the functional deterioration is due to one of these reversible factors rather than to actively progressing disease.

When the patient is experiencing functional deterioration on the basis of an active disease process, knowledge about the patient's prior disease course, response to medical treatments such as steroids or immunosuppression, and the level of residual disability due to previous exacerbations can be used to predict outcome from the current attack (see Table 6.4). If the patient has suffered multiple exacerbations with incomplete recovery and accumulating residual disability, it is unwise to predict full recovery to baseline. Although the patient may achieve the same functional level (e.g., independent mobility) it may be by wheelchair rather than by ambulatory means. Other patients with deterioration secondary to MS exacerbations, yet with a history of full or nearly full recovery from past relapses, may remit to baseline even if restorative therapies are not given. As a result, such a patient may not be an appropriate candidate for rehabilitation.

If recovery in these scenarios is uncertain, it is reasonable to project toward the conservative end of function so as not to find that discharge goals have been set too high and then need to be revised downward. Extending length of stay rarely will allow the patient to achieve goals set inappropriately high at admission or at the commencement of rehabilitation therapies. If goal setting is conservative, the patient has a greater chance of attaining the rehabilitation goals, experiencing the positive effect of success, and moving toward additional functional independence within the length of stay set for him or her at admission into the rehabilitation program.

Ultimately, goal setting and rehabilitation strategies must be function-oriented and tailored to meet the individual needs of each patient. More difficult challenges in prognosticating rehabilitation outcomes and setting goals come when the nature of the patient's MS is actively evolving and changing its character, as is the case when multiple relapses do not result in full recovery and the patient begins to accumulate disability. Predictions of outcome are also problematic in patients with slowly progressive disease who experience an abrupt deterioration in their functional condition in association with a medical or surgical illness. It can be difficult to judge whether the patient is suffering with increased disease activity in addition to the nonneurologic problems. Teasing out the symptoms and signs by a thorough history and physical is the most sound way to differentiate the various etiologies of deterioration. Gadolinium-enhanced MRI, looking for enhancing plaques and giving some idea of lesion load, may also be very helpful in assessing the patient's chances for functional recovery (49).

PROBABILITY OF IMPROVEMENT WITH TIME, REMEDIATION, OR COMPENSATION

Inpatient Rehabilitation

Most patients with MS are not admitted to an inpatient rehabilitation hospital until late in their disease, after they have accumulated substantial disability. Frequently, they are at the point in their disease progression where intensive restorative approaches are not effective. Relatively few situations will prompt the patient with MS to enter inpatient acute rehabilitation. The first is the case where the patient is experiencing an exacerbation of his or her relapsing-remitting disease. They may have received intravenous steroids in the acute care setting, or potentially be directly admitted to rehabilitation for both physical and steroid therapies. The patient is left with new neurologic deficits that may or may not recover completely with time.

Second is the patient whose MS is a secondary diagnosis, who is recovering from a fracture, surgery, or medical illness. The demyelination process is considered inactive, yet the patient with MS will likely progress through therapies more slowly than a patient without chronic neurologic disease. In addition, preexisting neurologic deficits may worsen as a result of the primary stressors and bed rest. These patients will generally return to their premorbid baseline after a rehabilitation stay.

A third group are those patients who deteriorate at home despite maximal community-based services. This may be the result of new or progressing urinary dysfunction, declining transfer or mobility skills, or cognitive impairments that have advanced to the point where the patient is no longer safe to be alone. These patients generally have either primary or secondarily progressive MS. Another group of patients who might be appropriate for inpatient rehabilitation are those who have intensive positioning, gait, or tone management needs following intrathecal baclofen pump insertion.

The final category contains those patients who are actively progressing from an ambulatory to nonambulatory state, or from independent to dependent transfer status. These two milestones are accompanied by severe psychosocial stress and financial drain as home services or the constant presence of a family caregiver become necessary in order to continue to dwell in the community. These situations present considerable opportunity for restorative approaches, but probably more important, they demand patient and caregiver education and creative compensatory strategies.

Outpatient Rehabilitation

Outpatient services available to patients with MS can take a variety of forms in terms of home-based services or traditional rehabilitation services in the outpatient setting. Also included may be some of the "alternative" therapies such as acupuncture and therapeutic massage, though their specific advantage in MS over other forms of therapy have yet to be established. Patients may be monitored on a monthly or bimonthly basis in order to assess the effectiveness of an independent program of structured, self-monitored exercise. Since patients who have mounting disability are frequently in the midst of their competitive employment years, they may dismiss the need for regular physical exercise as a trade-off for the gain in endurance and avoidance of fatigue that is required to perform at their jobs. Obviously some level of balance must be sought between the two opposing needs, and patient education again becomes an important therapeutic goal.

Deficits Amenable to Therapy

Table 6.5 lists the functional deficits seen in MS, defines the potential contributing factors for each, and specifies those that are remediable with compensatory or restorative approaches. Ataxia, some aspects of cognitive impairment, and sensory loss are fairly resistant to restorative approaches, though external compensations can be made to some degree. These might include weighted assistive devices or cuffs (50), memory logs, beepers, and rehearsal. External devices or schedules may enhance organization and recall, but the inability to understand abstract meaning and to demonstrate insight can only be addressed through caregiver education and understanding. Behavior management techniques can often be employed to deal with some of the troubling behavioral issues in MS such as poor safety awareness and judgement. Patients may benefit from therapeutic strategies if they need education about their functional capacities, require assessment and modification of their living environment, or need adaptive equipment or wheelchair seating systems. The areas where the least progress can be expected are ataxia and cognitive impairment (51,52). These same studies differ on whether significant gains in activities of daily living (ADL) skills are possible, but this may be a function of the restorative versus compensatory approach to rehabilitation.

Other areas of physical impairment that will likely respond to some form of physical management include spasticity, pain, incontinence, constipation, malnutrition, skin breakdown, disuse weakness, and cardiopulmonary deconditioning. Dysarthria, dysphagia, and cognitive difficulties may be made functional with compensatory communication devices, swallowing and food consistency precautions, and external aids to organization and planning. Gait disability and transfer

Table 6.5.   Functional Deficits and Amenability to Therapy

Area of Functional Disability	Components of Disability	
	Treatable	**Difficult to Treat**
Gait disorder	Disuse weakness Orthopedic issues Decreased range Spasticity Pain +/− Vestibular Sx Cardiopulmonary deconditioning Instruct assistive device	Neurogenic weakness +/− Vestibular Sx Sensory loss Spasticity Ataxia
Impaired transfer status	Weight gain Disuse weakness Spasticity Cardiopulmonary deconditioning Instruct assistive device	Neurogenic weakness Spasticity
Cognitive & affective disorders	Patient and family knowledge deficit Coping skills Time management skills Recall strategies Medication side effects Fatigue Vegetative or manic signs Sleep dysfunction	Progessive dementia Personality disorders
ADL impairment	Equipment needs Inappropriate energy expenditure Fatigue	Neurogenic weakness Cognitive impairment Sensory loss Visual loss +/− Fatigue Ataxia
Incontinence	Medication side effects Early dyssynergia Chronic drainage with Foley or SPT Laxatives/bowel regimen	Late DSD Severe detrusor spasticity
Pain	Range Spasticity Positioning Orthopedic or radicular Sx.	Somatization disorders
Skin	Malnutrition Pressure relief Positioning Patient/caregiver education	
Fatigue	Fatigue from medication trials Sleep disorder Depression Institute regular low-intensity aerobic exercise Malnutrition Medication side effect profile	Fatigue of MS

impairments may respond to restorative interventions if the etiology of the immobility is potentially reversible. This would be the case with orthopedic injury, postural problems like leg-length discrepancy, some spasticity problems, and disuse or deconditioning weakness. However, gait and transfer dysfunction on the basis of worsening ataxia, sensory loss, or progressive neurogenic weakness are unlikely to improve. Compensatory maneuvers, such as the use of sliding boards and walkers, may be of some help. Incontinence is nearly always manageable either with medication in some cases, intermittent catheterization in detrusor sphincter dyssynegia (DSD), or in-dwelling Foley in complex or advanced cases.

Assessment, Goal Setting, and Selection of Therapeutic Interventions

Assessment, goal setting, and selection of therapeutic interventions for patients with MS should be based on the natural history and pathophysiology of the disease.

Assessment

All areas of neurologic function should be assessed and potentially targeted for therapeutic intervention since the entire neuroaxis can be involved in MS, and its character and activity can change over time. This requires the clinician to be flexible and willing to continually reevaluate goals, treatment strategies, and outcomes along the way. The nature of the disease implies that patients can have setbacks through no fault of their own when disease activity flares or associated illnesses arise. Mobility, positioning, ADL skills, and cardiopulmonary condition need to be assessed on entry into the rehabilitation model. Admission cognitive evaluation will guide the clinician's expectations from the patient in terms of education, carryover, safety, and insight. Problems that require more than clinical examination are dysphagia assessment and urodynamic testing, since the clinical complaints and physical findings do not correlate with the pathology. Medical and nursing assessment of continence, sexuality, skin, and health problems should be accomplished early in the patient's rehabilitation encounter. Outpatient management needs to combine symptom management with modification and monitoring of the disease process. Coordination of medical and allied health resources in the outpatient setting can enhance the delivery of MS care. Timed outpatient visits, where the patients are screened in a preventive fashion by a multidisciplinary team, are a desirable model of preventive health care that should not be mistaken for "maintenance therapy" (53).

Therapeutic Strategies

Therapeutic strategies specific to the care of patients with MS are few. The more frequent clinical problems in the MS population include the management of tone, incontinence, fatigue, ataxia, mood disorders, and cognitive impairments. Useful therapy for any functional loss must be task driven and tailored to meet individual needs. For example, home settings should be re-created to the extent possible by bringing in the patient's wheelchair or motorized scooter for transfer training. The importance of even a few inches between transfer surfaces can make all the difference when it comes to getting patients to maneuver independently in their own homes. Gait training must consider the daily challenges for patients in their environments at home or work, and train them to task-specific levels of balance, endurance, and energy conservation. For example, limited energy reserves may be better utilized on toilet transfers than on long-distance ambulation training or by intermittent catheterization rather than on frequent ambulation to the bathroom. Continence training is imperative for patients with slow mobility or the inability to transfer alone. In some patients, practicality demands measures as advanced as an in-dwelling Foley catheter in order to remain in a community dwelling.

Other rehabilitative issues are generic and can be managed in the same fashion as they would be in any other patient population with the proviso that progress will be slower, cognitive or mood problems may interfere, and disease activity may flare and require realignment of goals and expectations. These clinical problems include deconditioning, skin and nutritional impairments, and musculoskeletal dysfunction. Treatment of adjustment disorder and management of psychosocial complications via psychopharmacologic agents, counseling, and vocational training are also areas in the rehabilitation of the patient with MS that require significant caregiver resources.

Specific interventions for *tone management* are discussed elsewhere (54–58), but the major determinants in the decision to treat are whether the spasticity is functionally useful and whether pain or hygiene issues exist. Secondary issues in treatment selection revolve around medication side effects, and surgical and technical considerations. The long-term effects of the newer therapies such as the intrathecal baclofen pump and botulinum A toxin injections are not yet known. Selective blocks of muscle or nerve using botulinum toxin or phenol may be superior to oral medication trials in terms of specificity of action and side-effect profiles. If patients are properly selected, local reduction in tone may be all that is needed to achieve control of spasticity and minimize direct therapy requirements and caregiver attention.

In the case of *adductor spasticity*, phenol blocks to the obturator nerve may relax the legs adequately for perineal access, improved gait patterns, and enhanced dressing ability. It may do so without the risk of inducing generalized weakness or sedation associated with antispasticity medications. It may even be less costly in the long run when compared to long-term medication needs. Bracing requirements and direct physical therapy services may also be decreased if selective blocks can be properly located and timed. Surgical therapies such as tendon lengthenings and transfers, though thought to be "last resort" options, may be more effectively used early if patients are appropriately evaluated and selected for treatment. Better positioning, skin integrity, and even pain relief may then be obtained without the need for ongoing physical therapies hamstrung by excessive spasticity or bony deformities.

Effective management of *urinary incontinence* involves accurate diagnosis of the specific bladder disorder, patient education, and ongoing periodic reassessment. The nature of the bladder disorder can change over time and though history and signs are important, they alone do not allow for accurate diagnosis. Aggressive treatment for urinary continence preserves the upper urinary tracts, allows for confidence and mobility within the community, and eases caregiver burden. Bladder assessment should be initiated early in the course of MS, prior to the stage of frequent urinary infections, and periodic reevaluation and monitoring of therapies is important.

Fatigue, cognitive impairment, and *mood disorder* will all potentially disrupt a patient's ability to participate in and benefit from therapy. They need to be considered when planning treatment in the rehabilitation setting. The decision to intervene with pharmacologic measures should be based on the patient's ability to participate in therapies and on the potential for medication side effects. In the case of *depression*, accurate diagnosis of all potential contributors is paramount for suggesting treatment strategies. The distinction between unipolar and bipolar depression must be clear, since the treatments are distinct for each condition. The presence or absence of concurrent complaints may help to influence medication selection. For instance, associated fatigue or slowed cognitive processing would sway the treatment decision toward selection of an activating antidepressant with few sedative side effects, such as fluoxetine (Prozac) or sertraline hydrochloride (Zoloft). Use of amphetamines might be considered appropriate in patients with fatigue, and decreased initiation, speed of cognitive processing, and sustained attention due to subcortical dementia (59). The serotonin reuptake inhibitors (Prozac, Zoloft), pemoline (Cylert), and ammantadine (Symmetrel) are all useful in fatigue; drug selection is guided by the presence of concurrent dementia, depression, or sleep disorder. If disorders of sleep initiation or bothersome parasthesias or urinary incontinence coexist with depression, the traditional tricyclics may be more helpful, but have their own set of significant side effects, including sedation, cardiac conduction delay, and acute urinary retention.

Ataxia is poorly responsive to pharmacologic management. The potassium channel blockers (4-aminodipyridine, 3,4-diaminodipyridine) may offer some improvement in heat-sensitive symptoms, including ataxia and neurogenic weakness, but are not yet commercially available. *Tremor* may be amenable to klonopin, methazolamide (60), or even botulinum A toxin, but treatment must be reserved for those tremors of the head that prohibit visual fixation and for limb tremors where underlying weakness and ataxia are not severe.

In summary, the decision to treat these difficult clinical problems must always be based on definable and measurable functional goals. Rehabilitation efforts should be directed at those issues that are actually amenable to treatment with pharmacologic or physical means and offer some reasonable chance of improvement.

Case Studies

Case 1

T.M. is a 37-year-old mother of three, admitted for emergency laporotomy and J-tube insertion to the acute hospital. She had a prior history of gastrointestinal (GI) motility disorder of unknown etiology requiring supplemental tube feedings. She had been diagnosed with MS only 2 years earlier, but admitted to symptoms for 8 years prior to that. There was no family history of MS. Her symptoms at onset included numbness below the waist and gait and balance difficulties. Prior to her acute illness, she had been a borderline ambulator; indoors, her walking was characterized by leaning on walls and furniture, and having difficulty on stairs. She was still driving and used a wheelchair for distances. She had been treated in the past with IV steroids for *ill-defined episodes of worsening*, and had been on betaseron for 6 months prior to admission with little effect on disease progression. She had managed her bladder with intermittent catheterization prior to admission.

On transfer to inpatient rehabilitation, she was nonambulatory, had been hospitalized 20 days, and required moderate assist of two to transfer. Her estimated expanded disability status scale (EDSS) prior to admission was 6 (unilateral assistance to walk 100 m), and at time of admission to rehabilitation, was 8 (essentially restricted to bed or chair, has some effective use of the arms, needs assist with transfers, retains some self-care functions). Medications included baclofen (80 mg/day), betaseron, and colace. Examination disclosed mild depression and cognitive slowing, mild left facial weakness, upper extremity (UE) power fair to good, lower extremity (LE) power trace proximally with strong extensor tone distally. She had no UE ataxia and moderate impairment in trunk control. In standing, she demonstrated no postural reactions and could not stand without the assist of two persons. A Foley catheter was in place.

In order to prognosticate, her disease history was analyzed and suggested a relapsing-remitting but secondarily progressive picture with a diminishing return in the past to steroid treatment. Disability was accumulating despite betaseron, and disease appeared active. In addition, precipitating factors in her functional decline included acute surgical emergency, possible malnutrition, prolonged bed rest in the acute hospital stay, potential worsening of leg weakness with baclofen, possible depression, and sleep disorder (to which the patient eventually admitted). In addition, there were signs of cognitive compromise, and family stressors were prominent, both in terms of intimacy and finances.

Goals set at the team meeting were first presented by the individual disciplines and then agreed on by the team. Her return to ambulation seemed unlikely, at least during her inpatient rehabilitation stay, due to her borderline ambulatory status PTA, the activity of her disease, and her increased tone and weakness problems. The weakness was felt to be multifactorial and included the effects of bed rest, disease activity, and possibly the baclofen.

Interventions included cognitive evaluation, with education for the patient and spouse as to the extent of deficits and what external compensations could be made; supportive counseling; and a sedating antidepressant to assist sleep. Individual and group therapies were designed to stress UE strengthening, wheelchair mobility, and trunk control. Ambulation goals were deferred. A urinary tract infection was identified and treated, and catheterization schedule commenced. Tone was treated with local measures that included inhibitory bivalved casts at night and an orthodigital device to prevent toe clawing in standing. Baclofen was decreased to 60 mg/day and scheduled to coincide with the times of her worst spasms and to avoid times when therapy was utilizing what leg power she had. Her bracing system was evaluated, and leather soles added to her shoes to enhance sliding of the feet in the face of excessive iliopsoas weakness. UE-assistive devices were prescribed for ADLs from the wheelchair level, and sliding board transfers instructed. Family teaching commenced, and, eventually, the patient opted for a suprapubic tube rather than intermittent catheter because her bathroom did not permit wheelchair entry and there was no place for a commode. Intravenous steroids were administered with only mild improvement in tone, but no other noticeable effect was seen. The betaseron was continued. At discharge, she remained nonambulatory, but independent in sliding-board transfers from bed to chair (but not commode), in wheelchair mobility, and in urinary and bowel continent with in-dwelling catheter and suppositories. EDSS at discharge was 7.0 (unable to walk 5m even with aid, independent in transfers, up in wheelchair for most of day).

Case 2

C.F. is a 47-year-old male with chronic progressive MS over a 20-year period who was admitted from home. Despite 202community-based services, the patient was constantly in pain, behaviorally acting out at his spouse and adult children, and unable to mobilize from his wheelchair. He had few environmental control systems in place. He had had a significant weight gain, and transfers by hoyer lift were becoming difficult for the caregivers. He had an in-dwelling Foley catheter and moved his bowels every fifth day. The patient's primary caregivers were his wife, who also worked full-time outside the home, and his college-aged children. His primary complaints on review of systems included lower extremity pain, which was most pronounced at night; inability to tolerate his wheelchair for more than an hour at a time due to low back pain; sleep initiation and maintenance difficulties; and fatigue. His EDSS at admission was not felt to be much different than baseline and was estimated to be 9.0 (helpless bed patient, can communicate and eat). He was admitted for a 1-week evaluative stay.

The potential for successful outcome was highly dependent on identifying treatable problems. His mobility and physical disability were nearly the worst score one can achieve on the Kurtske EDSS (10), and there appeared to be no indication that neurologic deterioration was occurring, since he was essentially quadraplegic and had little else left to lose. His chronic progressive disease was felt to be end-stage and probably burned out.

On the other hand, several remediable problems were identified; pain, sleep disorder, positioning difficulties, constipation, depression, poor coping strategies, caregiver education needs, inability to access community supports and use environmental controls were all identified as areas of need.

Interventions included positioning devices for his heels to decrease the burning pain due to pressure. The seat back insert on his wheelchair was revised. He was started on Prozac at 20mg/day for his depression, aggressive outbursts, and fatigue. Neuropsychologic evaluation, a behavioral management program, and counseling for the patient and family for coping strategies were begun. Referral to appropriate community agencies for counseling and personal care attendants was made. A home visit was accomplished by the occupational and physical therapists to address architectural barriers. A bowel program was devised after disimpaction was accomplished. Discharge EDSS remained at 9.

References

1. Anderson DW, Ellenberg JH, Leventhal CM, et al. Revised estimate of the prevalence of multiple sclerosis in the United States. Ann Neurol 1992;31:333–336.
2. Compston DAS, Ebers CG. The genetics of multiple sclerosis. In: Cook S, ed. Handbook of multiple sclerosis. New York: Marcel Dekker Inc., 1991:19.
3. Sadovnick AD, Baird PA, Ward RH. Multiple sclerosis: updated risks for relatives. Am J Med Genet 1988;29:533–541.
4. Sadovnick AD, Ebers CG. Genetics of multiple sclerosis. Neurol Clin 1995;13:99–118.
5. Hafler DA, Weiner HL. Immunologic mechanisms and therapy in multiple sclerosis. Immunol Rev 1995;144:75–105.
6. Hafler DA, Matsui M, Wucherpfennig KW, et al. The potential of restricted T-cell recognition of myelin basic protein epitopes in the therapy of multiple sclerosis: antigen and clone-specific immuno-regulation. Ann N Y Acad Sci 1991;636:251–265.
7. Hafler DA, Weiner HL. Immunologic mechanisms and therapy in multiple sclerosis. Immunol Rev 1995;144:75–105.
8. Owens T, Sriram S. The immunology of multiple sclerosis and its animal model, experimental allergic encephalomyelitis. Neurol Clin 1995:13: 51–73.
9. Katz D, Taubenberger JK, Canella B, et al. Correlation between magnetic resonance imaging findings and lesion development in chronic, active multiple sclerosis. Ann Neurol 1993;34:661.
10. Weinshenker BG, Ebers GC. The natural history of multiple sclerosis. Can J Neurol Sci 1987;14:255–261.
11. Kurtzke JF. Rating neurologic impairment in multiple sclerosis: an expanded disability status scale (EDSS). Neurology 1983;33:1444–1452.
12. Keith RA, Granger CV, Hamilton BB, Sherwin FS. The functional independence measure: a new tool for rehabilitation. In: Fuhrer MJ, ed. Rehabilitation outcomes: analysis and measurement. Baltimore: Brookes, 1987:137–147.
13. Bradley WG, Daroff RB, Fenichel GM, Marsden CD, eds. Neurology in clinical practise. Vol II. Boston: Butterworth-Heinemann, 1991:1154.
14. Miller DH, McDonald WI, Blumhardt LD. Magnetic resonance imaging in isolated noncompressive spinal cord syndromes. Ann Neurol 1987;22:714–723.
15. Birk K, Ford C, Smelter S, et al. The clinical course of multiple sclerosis during pregnancy and the puerperium. Arch Neurol 1990;47:738–742.
16. Nisipeanu P, Korczyn AD. Psychological stress as a risk factor for exacerbation of multiple sclerosis. Neurology 1993;43:1311–1312.
17. Grant I, Brown GW, Harris T, et al. Severely life threatening events and marked life difficulties preceding the onset or exacerbation of multiple sclerosis. J Neurol Neurosurg Psychiatry 1989;52:8–13.
18. Franklin GM, Nelson LM, Heaton RK, et al. Stress and its relationship to acute exacerbations of multiple sclerosis. J Neurol Rehabil 1988;2:7–11.
19. Weinshenker BG, Bulman D, Carriere W, et al. A comparison of sporadic and familial multiple sclerosis. Neurology 1990;40:1354–1358.

20. Sadovnick AD, Ebers GC, Wilson RW, et al. Life expectancy in patients attending multiple sclerosis clinics. Neurology 1992;42:991–994.
21. Weinshenker BG, Ebers GC. The natural history of multiple sclerosis. Can J Neurol Sci 1987;14:255–261.
22. Kurtzke JF, Beebe GW, Nagler B, et al. Studies on the natural history of multiple sclerosis VIII: early prognostic features of the later course of the illness. J Chron Dis 1977;30:819–830.
23. Shapiro R. Multiple sclerosis: a rehabilitation approach to management. New York: Demos, 1991:7.
24. Bauer HJ, Firnhaber W, Winkler W. Prognostic criteria in multiple sclerosis. Ann N Y Acad Sci 1965;122:542–546.
25. Beatty WW, Blanco CR, Wilbanks SL, et al. Demographic, clinical, and cognitive characteristics of multiple sclerosis patients who continue to work. J Neurol Rehabil 1995;9:167–173.
26. Scheinberg L, Holland N, La Rocca N, et al. Multiple sclerosis: earning a living. N Y State J Med 1980;August:1395–1400.
27. Frankel D. Long term care issues in multiple sclerosis. Rehabil Literature 1984;45:282–285.
28. Isaac C, Li DKB, Genton M, et al. Multiple sclerosis: a serial study using MRI in relapsing patients. Neurology 1988;38:1511–1515.
29. McFarland HF, Frank JA, Albert PS, et al. Using gadolinium-enhanced magnetic resonance imaging lesions to monitor disease activity in multiple sclerosis. Ann Neurol 1992;32:758–766.
30. Beatty WW, Scott JG. Issues and developments in the neuropsychologic assessment of patients with multiple sclerosis. J Neurol Rehabil 1993;7:87–97.
31. Rao SM, Leo GJ, Bernadin L, Unverzagt F. Cognitive dysfunction in multiple sclerosis I: frequency, patterns, and prediction. Neurology 1991;41:685–691.
32. Beck RW, Cleary PA, Trobe JD, et al. The effect of corticosteroids for acute optic neuritis on the subsequent development of multiple sclerosis. New Engl J Med 1993;329:1764–1769.
33. Abraham S, Scheinber L, Smith T. Disordered deglutition and dysphonia in multiple sclerosis. Neurology 1994;44(suppl 2):A185.
34. Herrera W, Zeligman BE, Gruber J, et al. Dysphagia in multiple sclerosis: clinical and videofluoroscopic correlations. J Neurol Rehabil 1990;4:1–8.
35. Appel RA. Evaluation and management of urologic disorders in multiple sclerosis. Multiple Sclerosis Clin Issues 1995;2:6–9.
36. Fowler CJ. Bladder dysfunction in multiple sclerosis: causes and treatment. Int MS J 1994;1:99–107.
37. Lilius HG, Valtonen E, Wilkstrom J. Sexual problems in patients suffering from multiple sclerosis. Scand J Soc Med 1976;4:41–44.
38. Inderhoud JM, Leemhuis JG, Kremer J, et al. Sexual disturbances arising from multiple sclerosis. Acta Neurol Scand 1984;70:299–306.
39. Stone B, Melman A. Management of sexual and bladder dysfunction in multiple sclerosis. J Neurol Rehabil 1989;3:167–175.
40. Stefoski D, Davis FA, Faut M, Schauf CL. 4-aminopyridine in patients with multiple sclerosis. Ann Neurol 1987;21:71–81.
41. Krupp LB, Alvarez LA, LaRocca NG, Scheinberg LC. Fatigue in multiple sclerosis. Arch Neurol 1988;45:435–437.
42. Smeltzer SC, Utell MJ, Rudick RA, Herndon RM. Pulmonary function and dysfunction in multiple sclerosis. Arch Neurol 1988;45:1245–1249.

43. Schiffer RB, Wineman NM, Wetkamp LR. Association between bipolar affective disorder and multiple sclerosis. Am J Psychiatry 1986;143:94–95.

44. Schiffer RB, Weitkamp LR, Wineman NM, Guttormsen S. Multiple sclerosis and affective disorders: family history, sex, and HLA-DR antigens. Arch Neurol 1988;45:1345–1348.

45. Berman AL, Samuel L. Suicide among people with multiple sclerosis. J Neurol Rehabil 1993;7:53–62.

46. Minden SL. Psychotherapy for people with multiple sclerosis. J Neuropsychol 1992;4:1–16.

47. Ritvo PG, Fisk JD, Archibald CJ, et al. A model of mental health in patients with multiple sclerosis. Can Psychol 1992;33:391.

48. Kahana E, Leibowitz U, Acter M. Cerebral multiple sclerosis. Neurology 1971;21:1179–1185.

49. Miller DH. Magnetic resonance in monitoring the treatment of multiple sclerosis. Ann Neurol 1994;36(suppl):91–94.

50. Aisen ML, Arnold A, Baiges I, et al. Effect of mechanical damping loads on disabling action tremor. Neurology 1993;43:1346–1350.

51. Greenspun DO, Stineman M, Agri R. Multiple sclerosis and rehabilitation outcome. Arch Phys Med Rehabil 1987;68:434–437.

52. LaRocca NG, Kalb RC. Efficacy of rehabilitation in multiple sclerosis. J Neurol Rehabil 1992;6:147–155.

53. Winters S, Jackson P, Sims K, Magilvy J. A nurse-managed multiple sclerosis clinic: improved quality of life for persons with MS. Rehabil Nurs 1989;14:13–22.

54. Shapiro RT. Multiple sclerosis: a rehabilitative approach to management. New York: Demos, 1993:19–32.

55. Smith CR, LaRocca NG, Giesser BS, Scheinberg LC. High dose oral baclofen: experience in patients with multiple sclerosis. Neurology 1991;41:1829–1831.

56. Coffey RJ, Cahill D, Steers W, et al. Intrathecal baclofen pump for intractable spasticity of spinal origin: results of a long-term multicenter study. J Neurosurg 1993;78:226–232.

57. Snow BJ, Tsui JKC, Bhatt MH, et al. Treatment of spasticity with botulinum toxin: a double blind study. Ann Neurol 1990;28:512–515.

58. Smith C, Birnbaum G, Carter JL, et al. Tizanidine treatment of spasticity caused by multiple sclerosis: results of a double-blind, placebo controlled trial. Neurology 1994;44(suppl 9):34–43.

59. Krupp LB, Sliwinski M, Masur DM, et al. Impact of fatigue treatment on cognitive functioning in multiple sclerosis. Poster presentation, ANA 1993. Ann Neurol 1993;34:248.

60. Goldhammer G, Giladi N, Honigan S. Low dose methazolamide in essential tremor. Neurology 1994;44(suppl 2):A214.

Use of the Neurologic Rehabilitation Model in Assessment and Treatment

Virginia M. Mills, Douglas I. Katz, and John W. Cassidy

The ultimate goal of this text is to evolve the practice of rehabilitation and ultimately the care provided to patients with neurologic disabilities. To that end, this chapter will illustrate how understanding the principles of neurologic rehabilitation can improve treatment planning and service delivery to this patient population. The requisite underpinnings have been developed in earlier chapters and assume a complete understanding of the natural history of the basic neuropathologic process in order to properly formulate a course of treatment. These fundamentals apply in other medical conditions, but seem somewhat more intuitively obvious in those situations. For example, in a pathologic process as elemental as a fracture of a long bone, it seems apparent that the natural evolution of healing bone delimits the constraints of the rehabilitative process. This natural history determines when weight bearing can occur, how much weight can be borne, and when casting becomes unnecessary. These parameters are well known and consistently applied in nearly all rehabilitative organizations. In a more complicated condition, that of myocardial infarction, it is cardiovascular physiology that drives treatment. No one presumes to begin treadmill training until the Swan-Ganz catheter has been removed. Furthermore, clearly the patient must understand his current functional limitations, the time course in which these limitations will evolve, and what should be done along the way to facilitate recovery. The same kind of information about specific neurologic diagnosis and natural history should apply in planning treatment for neurologic disorders; yet this approach is not routinely practiced in most rehabilitation settings. A probable explanation is that neurologic principles, unlike orthopedic ones, seem too complicated to apply in clinical settings. While not necessarily making neurology any easier to understand, this chapter should dispel such notions.

In traditional rehabilitation practice, it is the observable manifestations of the disorder that largely constitutes the working diagnosis. For example, typical rehabilitation diagnoses would be "right hemiparesis" or "agitation." This conceptualization of diagnosis then leads to treatment planning designed to address these observable problems. Commonly, these treatment plans enumerate a list of impairments evident at the time the initial multidisciplinary evaluations are performed, usually on admission to the program. The treatment plans generated from such a list are often discipline-specific with each problem given equal remedial effort. Each discipline is assigned a problem or part of a problem to work on and generally reports back to the team every other week on its progress or lack thereof toward its remediation (1–3). This kind of service delivery fails to respect the role of natural history, for some impairments improve without any intervention and others never recover no matter how much "therapy" is directed toward them. Furthermore, this unawareness leads to the implementation of empirical, "trial and error" treatment strategies that assume the method is wrong when improvement is not forthcoming rather than acknowledging that some deficits may not be remediable. In these situations, therapists often overemphasize the role of direct treatment in the recovery process, believing that each of a patient's problems can be "fixed." Finally, this belief assumes that rehabilitative efforts will generalize and lead to improvement in the patient's ability to perform "real life" tasks when such optimism is not justified.

Treatment planning using the traditional approach lists a variety of strategies designed to facilitate recovery. Generally these strategies include the following:

1. Direct treatment of the problem (e.g., stretching or casting for a contracture)
2. Teaching a method of compensation for a deficit area (e.g., using a memory notebook for problems with memory and planning)
3. Repetitive practice or exercise to strengthen, retrain, or reinforce a particular movement or activity (e.g., lifting weights to increase strength)

4. Learning or relearning a movement pattern or skill (e.g., relearning a normalized gait pattern)
5. Using an assistive or augmentative device to improve functions (e.g., walking with a cane)
6. Lessening environmental obstacles (e.g., creating a wheelchair accessible environment)

What does the neurologic model of rehabilitation add to the traditional approach? The specific neurologic diagnosis conveys information about the neuropathology, the patient's impairments, natural history, and prognosis. The model directs clinicians to look at other premorbid and comorbid problems and the relationship of other factors, such as age, in formulating the patient's anticipated outcome. Although the specific neurologic diagnosis cannot predict with certainty the exact outcome for any individual patient, it can offer statistical evidence to suggest its trajectory and time frame. Recovery and therefore outcomes are based on the probability of improvement for the disease process under consideration; this probability is based on studies of many people with the same, or very similar, diagnostic and clinical characteristics. Thus the neurologic model gives clinicians an actuarial framework to use when formulating any individual's anticipated outcome.

The neurologic model provides a theoretical framework to understand which problem areas to target for treatment. For example, if a patient with mild brain injury presented with attentional deficits at 1 year post injury, the clinician would not necessarily assume that this inattentiveness was due to the brain injury per se, but rather would suspect depression or chronic pain. Similarly, if a patient with anoxic brain injury is unable to shave and has no weakness, apraxia cannot be assumed, but other problems such as agnosia must be explored. Thus, the neurologic model focuses treatment in the following three ways:

1. The specific neurologic diagnosis identifies the underlying etiology of the problem causing the impairment.
2. Prognosis forms the basis for developing realistic outcome goals for treatment and suggests treatment strategies that respect the natural history of the disorder and the expected limitations of recovery.
3. The disorder's natural history helps clinicians anticipate the length of hospitalization, outpatient treatment, and the expected need for environmental prostheses at the conclusion of formal treatment.

This paradigm also permits clinicians to set reasonable limits for the accomplishment of their goals. For example, if a patient has a hemiparesis from a right middle cerebral artery infarct that involves the deep periventricular white matter interrupting the descending pathways of the pyramidal motor pathways, the therapist should be able to anticipate a prognosis for a functional hand. In the same way, the therapist can anticipate the patient's prospects for walking and how much assistance he or she will require as recovery proceeds. Thus, clinicians are better informed to predict the patient's potential to develop a functional hand or walk with independence, as they can now rely on a well-established framework to provide such answers. This improved predictability permits cost containment by more accurately knowing the extent of the resources necessary to produce an expected patient outcome.

As reviewed in prior chapters, a considerable amount of knowledge about how the central nervous system (CNS) recovers from various exogenous and endogenous insults currently exists. The remainder of this chapter will be dedicated to outlining illustrations of how the neurologic model provides a theoretical framework for assessment, treatment planning, and goal setting in this patient population.

In regard to the last item, goal setting, the following are examples of goals that were taken verbatim from the medical records of patients in traditional rehabilitation centers:

- The patient will perform to the satisfaction of the therapist
- Maximize the patient's potential
- Positively assess the effect on the central nervous system environment

It is unclear how these goals relate to rehabilitation, as they are at best idiosyncratic and vague and at worst, incomprehensible. They provide no information about the therapeutic process or its time frame. They could not be translated to another treatment team and are devoid of any true functional understanding of the patient's disabilities.

CASE STUDIES

The following example was taken from a textbook used for training physical and occupational therapists in the management of motor and cognitive problems.

Case 1

The author describes a 21-year-old woman who is now in treatment 4 months following a brain injury that was the result of a motor vehicle accident. The patient's cognitive assessment recorded that she had problems with attention and difficulty with "choice reaction" tasks of increasing complexity. She also presented with *astereognosis* (inability to identify objects by tactile choice, despite normal elemental sensation) and was combative during therapies. The goals and treatment plan outlined below were derived from the problems listed above.

- To treat the attention problem, the patient was to draw lines through a maze with five or fewer errors, and she was to mimic 10 upper extremity activities without being distracted.
- To improve astereognosis, the patient was to match three-dimensional (3-D) forms with tactile cues with 75% accuracy.
- To improve choice reaction times, the patient was to place a hat on her head with either her left, or right, or both hands, with 50% accuracy based on the therapist's cues.
- To improve the patient's behavior, clinicians were to implement a behavior modification program with the patient.

At first glance, these goals may seem reasonable and appropriate, as various cognitive problems were identified and acceptable treatment plans were proposed. However, this approach to assessment and treatment does not provide a framework for understanding what is really wrong with this patient or how the identified problems fit into the larger context of her illness. As such, the goals do not outline a functional outcome that should be anticipated given the patient's handicaps.

The text states that the patient performs poorly on tests of astereognosis; however, nowhere is the etiology of the problem considered. Therefore, it is possible that the patient's nonsensory, processing problem is a consequence of her attentional disturbance, not astereognosis. Even if the problem is truly astereognosis, can treatment affect this impairment and does its continuing existence produce a functional disability for the patient at this point in her recovery? If the neurologic model had been used it would have informed this therapist that even if astereognosis were the problem, it usually diminishes on its own during recovery, without therapeutic intervention, especially in the absence of focal parietal brain damage (see below). Therefore, the proposed exercises are not an efficient or cost-effective use of a therapist's time and the patient's resources.

Regarding the attentional problem, it has not been demonstrated that attention deficits can be treated directly with exercises. There is evidence that patients can proceduralize skills while in a confusional state, but having a patient draw lines in a maze will not generalize and improve the patient's attentional abilities on a day-to-day basis. Further, this patient's attention disturbances will likely improve on their own as her recovery evolves beyond the confusional stage.

The same is true of trying to enhance the patient's choice reaction time by having her perform a motor activity with a hat. The therapist may be able to improve the patient's performance in this task during therapy, but it will not generalize to other tasks that are required for her to function in her environment. The task of having the patient place a hat on her head with greater and greater accuracy is useless and has no apparent real-life value. Training in a task of immediate value to the patient's functioning (e.g., activity of daily living [ADL]) would have been much more practical, even in the absence of generalization to other tasks.

The reader is also informed that this patient had behavioral problems ("combative during therapies"). Again, her behavior must be viewed in the context of an evolving confusional state. Most patients demonstrate improved behavioral regulation as they emerge from their confusional state. It is improvident to establish an elaborate behavior modification program during this phase of her recovery. Her behavior dysregulation can be far better managed by environmental manipulation and prosthesis by simplifying the environment and by training her treatment staff to proactively manage behavior that might escalate out of control.

Let's now approach this patient using the neurologic model of rehabilitation. First, the model would insist on formulating an accurate neurologic diagnosis, which in this case can be derived from the information provided in the text. It would be explicitly stated as: "profoundly severe, diffuse axonal brain injury, without focal injury or secondary CNS complications, produced by a significant acceleration/deceleration mechanism." How is this determined? This patient lost consciousness immediately upon impact (consistent with diffuse axonal injury) and was decerebrate (arms and legs in tonic extension = best motor response of only 2 on a scale ranging from 1 to 6) on admission, with a Glasgow Coma Scale score of 4 (range 3 to 15, 3 to 8 by definition = severe injury), and remained unresponsive to commands for 2 months. The initial brain CT scan revealed a small intraventricular hemorrhage, but no focal hemorrhagic or contusional injuries. This history and associated neuroimaging findings are consistent with the diagnosis of severe diffuse axonal injury. At 4 months post injury when the patient was first evaluated, it was clear that she was still in a confusional state and had continuing post-traumatic amnesia (PTA). During this phase of recovery, it is expected that she will have very poor attention, problems with new learning, and, as a consequence, behavioral dysregulation.

The next step under this paradigm is to use knowledge about the natural history of diffuse axonal injury to determine what problems should be treated at 4 months post injury. The natural history informs us that this patient is still in an early phase of recovery where global problems with arousal and attention obscure more localizable deficits and are the progenitors of many of the problems noted during the initial clinical assessments. Furthermore, this awareness would predict that she will pass through this stage of recovery at a fixed rate despite therapeutic interventions. The evolution of these early phases of recovery is inevitable; although improper treatment can retard this progression, little can be done to advance it. Directed therapies cannot make a confused patient lucid. Some pharmacologic agents, such as dopamine agonists, may help focus attention, but there is little evidence that these agents alter the stages of recovery. During the confusional state, the overall goal of the team should be to manage the patient's symptoms and her environment to permit this stage to safely pass. Thus, the initial assessment would explicitly state that the patient's primary problem is confusion, and the treatment plan would focus on providing a prosthetic environment. Although this may sound like a simple goal, it is not. These modifications involve a considerable amount of staff education in areas that are usually deficient in their training.

The model also predicts that during the confusional state, the patient's declarative, or explicit, learning is severely impaired. Patients can relearn functional tasks, such as toileting, while in a confusional state; however, they do so by using preserved procedural or implicit learning, involving extensive repetition of the task to be learned. Therefore, this is the learning modality that clinicians must exploit in therapy during this phase of recovery. It is a tedious process for which there is no adequate substitute. A treatment plan would thus reflect a toileting schedule that involved staff supervision and patient procedural training every 2 hours while she was awake. Transfers would be trained by repeated practice of the elements of the task, without relying on any explicit recall of the procedure. Other important functional skills such as feeding, bathing, and dressing could be proceduralized in a similar manner. Thus, the patient could be helped to proceduralize her daily routine on the treatment unit, attempting to have her do more and more for herself. Retraining more difficult tasks such as cooking, money management, academic, or vocational skills will need to wait until the post-confusional stage, where more declarative strategies of learning can be successfully employed. Given the severity of the patient's injury, a full return of declarative memory function, even after the confusional state resolves, cannot be expected.

The patient's behavior may be a continuing problem for her until confusional state clears. Given the patient's amnesia, an elaborate behavior management program, such as a token economy, would not be appropriate given that she is unable to recall behavioral expectations or retain information about the back-up reinforcers. As alluded to earlier, environmental modification coupled with staff and family training are the best strategies to manage behavior dysregulation during this phase of recovery.

The neurologic model of rehabilitation would change this patient's management, recommended treatments, and her outcome. It also helps predict the trajectory of her recovery, alerting her treating clinicians that she is likely to have a protracted confusional state, averaging 6 to 7 months (see formula in Natural History section in Chapter 4). This paradigm promotes having the patient perform therapeutic activities that are ecologically consistent with skills she will need to perform to be discharged to a less restrictive setting. Therefore, the activities used in therapy should be "real" and focus on important tasks such as toileting, washing, dressing, and eating. Consistent chaining hierarchies should be developed and stereotypically practiced by the patient with staff supervision many times a day. For example, if showering remains a problem area, it should be rehearsed more than once a day. The model promotes teaching a patient to assist in performing meaningful activities safely and as independently as possible within the limits of her disability. Goals of treatment can be specific; for example, learning how to perform a squat and a pivot transfer and to maintain non-weight bearing on a fractured leg 100% of the time, or to "initiate showering with one staff cue and complete chaining hierarchy by checking off each item with a grease pencil, performing 75% of the steps independently."

There are many illustrations of how goal setting can be enhanced by using the neurologic model. Memory impairment will be used as an example because it is a significant problem for patients following many types of CNS insults. There are a number of generic exercises designed to "help" memory: computer memory exercises; requiring the patient to remember words, items, or a story and to answer questions; or individual training in the use of a memory book. The real question becomes, which strategy to use, if any? The answer to this question could be very different depending on the specific neurologic diagnosis and time post insult.

Case 2

An amnestic 23-year-old man, who is 5 weeks post injury following a motor vehicle accident resulting in severe diffuse axonal injury, has a memory problem that is a manifestation of his post-traumatic amnesia. It is known that the patient's memory problem will improve over time, and as such requires no specific treatment at this stage of his recovery. As noted earlier, it might be useful to use procedural learning strategies to help the patient relearn basic ADLs and his daily routine.

Case 3

Our third patient is a 36-year-old man, who is 3 months post cardiac arrest and has an anoxic encephalopathy. He is no longer confused, and his attention is good. As his attentional mechanisms recovered, his episodic (day-to-day) memory did not improve. Given these clinical circumstances, it is likely that he has sustained bilateral hippocampal damage. He will have a persistent memory disorder, and the prognosis for improvement is poor. In this case, rather than wait for improvement that will never come, the treatment team would want to start teaching the patient to compensate for his memory problems as soon as possible. It would be expected that the patient would need to use a memory aid for the remainder of his life. With this patient, the clinicians would, again, want to exploit preserved procedural learning to improve his ADL skills. This patient will have long-term deficits, which can be recognized early in his recovery; appropriate treatment can be directed toward compensation.

Following are four more examples of how this model can be used to produce a coherent treatment plan for patients with motor deficits. The most common motor problem in this population is hemiplegia with spasticity and a nonfunctional arm and hand.

Case 4

This patient is a 19-year-old woman 7 weeks post traumatic brain injury (TBI) with a dense right hemiplegia. She sustained severe diffuse axonal injury and a small, left thalamic hemorrhage demonstrated by CT scan (Figure 7.1). The left thalamic hemorrhage involved the ventral posterior lateral nucleus of the thalamus, an important relay between somatosensory areas of the cortex. The lesion did not completely involve the posterior limb of the internal capsule, where motor information descends from the motor cortex. Because the location of the lesion spared much of the posterior limb of the internal capsule and it was hemorrhagic rather than ischemic, a more favorable outcome for return of motor function would be anticipated. Within 1 month following her injuries, she had good arm, hand, and leg function. However, she had some remaining sensory loss and a central pain syndrome associated with the residual thalamic lesion. Early goal setting for upper extremity function in this patient should reflect a favorable prognosis for arm and hand function.

Case 5

Case 5 is a 65-year-old woman, who is 1 month post embolic middle cerebral artery stroke, with involvement of the deep lenticular-striate artery territory structures. This patient also presented with a dense hemiplegia, spasticity, and a nonfunctional hand. The brain CT scan showed a deep white matter lesion near the lateral ventricle, which involved almost all of the descending motor pathways (Figures 7.2 and 7.3). This lesion signifies a poor prognosis for motor function, particularly fine motor control and extensor movement of the upper extremity. This "deep" lesion is much more debilitating than a superficial cortical lesion involving the primary motor cortex alone.

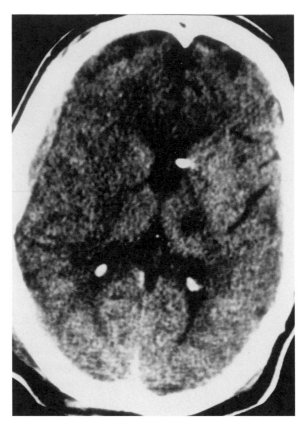

Figure 7.1 *CT scan of a 19-year-old woman 7 weeks after a TBI, showing a lesion in the left lateral thalamus, the remnant of a post-traumatic deep hemorrhage. Primary motor pathways running in the posterior limb of the internal capsule were not completely involved so prognosis for recovery of right hemiparesis was favorable.*

Treatment goals for this patient need to anticipate a poor prognosis for recovery of arm function; thus, they should focus on training her to use one-handed techniques in ADLs and should incorporate the use of adaptive equipment. Despite the similarity of their initial presentations, the prognosis for upper extremity recovery in Case 4 and Case 5 is extremely divergent. Yet, in many rehabilitation centers these two patients could easily have the same treatment plans written for them.

The following two cases have similar problems in the performance of ADLs; however, their underlying neuropathology is very different.

Case 6

Case 6 is a 62-year-old man who is 2 weeks out from having survived a left parietal stroke (Figure 7.4). He was unable to get through his

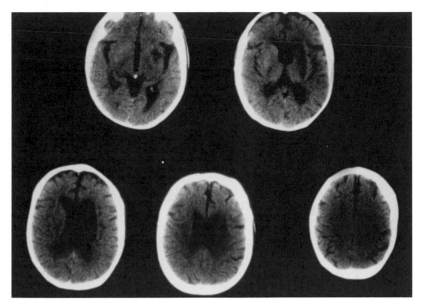

Figure 7.2 CT scan of a 65-year-old woman 1 month after an embolic stroke. The lesion involves most of the descending primary motor (pyramidal tract) pathways at the level of the periventricular white matter adjacent to the lateral ventrical. (The putamen and possibly some of the internal capsule is involved in the lower sections.)

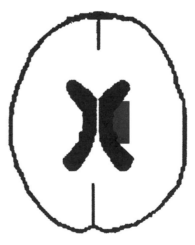

Figure 7.3 Schematic diagram illustrates the location of the primary motor pathways. (Modified from Naeser MA et al [4].)

morning ADL routine, despite the absence of motor or learning difficulties. His neurologic assessment revealed a fluent aphasia, with moderate comprehension deficits and a severe ideomotor apraxia. Based on this assessment, treatment strategies should include teaching his caregivers to use short, simple, declarative instructions and to avoid using

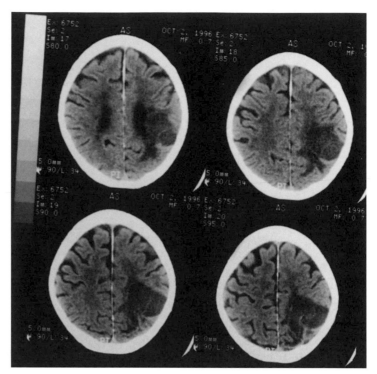

Figure 7.4   CT scan of a 62-year-old man 2 weeks after a left MCA territory stroke. The lesion involved primarily posterior temporal and parietal areas. (The parietal portion of the stroke is illustrated.) The patient had moderate language comprehension deficits and severe ideomotor apraxia for limb movements. Primary motor function had recovered well.

complex language. Demonstration of functional activities should use contextual cues and real objects. The patient's apraxia would be best managed by having the patient perform everyday activities with real objects in as natural a context as possible.

Case 7

Case 7 involves a 48-year-old man 3 weeks after a right parietal-occipital border-zone stroke (Figure 7.5). The neurologic assessment revealed that he had left neglect with impaired facial recognition and body orientation. The patient had topographic disorientation and was unable to find his way around the treatment unit. He had a dressing apraxia as evidenced by his inability to orient his clothes properly to his body. In this case, treatment strategies should focus on environmental prostheses; for example, his food and utensils should be placed on his "good side," where visual attention continues. Caregivers should be instructed to stand in the visual field to which he attends

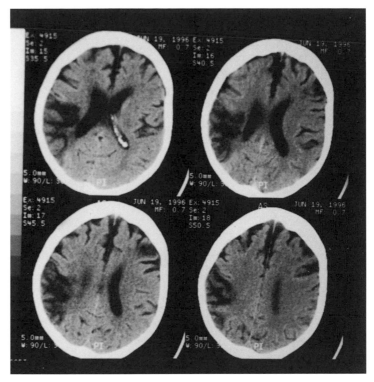

Figure 7.5   *CT scan of a 48-year-old man 3 weeks after a right hemisphere parietal-occipital stroke. The patient had topographic orientation problems, body orientation difficulties, dressing apraxia, and left hemispatial neglect.*

when speaking to him and to perform therapies from that side of his body. During therapy, attention should be drawn to his impaired side. Objects and clothing should be given to him oriented properly to his body. The environment should be laid out to give him contextual cues to orient himself. It should be clear that Case 6 and Case 7 had a different neuropathologic substratum—that is, in Case 6 it was language and apraxia, and in Case 7, it was visual neglect—and as such each patient needed a distinct therapeutic approach.

CONCLUSION

In conclusion, this text asserts that there are general principles clinicians should use in treatment planning and goal setting.

1. The goals of treatment should be consistent with the patient's underlying neurologic diagnosis and expected ability to recover. The clinician should know the etiology of the impairment he or

she is treating. The natural history of the disorder permits prediction of outcome and its time frame and directs treatment.

2. Treatment goals should recognize spontaneous recovery and therefore avoid unnecessary treatments.

3. Not all of the patient's deficits require treatment because some will not be handicapping to that individual.

4. Treatment goals should reflect areas where poor recovery is expected and recognize that not all impairments are amenable to treatment. In such circumstances, goals need to emphasize teaching compensatory strategies.

5. The goals of treatment should focus on functional skills that are meaningful for the patient. If the patient's access to rehabilitation is limited, rehabilitation efforts should focus on goals that are going to be useful to the patient.

For patients who are going home, treatment goals should attempt to return the patient to his or her own environment, community, and social network as early as possible. It is better to train new skills or compensatory skills in the environment where the patient will be living. Hospitals are artificial environments, and many training procedures learned in the hospital are not transferable to the patient's own living environment. For those patients who cannot return home, treatment goals should focus on assisting the patient to have the highest quality of life in the least restrictive environment possible and should permit as much independence as possible. As much as we rehabilitation clinicians hate to admit it, not all patients are capable of true independence; many will require assistance for the remainder of their lives.

References

1. Strasser DC, Falconoer JA, Marino-Saltzmann D. The rehabilitation treatment team: staff perceptions of the hospital environment, the interdisciplinary team environment, and interprofessional relations. Arch Phys Med Rehabil 1995;75:177–182.

2. Keith RA. The comprehensive treatment team in rehabilitation. Arch Phys Med Rehabil 1991;72:269–274.

3. Diller R. Fostering the interdisciplinary team, fostering research in a society in transition. Arch Phys Med Rehabil 1990;71:275 278.

4. Naeser MA, Alexander MP, Stiassny-Eder D, et al. Real versus sham acupuncture in the treatment of paralysis in acute stroke patients—a CT lesion site study. J Neurol Rehabil 1992;6:163–173.

Assessment of Impaired ADL/Functional Activities: An Activities Assessment Algorithm

Michael P. Alexander

Many patients who suffer a stroke are left with some limitation in cognitive abilities. Aphasia, visuospatial neglect, and apraxia are each present in 25% to 30% of acute testable stroke patients. Substantial improvement occurs in many but not all, and improvement may take several weeks to months during which the patient may be in inpatient and outpatient intensive rehabilitation. Smaller numbers of stroke survivors have lesions that produce amnesia or agnosia, but their recovery is often less complete. Larger number of stroke patients have a more restricted learning deficit, impaired executive functions, or depression, and these problems can be both subtle and persistent. Thus, many stroke survivors may be limited in some manner in cognitive or communicative functions, often most severely during the post acute epoch when they may be receiving rehabilitation services.

How should individual therapists and the rehabilitation team address and approach these problems? Currently, responsibility for the patient tends to get divided along discipline "turf" boundaries. Speech pathologists perform aphasia testing, often assess apraxia, and may evaluate attention, memory, or other cognitive domains "associated" with communication. Occupational therapists may perform a variety of cognitive tests that purport to be directly functional: money management, figure-ground discrimination, etc. Neuropsychologists may perform a more comprehensive cognitive assessment utilizing a variety of standardized tools.

There are many reasons to be dissatisfied with this approach. The tests used may be informative to the appropriate specialist (e.g., a standardized aphasia test to Speech Pathology or a card sorting test to Neuropsychology) but meaningless regarding real-life functions to anyone else on the treatment team. The tests may be homegrown measures without any demonstrated reliability or validity, except presumably face validity. The cognitive assessments used by therapists are often an amalgam of homegrown tests, various tests or subtests borrowed from neuropsychology, and functional tasks that are highly overdetermined. The test results are more often a description of the patient's symptoms or impairments. Translating these test "results" into a clear picture of how or why patients might fail an activities of daily living (ADL) task due to their cognitive or communicative impairment is often difficult or impossible.

ACTIVITIES ASSESSMENT ALGORITHM

I propose an entirely different approach for therapists to use to determine how and why cognitive/communicative deficits impair the patient's performance in ADL. It uses a cascade of questions that focuses on possible limitations of function and guides the therapist to specific probes of cognition, to observations of behavior that will illuminate cognition, to other clinicians who might offer additional assistance, or to treatment recommendations. Because it focuses on functional activities and provides a management algorithm, I propose the name Activities Assessment Algorithm (A^3).

Figure 8.1 summarizes the A^3. There are eight questions that could be asked of any functional task failed apparently because of cognitive deficits.

A^3-1: Attention (Figure 8.2)

Is the patient's global attention adequate for the task? There are three related problems here. First, the problem could be inadequate arousal if the patient is drowsy or stuporous. Second, there could be inadequate activation; the patient is awake but does not seem to respond at all,

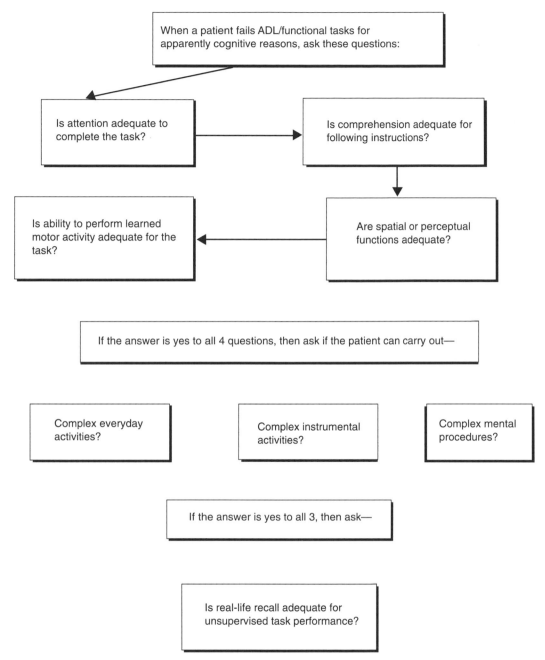

When a patient fails ADL/functional tasks for apparently cognitive reasons, ask these questions:

Is attention adequate to complete the task?

Is comprehension adequate for following instructions?

Is ability to perform learned motor activity adequate for the task?

Are spatial or perceptual functions adequate?

If the answer is yes to all 4 questions, then ask if the patient can carry out—

Complex everyday activities?

Complex instrumental activities?

Complex mental procedures?

If the answer is yes to all 3, then ask—

Is real-life recall adequate for unsupervised task performance?

Figure 8.1 *Activities assessment algorithm for analysis of ADL deficits that seem to have a cognitive basis.*

responds only after a long latency, or responds only with maximal prompting. Third, concentration, sustaining attention, dividing attention, or inappropriate loss of attention may be present in various mixes (1). The patient would be awake and responsive but distractible or

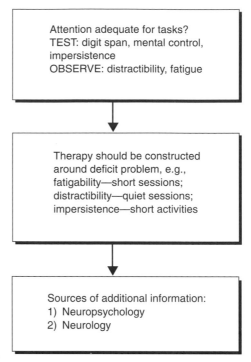

Figure 8.2 *Algorithm and management suggestions for attentional deficits.*

preseverative or rapidly fatigued. A³-1 would be tested with digit span (normal 5–9 forward) or any task that requires more complex attention, so-called mental control, such as recitation of overlearned series (e.g., numbers, months, days) in reverse order, serial subtractions, etc., keeping the tests easy so any difficulty can be presumed abnormal. Recall that even mild aphasia may make these tasks impossible despite normal attention. Another approach is to ask the patient to hold a complex arbitrary posture for 15 seconds (e.g., good arm above head, eyes closed, and tongue protruded). Inability to maintain the position is called *motor impersistence*. It is a failure of sustained attention and is associated with a poor functional outcome. Even aphasic patients can be tested if they can be modeled into posture.

If these tasks and observed behaviors are normal, there is no likely effect of global attentional impairments on treatment. If problems are observed, additional clarification may be obtained regarding cognitive deficits from neuropsychology. Neurology may be able to predict near-term prospects for improvement based on medical factors. If there are deficits, therapy should be constructed around the deficit problem. For instance, fatigability requires short sessions, while impersistence requires short activities, and distractibility requires simplified, sequenced activities and quiet room treatment.

A³-2: Language (Figure 8.3)

For most functional tasks, comprehension of commands and instructions is the performance-determining language ability. Even assuming that clinicians are experienced and present instructions in a straightforward manner, successful completion of tasks requires substantial language ability. This could be probed directly by any clinician (2). If presented with an array of common ADL objects (e.g., comb, razor, toothbrush), can the patient pick up the correct one when named? Can the patient move or indicate a named body part? If the answers are no, then much ADL intervention will be useless unless set and task are established nonverbally. Can the patient carry out simple placement and movement commands using body parts whose names he or she recognizes, such as "lift your arm"? Can the patient reliably indicate yes or no to straightforward questions about family or personal information? If not, then answers to questions about needs, feelings, motivations, and pains will surely be meaningless.

If comprehension in these tasks is good, then there will not be any likely communication impediment to ADL assessment and manage-

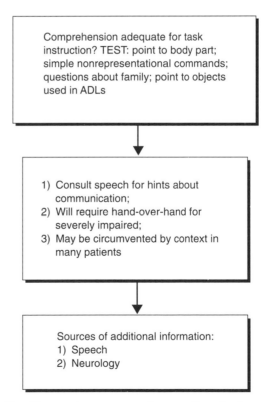

Figure 8.3 *Algorithm and management suggestions for language deficits.*

ment. More complex tasks of function, money management, shopping, etc. may still be profoundly limited because of aphasia even in a patient who passes this screening. Whether patients can recognize and correctly use objects in their own care when comprehension of a request is impaired will be probed below under apraxia. If there are deficits in the comprehension screening, Speech Pathology may be able to suggest some compensatory approaches to communication. Neurology may be able to predict at least short-term prognosis. Therapy should be constructed around the deficits in communication. Some patients may require hand-over-hand modeling of ADL activities before a request is "understood." Many patients simply need context, and they will perform much better. For a patient dressed in pajamas at 9:00 P.M., a toothbrush in the bathroom may represent a much less ambiguous request than the same toothbrush presented in mid-morning to a patient who is fully dressed.

A³-3: Spatial Attention and Perceptual Function (Figure 8.4)

Patients with or without general attentional impairments may have difficulty attending to either the right or left half of space. Significant so-called *hemispatial neglect* much more commonly affects the left hemispace (3). Hemispatial neglect often improves substantially over a few weeks, but it can play a limiting role in rehabilitation interventions. Persistent left hemispatial neglect has a poor prognosis for functional recovery or compensation. Hemispatial neglect may be apparent when observing patients' behavior—for example, failing to attend to speakers on their left side or failing to eat off of the left side of the meal tray. It may be more subtle. Simple screens for neglect could include using the same ADL objects used to test word comprehension. Spread them out from far left to far right and ask the patient to locate them. If problems are observed, clarification about severity and prognosis might be available from Neuropsychology or Neurology. There is no definitive medical treatment for neglect. Numerous behavioral manipulations may reduce apparent severity. Have the patient perform all tasks with head deviated to the left. Place a salient stimulus (large plastic yellow flower) on the left margin of the attended stimulus, whatever it may be—a book, a dinner plate, a pile of clothes, etc. If the patient is able to move the left arm, patting the left hand or opening and closing the fist may improve attention to the left.

Patients with extensive damage to parietal, occipital, and inferior temporal lobes may have various perceptual and recognition disorders (4). These may be suggested by the patient's behaviors such as inability to reach for an object that he or she can see with the good arm (*optic ataxia*), difficulty directing gaze to a particular object (*optic apraxia*),

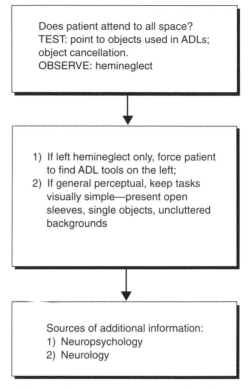

Does patient attend to all space?
TEST: point to objects used in ADLs;
object cancellation.
OBSERVE: hemineglect

1) If left hemineglect only, force patient
   to find ADL tools on the left;
2) If general perceptual, keep tasks
   visually simple—present open
   sleeves, single objects, uncluttered
   backgrounds

Sources of additional information:
1) Neuropsychology
2) Neurology

Figure 8.4 *Algorithm and management suggestions for perceptual deficits.*

inability to recognize familiar faces (*prosopagnosia*) or objects (*visual agnosia*) despite adequate vision, etc. These can all be screened for by systematic testing of the behaviors, but clarification of the nature of the deficit—perceptual or discriminative or naming—probably requires neuropsychologic assessment. The management implications are transparent. Do not utilize test items that the patient cannot recognize. Keep tasks visually uncluttered. Keep the patient's sleeves and cuffs rolled back. Keep backgrounds simple.

A³-4 Praxis (Figure 8.5)

Praxis is surely one of the most incorrectly used terms in rehabilitation. There are two levels of limb apraxia of clinical importance (5). *Ideomotor apraxia* is the inability to carry out a learned motor task in response to a direct request, either spoken or gestured. The task is contextless, even if the object typically used in the task (e.g., a toothbrush) is not present. Correct performance requires recruiting the particular movement that characterizes the task as well as representing the absent object in abstract space. For example, told to pretend to brush teeth, the

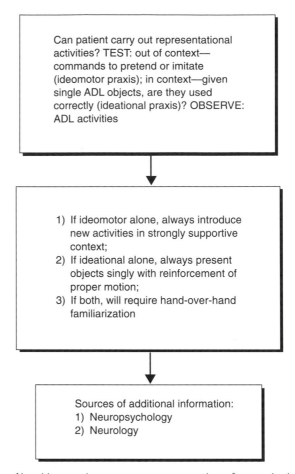

Figure 8.5 *Algorithm and management suggestions for praxis deficits.*

correct brushing motion requires the hand to be loosely fisted, inches from the angle of the mouth, ulnar deviated at the wrist, pronated at the elbow, with rapid wrist flexion and extension while maintaining a gap for the absent toothbrush. The more context the patient is given— a model to imitate, a real toothbrush, a bathroom at night in his pajamas, etc.—generally the better the performance. Thus, the finding of ideomotor apraxia may have no real functional consequence.

Ideational apraxia is the inability to use in the correct manner a tool whose use is clearly recognized. Patients with perceptual problems who do not recognize objects may be mistakenly thought to have ideational apraxia. This deficit is recognized by observing the patient perform ADL tasks; for example, an awkwardly positioned comb, poorly oriented for its purpose and moved orthogonal to intention would suggest ideational apraxia.

Many patients with large left-sided strokes will have severe word comprehension deficits, ideomotor apraxia, and ideational apraxia simultaneously. Establishing the level at which performance in ADLs is abnormal may require collaboration with Speech Pathology, Neuropsychology, and Neurology. If patients have ideomotor apraxia alone, there are only two management issues: 1) be certain that failure to carry out some complex limb command is not apraxia as opposed to poor comprehension; and 2) when introducing new activities always provide maximal context. If patients have ideational apraxia alone, always present ADL objects singly and in context with tactile and verbal reinforcement of correct movement. If both are present, hand-over-hand repetition will probably be required.

The next three levels of the A^3 are variations on a theme. They all require the capacity to carry out more complex, often multistep activities. Few patients will receive inpatient treatment at this level, but there will be occasional inpatients and many outpatients who can do all their self-care but fail homemaking, instrumental ADLs, or cannot access the community, thus leaving the patient with requirements for supervision. The assessments of these problems have some similarities.

A^3-5: Organizing ADL Action Plans (Figure 8.6)

Can the patient carry out complex everyday activities? Many patients can get dressed independently if they are handed items one at a time. Preparing a mental plan to go to the bureau and the closet, lay out appropriate clothing, and don the items in correct order is another level of function. Organizing all morning bathroom activities, gathering items for dressing, and eating a large meal are examples of activities that require an ADL action plan. Observing the patient may illuminate an action plan deficit; for example, the patient uses items correctly but in the wrong order, omits one step or item, uses an item as though it were another item. These action plan deficits are believed to be secondary to frontal system lesions (6).

The first intervention when they are observed is to reanalyze the lower-level operations—attention, praxis, etc. If no lower-level deficit accounts for the problem, reconsideration of error types suggests treatment. Use of incorrect object within the complex multistep action (e.g., stirring coffee with napkin) or using an object correctly on the wrong target (e.g., successfully buttering the breakfast sausage) suggests presenting tasks sequentially on an uncluttered background. Perseverative use of objects suggests clearing objects after their use. Inability to maintain order of actions suggests laying out tools in correct (and self-cuing) order.

Neurospychology and Neurology may assist with clarification of the deficit pattern, with specifying the "frontal" impairments underlying disrupted organization, and perhaps with prognosis by analysis of CT or MRI lesion.

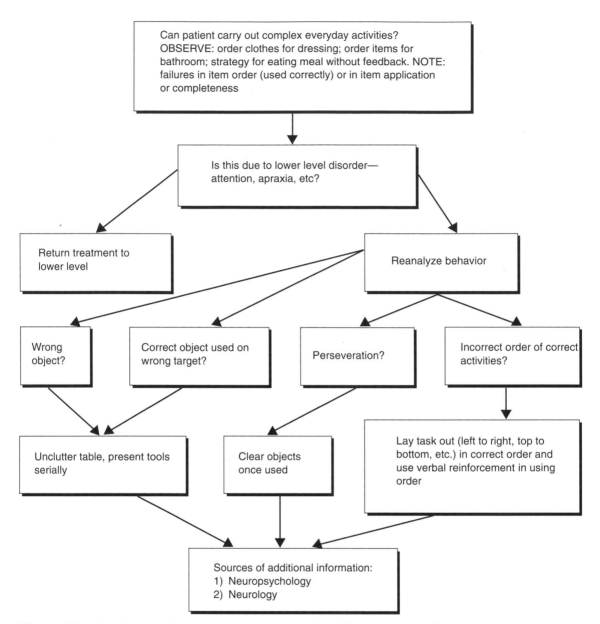

Figure 8.6   *Algorithm and management suggestions for ADL action plan deficits.*

A³-6: Organizing Complex Instrumental Action Plans (Figure 8.7)

Many patients can get dressed independently, but are unable to manage the weekly laundry or successfully run the washing machine. They may eat independently but be unable to prepare a menu or a meal or do the requisite shopping (7). This is a higher level of organizing

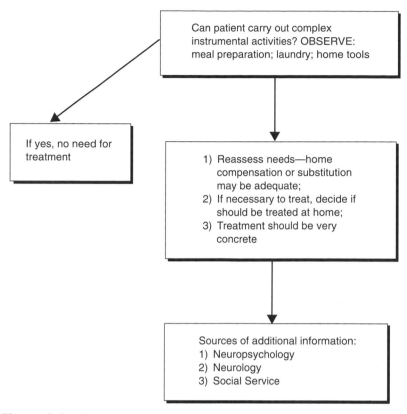

Figure 8.7   *Algorithm and management suggestions for complex instrumental activity deficits.*

action plans, and assessment and characterization are similar to A^3-5. Neuropsychology and Neurology may be helpful for the same reasons as above. It is possible a patient does not require treatment at this level because his or her supervision at home may be so good that the patient will never get into an arena where trouble could develop. All treatments should be delivered at home or in a residential or community-based outpatient setting for two reasons: 1) If patients are independent in dressing, toileting, and feeding, they do not need inpatient hospital or skilled nursing care, no matter how addled their organizational capacities; and 2) Performance should be reinforced at the stove, washer, or other real-world setting that the patient will actually be using.

A^3-7: Complex Mental Action Plans (Figure 8.8)

Can the patient carry out complex mental procedures? Many patients can get dressed independently and do the weekly wash, but they cannot organize shopping trips, plan the clothing budget, or manage

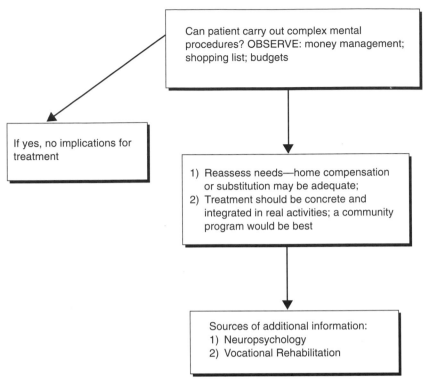

Figure 8.8 *Algorithm and management suggestions for mental procedural deficits.*

their money. (To be sure, many neurologically intact people cannot do these either.) This is another, yet higher, plane of impaired action plans (7). The first step in assessment is to reevaluate lower-level deficits to be certain that there is not a more direct cause of impairment. Mild aphasia, alexia, acalculia, or memory impairment may derail the locomotive of budgeting, checkbook balancing, etc. without a true action plan deficit.

Again, for a well-supervised patient who is otherwise independent, treatment for these higher-plane impaired action plans may be unnecessary because the patient may not have to perform ADL independently in his or her home setting. Before attempting treatment, the patient should have a thorough analysis by Neuropsychology, and the extent (and implicitly, the probability of improvement) of the brain lesion should be reviewed by Neurology. The practical assessment of the deficits should again focus on characterizing the error patterns—distractibility, fatigue leading to incomplete performance, substitution of subtasks in the wrong order of performance, etc. Treatment should be practical and immediately related to the patient's needs. The treatment setting should be the patient's home and community environment. There does not seem to be a role for abstract, table-top "cognitive therapy" that does not generalize improved functional performance to the patient's real living environment. Treatment is probably best delivered in an integrated family, community, school, or workplace setting where the tasks are germane to the individual patient's life requirements.

A³-8: Memory (Figure 8.9)

Much of the above presumes that the patient is able to learn (or relearn) skills and can recall from session to session the purpose and goals of treatment. Significant memory or learning problems can impair and prolong even a well-designed treatment strategy. I recommend that therapists leave formal memory testing to Neuropsychology and concentrate on functional manifestations of learning impairment (8). Is the patient oriented? Does the patient know or recall the purpose of the therapy? Can the patient recall day to day the role and identity of the therapist? Over time, are there savings (i.e., improved performances) on tasks? If the answer is no, some reassessment is essential before proceeding. First, what level of function does the patient require for home discharge? He or she may be able to recapture old abilities for ADL that may be sufficient. If neuropsychologic testing demon-

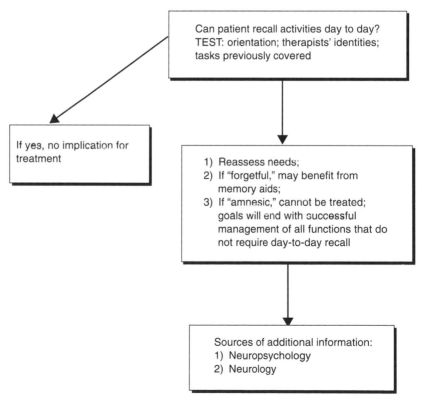

Figure 8.9 *Algorithm and management suggestions for memory deficits.*

strates that the patient is not amnesic but has inefficiencies in recall, well-designed external memory aids may be helpful. Inefficiencies in rate of learning with reasonable delayed recall of whatever has been learned may benefit from errorless repetitions. Classical (totally) amnesic patients cannot be successfully treated with repetitions and cues, at least not in a practical manner for the high-functional level we are considering here. Neurology consultation may clarify whether this is a disorder with likely improvement (9).

After home discharge, the patient may continue rehabilitation in his or her home or in a community setting where problems with meal preparation, laundry, money management, shopping, and other ADLs can be addressed. Treatment should be concrete and directly relate to what activities the patient needs to routinely perform in his or her individual living situation.

CAVEATS

Much of the above has presumed that therapists should do what they do well: Assess function and characterize deficit patterns. I do not recommend they devise or borrow tests from Neuropsychology to put a more sophisticated patina on their assessment efforts. I have assumed that therapists have two resources that, in fact, they may not. There has been repeated encouragement to utilize neuropsychologists and neurologists who work in rehabilitation to clarify prognosis and impairments. Both must, however, ask the correct questions. There is nothing more discouraging than a carefully done neuropsychologic assessment of a severely aphasic patient demonstrating that he has poor Block Design, impaired Trails-B, and perseverative card sorting. This set of observations is useless for the treatment team. Cookbook neuropsychologic assessment in most stroke survivors has little information to assist therapists to design treatment programs. If therapists bring specific and limited questions to a neuropsychologist, however, they should get helpful information. For example, the neuropsychologist should be able to give a more definitive description of attentional problems, clarification between perceptual and recognition deficits, precise characterization of memory processes, and more.

In a similar manner, if your neurologic consultant can only provide diagnostic information about the stroke—an embolic infarct involving the frontoparietal convexity, for example—but cannot see through the lesion into functional prognoses, the value of this consult for rehabilitation planning is minimal. Is this a pattern of lesion usually associated with recovery of comprehension, of arousal, of agnosia, etc? Does the amnesic patient have unilateral or bilateral limbic lesions? There is an art to using Neurology to guide—not prescribe or proscribe—an approach that many Neurologists simply never learn. But therapists should not attempt to compensate for uninformative Neuropsychology or Neurology by imitating neuropsychologic assessment procedures. Do what you do best! Observe and remain practical and functional.

References

1. Stuss DT, Shallice T, Alexander MP, Picton TW. A multidisciplinary approach to anterior attentional functions. Ann NY Acad Sci 1995;769:191–211.
2. Alexander MP. The aphasias and related disorders. In: Joynt RJ, ed. Clinical neurology. vol. 1. Philadelphia: Lippincott-Raven, 1991:1–58.
3. Heilman KM, Watson RT, Valenstein E. Neglect and related disorders. In: Heilman KM, Valenstein E, eds. Clinical neuropsychology. New York: Oxford University Press, 1985:243–293.
4. Alexander MP. Higher-order visual impairment. In: Samuels MA, Feske S, eds. Office practice of neurology. New York: Churchill Livingstone, 1996:722–728.
5. De Renzi E. Apraxia. In: Boller F, Grafman J, eds. Handbook of neuropsychology. vol. 2. Amsterdam: Elsevier, 1989:245–263.
6. Schwartz MF, Mayer NH, Fitzpatrick EJ, Montgomery MW. Cognitive theory and the study of everyday action disorders after brain damage. J Head Trauma Rehabil 1993;8:59–72.
7. Burgess PW, Shallice T. Deficits in strategy application following frontal lobe damage in man. Brain 1991;114:727–741.
8. Wilson B, Cockburn J, Baddely A. The Rivermead behavioural memory test. Reading (UK): The Thames Valley Test Company.
9. D'Esposito M, Alexander MP. The clinical profiles, recovery and rehabilitation of memory disorder. Neurorehabilitation 1995;5:141–159.

9

The Use of the Neurologic Rehabilitation Model in the Assessment and Treatment of Patients with Balance Impairments

Eileen Wusteney and Kathy Joy

The task of the nervous system in regulating balance is to acquire and integrate sensory information from the visual, somatosensory, and vestibular systems. Then, coordinated postural reactions must be selected and generated to keep the body aligned and ready to perform motor activities. In order to understand balance and its disorders, it is critical to have knowledge of the many systems in the body that normally contribute to its production. As such, this chapter is devoted to providing an overview of the basic parameters of balance. This is followed by an introduction to the associated balance impairments related to the neurologic diagnoses reviewed throughout the text. We have provided tools for assessment and treatment planning based on the framework of the neurologic rehabilitation model. Its use, combined with expert assessment, guides clinicians in designing and implementing the most effective rehabilitation treatment plans for their patients with this disability.

CRITICAL PARAMETERS OF BALANCE

Definitions

In the rehabilitation literature different meanings can be used for the same term. This can lead to substantial misunderstanding. Therefore, for the purposes of this chapter, the following definitions are provided to establish a common terminology.

Balance

Balance refers to the ability to control one's *center of gravity* over any given base of support within varied sensory environments, producing the appropriate postural responses to accomplish functional tasks (1–3).

Center of Gravity (Alignment)

Research suggests that the central nervous system (CNS) uses information related to center of gravity to determine the level of stability and then to generate the postural responses necessary to maintain balance (1,4). Technically, the body's center of gravity can only be determined by summing discrete measurements of the area and weight of each body segment (5). Anthropometric research has generally found the anatomic position of the center of gravity in standing to be slightly anterior to the midline of the body at approximately 55% of the total body height (5–7). Clinically, the center of gravity can be thought of as an imaginary point in the center of the body at the height of the umbilicus. If one projects a vertical line down from this point, it would fall approximately in the middle of the base of support.

Postural Alignment

Postural alignment refers to the proper biomechanical alignment of the individual body segments, for example, the head, neck, trunk, and limbs. Historically, clinicians have assessed posture for the purposes of correcting individual alignment deviations, not center of gravity alignment. In balance control, it is imperative to relate postural alignment to center of gravity alignment.

Limits of Stability

Limits of stability refers to the area in which one's center of gravity can be moved without changing the base of support (8). These limits represent the distance one can lean in each direction without stepping or falling. The limits of stability depend on the individual's height and base of support. Normally, in quiet standing with the feet even and hips-width apart, one can lean 6.5° forward, 4.5° backward, and 8° each side (4,8,9). These limits are dynamic. They are determined by some obvious external circumstances. If the support surface does not offer sufficient resistance to apply forces against, the ability to maintain balance will be more difficult and the degrees of movement lessened. If the base of support is very narrow, the ability to lean in the narrowed direction(s) would again be lessened. There are internal constraints that could reduce the limits at which a fall might occur. Biomechanical limits of stability can be altered by musculoskeletal or neuromuscular deficits, such as joint range of motion, muscle flexibility, tone, strength, sensation, coordination, and pain. In an individual without impairment, the biomechanical limits of stability are consistent with the perceived limits of stability. Certain types of neurologic lesions can cause people to perceive their limits of stability to be more or less than their actual biomechanical limits of stability. Abnormalities in perceived limits of stability can create abnormalities in balance stability and/or control in the absence of biomechanical deficits.

Automatic Postural Response

An automatic postural response may be thought of as an overlearned, repeatedly practiced, multisynaptic "long loop" response in the nervous system that allows the individual to rapidly respond to the continuous demands of balance and movement through space (10,11). They are commonly referred to as *ankle, hip, and step strategies*. Most research to date deals with automatic postural responses in the anteroposterior plane. It is hypothesized that there are similar strategies for lateral movements. The *ankle strategy* is our first line of defense to prevent loss of balance (Figure 9.1A,B). Forces are applied by the muscles around the ankles first to develop rotations or torques that move the center of gravity in a fore and aft plane. This requires that the two joints (knee and hip) that lie between the ankle and the center

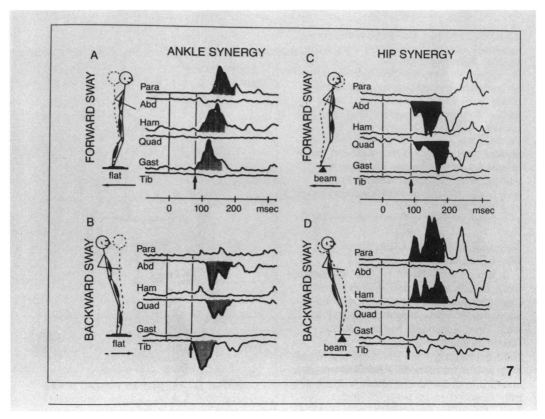

Figure 9.1   EMG responses associated with ankle and hip movement strategies. Muscles on the figures to the left correspond to those named on the graph. Solid-line figures depict position after movement of the support surface; dashed-line figures depict the target return to equilibrium position. The vertical line farthest left is the onset of the translation, and the vertical line to the right (with arrow) shows the time that the muscles begin to contract. (Reproduced with permission from Lewis M. Nashner, PhD.)

of gravity be stabilized during the movement. An ankle strategy is useful for relatively small perturbations that occur when the center of gravity is not very close to the limit of stability, and when the individual is standing on a support surface that is firm and wide enough to allow forces to be effectively applied at the foot. This strategy is commonly used when standing and walking on indoor surfaces.

The *hip strategy* calls on the muscles around the hips first to generate flexion and extension movements to elicit a more direct movement of the center of gravity (Figure 9.1C,D). When the center of gravity is moving rapidly toward the limits of stability, or if the perturbation occurs while the center of gravity is close to the limits of stability, it is hard to generate effective torques in the ankle to bring the center of gravity back to midline. When a person is standing on a support surface that is compliant (soft) or smaller than his or her feet (e.g., a balance beam), ankle movements will not generate effective torques because the support surface does not offer enough support resistance to the base of the foot. An example is someone standing on a rail of a fence: movements occur around the hips to maintain the center of gravity within the base of support while the feet remain relatively still.

The *step strategy* is the last of the automatic postural strategies and is elicited as a final strategy to maintain balance by widening the base of support by taking a step in the direction of the center of gravity displacement. A step strategy is used when the center of gravity is rapidly brought beyond the person's limits of stability, and the ankle or hip strategies are no longer effective.

Sensory Parameters

The first and most obvious contribution of the sensory systems to balance is in providing information on where the center of gravity is positioned. If the nervous system has an inaccurate sense of the position of the center of gravity relative to the base of support, it might not perceive that a fall is about to happen, and thus, no automatic postural response using an ankle, hip, or step strategy will occur. If movement of the center of gravity is perceived after a delay, the response, even though it might be correct, will occur late and be ineffective. The wrong strategy would be chosen if the nervous system had a misperception of the orientation of center of gravity. If, for instance, the sensory systems do not perceive that the center of gravity is moving rapidly toward the limits of stability, an ankle strategy, as opposed to the necessary hip or step strategy may be generated and therefore be ineffective in preventing a fall. In general, the contribution of sensation to the production of balance is to provide continuously accurate orientation information, so that an appropriate motor response can be chosen and timed. Each individual sensory system has a specific role in the control of balance (12).

In order to maintain balance, the nervous system must assemble data to understand the relative position of the center of gravity and the limits of stability. This is achieved by the creation of an internal sensory map, an inner "picture" resembling a stick figure, which must include certain parameters (13). At any point in time, the nervous system must know the position of all body segments relative to one another. The nervous system must also know the position of the body relative to the support surface and to the earth's vertical. In addition, moment-to-moment data about the immediate environment, combined with prior experience, is needed to compute a person's limits of stability. To create this map, the brain has three sources of data: proprioceptive, vestibular, and visual inputs. Given these three systems, there is some redundancy, but each system has a particular specialized role. It is believed that the integration of this data with the internal sensory map occurs in the parietal lobe of both hemispheres (13).

Proprioceptive Input

The nervous system uses all sources of somatosensation, including touch, pressure, and vibration, to determine the body's position in space. Proprioception has a critical role in telling the body the relative position of all the body segments (14,15). If the body does not have reliable information about these body segment alignments, accurate motor activity cannot be planned or generated. Proprioception is the sole source of that data. Proprioception is critical to the production of ankle strategies (10). People who lose proprioception, especially if it is bilaterally absent, will be markedly deficient in the generation of ankle strategies. Proprioception also has a specific role in terms of generating rapid postural corrections for changes in position of the body relative to the support surface. If there is a perturbation generated between the support surface and lower extremities, the body usually relies on proprioception to sense the perturbation and generate a rapid postural correction. Examples include tripping or stepping on an uneven obstacle encountered on a support surface (17).

Peripheral neuropathy is perhaps the most common disorder that causes bilateral, distal loss of proprioception. If the loss is primarily distal, the brain retains a large degree of information about the relationship of body segments. People who lose distal proprioception, but have intact proprioceptive information from the remainder of the legs and body, will be able to generate postural responses, albeit somewhat delayed and less than coordinated. In contradistinction, many neurologic syndromes produce unilateral sensory loss from proprioceptive pathways. Here, the nervous system may lose all reliable information regarding the relative position of the limbs and trunk on that side. Unilateral loss is not nearly as devastating as bilateral. Disruption of the postural responses will, in general, occur only when the affected limb is bearing a significant proportion of the responsibility for postural control. That is why patients who have loss of proprioception on one side, with everything else intact, will do their best to shift all of their weight onto the unimpaired side. The only time they will have difficulty is when they weight-shift onto the involved side, have to perform single-support activities on that side, or during the stance phase of gait on that side. The usual compensation seen is a shortening of the stance phase on the involved side. If a patient has very severe loss of proprioception on one side, the brain's sensory map of the position of all body segments on that side is going to be distorted. As the segmental body relationships change with movement, the brain's map of the relationships will remain inaccurate. Therefore, all postural motor responses that are planned, based on that inaccurate sensory map, will be deficient.

Vestibular Input

The vestibular system has many roles in producing postural control (18). The most important for the purpose of this discussion is its functioning as an inertial guidance system or gyroscope. It tells the nervous system at all times where the earth's vertical is by detecting gravity. The vestibular system is the only sensor that can reliably determine where the vertical (i.e., up and down) is under all situations where the body experiences gravity. Therefore, impairments in vestibular input result in a loss of body orientation in the vertical plane. When vestibular inputs are lost or deficient from one side of the body, there is a perceived tipping in the lateral plane. The nervous system now perceives the earth's vertical as being tipped to one side. If one loses vestibular inputs from the left labyrinth, regardless of where the loss occurs within the nervous system, one tends to believe that the earth's vertical is tipped to the left. One will then orient himself or herself and generate all postural responses based on the perception that the body is tipped to the left, relative to the true earth's vertical. On a consistent moment-to-moment basis, the brain cannot use vision and proprioception to correct for the perceptual and postural bias. However, patients can use vision and proprioception on a longer term basis for relearning the proper perception of the earth's vertical. An acute, unilateral vestibular loss results in a significant bias in the perception of center of gravity and shifts the limits of stability off to one side. This fact is important for clinicians to recognize in their attempts to properly treat patients with neurologic syndromes presenting with balance problems and yet, historically, it has been ignored.

In addition to contributing to accurate orientation of the center of gravity, the vestibular system is critical to the generation of hip strategies (19,20). Patients who have vestibular loss will not generate hip strategies. Therefore, a major component of the repertoire of postural responses will be missing. Patients will be deficient in the situations in which hip strategies are critical to maintain balance.

Vision

Common experience tells us that vision is not critical to postural control because eye closure does not produce a dramatic loss of balance. Vision is a modulator of postural motor responses (21). Loss of vision will slow down postural responses in certain settings and make them less accurate, but vision is not critical to the production of any of these postural responses. Vision tends to make postural responses more efficient and can be a source of sensory data that helps to improve the inputs from other sensors when they are less than perfectly reliable. Vision can be used by patients to compensate for other sensory impairments following neurologic illness. If vision is no longer available as a substitute for the loss of other balance sensors, the compensatory ability of the patient will be limited.

Sensory Organization

As discussed, the brain assembles data from the various sensors to create an internal sensory map representing postural orientation. In addition to taking into consideration the specific characteristics of each of the sensory systems, the brain also must consider the quality of the environment and ongoing changes in the environment. Environmental changes can occur quickly in a way that makes the information from a particular sensor more or less useful for postural orientation (22). Vision and proprioception are relative sensors; that is, they provide data about the relationship between the individual and the outside world, but they are not always reliable. For example, if you are standing or walking in a room in which the walls are clearly seen and the floor is flat, you can use vision for postural orientation because the walls and floor provide high quality, reliable information. If you suddenly find yourself in a situation where a good deal of the visual environment is moving, vision is no longer reliable for postural orientation. From one moment to the next, vision can change from being reliable to being useless to you for postural orientation. The same is true for proprioception. If the support surface is flat and stable, proprioceptive cues are reliable inputs for determining the earth's vertical. Any change in ankle position detects a change in the earth's vertical. If, however, you begin to walk on a surface that is unpredictably uneven, vertical orientation is impossible to determine based upon ankle joint position alone.

The vestibular system is different. It is not relative to anything but gravity. It will always tell you the location of the earth's vertical (18). The problem is that the vestibular system is not as rapid as proprioception and vision in providing the needed data. As a result, the brain has developed a two-tiered response system. It initially responds to vision or proprioception, and, shortly thereafter when vestibular inputs are available, it corrects an inappropriate response or allows an appropriate response to be completed (12). For example, if you are walking on a stable support surface and you generate postural responses based on accurate proprioceptive cues, the vestibular inputs arriving at the brain a short time thereafter will agree. If, however, you are walking on an uneven support surface, and your foot is tipped up by a rock, proprioception alone will signal a falling back of the center of gravity. This will generate postural responses to bring the center of gravity forward, which will actually make you unsteady. The foot tipping up may not, however, cause a falling back of the center of gravity because the ankle may dorsiflex enough to compensate. In this situation the erroneous signal will be corrected when vestibular cues arrive in the nervous system.

This two-tiered system is a fundamental concept in understanding the pathology of postural control. The implication is that pathology involving the vestibular system will result in a situation in which patients will respond to orientationally inaccurate visual or proprioceptive cues. For example, vestibularly impaired patients who find themselves on an uneven support surface may generate totally inappropriate postural responses based on the data they receive from intact proprioceptors. This type of patient is termed *support surface dependent* (23) and uses proprioception even when the data is inaccurate for postural orientation. *Visual dependence* can occur when a patient utilizes intact visual input that is inaccurate for overall postural orientation. This type of problem is termed a *sensory organization deficit*. The phenomenon, described earlier, in which the vestibular system is used as the final arbiter when sensory information is conflicting is called the process of *sensory selection* (23). Therefore, patients may have a problem with sensory selection when the most accurate sensory data within a setting is inaccurate.

MOTOR PARAMETERS

How does the motor system respond to maintain postural balance? In order to answer this question, several aspects of postural control must be understood. When balance is disturbed, the motor system responds in a stereotyped, preprogrammed fashion (11). Using nonrandom, preprogrammed strategies tends to be the most efficient way to effect a postural response. For the multitude of situations that might result in a loss of balance, the nervous system needs few patterns of muscle response to regain balance. With only a few responses to pick from, the motor system can make postural adjustments to the environment extremely fast. Ample physiologic evidence exists to support that there are only three patterns of muscular postural response, or strategies, necessary to maintain balance. As defined earlier in the chapter, these strategies are the ankle, hip, and step strategies. Each of these preprogrammed strategies is ideal for a particular type of demand made on our postural system in common environmental situations.

Lesions of the nervous system can effect the motor system's ability to generate these strategies. The organization of the synergy patterns (preprogrammed groupings of muscle responses within the nervous system) can be broken up or distorted so that the postural response, instead of being well-timed and well-coordinated, becomes uncoordinated. The strategy chosen to respond to a given situation can be inappropriate.

Ankle Strategy

What is the normal ankle strategy? The goal of a normal ankle strategy is to generate forces about the hip, knee, and ankle joints to keep the legs straight and to control the center of gravity within the base of support. The torque generated at each joint has to be well timed, and the force must be sufficient to complete the goal. If the joints are not stabilized, they may flex or even buckle, and the force will not control the center of gravity, causing excessive movement or postural sway.

The makeup of the ankle strategy takes all of these factors into consideration. For example, if an individual's center of gravity is being thrown backward, in order to maintain balance the leg muscles must contract in a sequence that pushes the center of gravity anteriorly (see Figure 9.1B). If an ankle strategy is used because the perturbation is minimal and the center of gravity is not too close to the limits of stability, the first response is the contraction of the anterior tibialis muscle. The second response is a contraction of the quadriceps muscle across the knee joint to stabilize it. And the third response is a contraction of the abdominal and hip flexor muscles across the hip joint. The two latter contractions have the sole purpose of stabilizing those joints that lie between the ankle and the center of gravity.

Hip Strategy

A hip strategy is utilized when the surface under the feet does not offer enough resistance to generate sufficient torque about the ankles. Examples of this are standing on a narrow beam or on a thick foam surface. A hip strategy is also needed when the center of gravity is brought too close or too quickly to the limits of stability. Under these conditions, the same posteriorly directed sway of the center of gravity will elicit muscle contractions in a proximal to distal sequence. The antagonistic trunk and leg muscles (paraspinals, hamstrings, and gastrocnemius) to those contracting in the ankle strategy will be stimulated. This pattern of muscle contraction extends the hips and flexes the knees, bringing the center of gravity forward and to midline.

Mixed Responses

Automatic postural responses are not always purely synergistic responses. There are environmental conditions in which there is an overlap in postural requirements calling on the nervous system to mix the strategies (hip, ankle, and step). The synergies cannot occur simultaneously, for if they did, the joints would be frozen because the agonist and antagonist muscles would try to contract at the same time.

All Responses

There are some important factors that are necessary for all of the automatic postural responses to be effective. There must be normal latency and amplitude of the muscle responses for a normal postural response to occur. Postural responses occur within 100 to 120 milliseconds after a perturbation, which is a much shorter time delay than the time it takes from the initiation of a volitional motor response to the completion of a voluntary motor movement (24). Postural responses have a rapid buildup in muscular force and amplitude because motor units are recruited rapidly.

The postural responses must occur in a properly timed fashion after the initial perturbation. In the ankle synergy, the hamstring stabilizes the knee joint against forces that are generated distally. There must be a very short, but well-timed delay between the activation of the hamstrings and the muscles activated across the hip in order to stabilize proximally. If any of these factors are disrupted in a patient's postural response, the clinician observes the patient producing an inefficient postural response, unstable center of gravity, unstable knee joint, and falling.

CLINICAL SYNDROMES

Vestibular System Lesions

In many neurologic conditions, a lesion in the vestibular system is totally unsuspected, yet it turns out to profoundly affect balance. The source of vestibular input is located in the inner ear (Figure 9.2). The next center is the vestibular nucleus in the medulla. Pathways then cross over to the medial brainstem, ascending through the medial brainstem, the pons, and midbrain. From there, the information travels through the thalamus and ascends to certain areas in the parietal lobe, particularly the parietal insula region (18). The parietal insula is where the internal sensory map is created. If vestibular pathways are disrupted anywhere along this pathway, there will be an impaired sensory map. If the disruption is in the inner ear or the medulla, the person will have a postural bias toward the side of the lesion. If the disruption is anywhere above the medulla, the person will be biased away from the side of the lesion.

Motor System Lesions

How do the individual parts of the nervous system contribute to the postural responses as we have defined them? The *pyramidal system* is

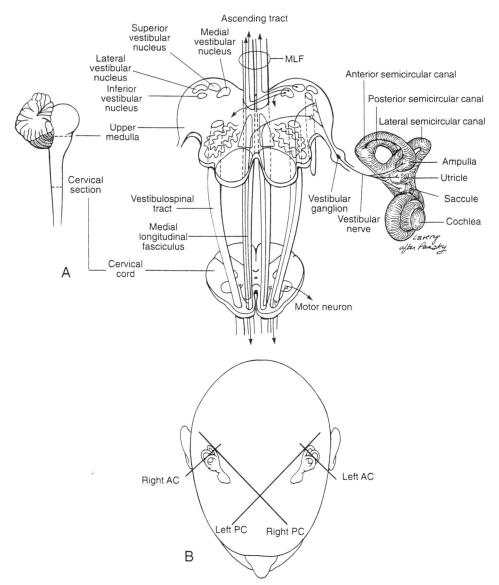

Figure 9.2 Vestibular system. (A) Schematic drawing of the membranous labyrinth (otoliths and semicircular canals) and the central connections of the vestibular system. Shown are the ascending vestibular inputs to the oculomotor complex, important for stabilizing gaze, and the descending vestibulospinal system, important for posture and balance. (B) Location of the paired semicircular canals within the temporal bone of the skull. AC = anterior canal; PC = posterior canal. (Reproduced with permission from Shumway-Cook A, Woollacott M. Motor control: theory and practical applications. Baltimore: Williams & Wilkins, 1995.)

the primary motor pathway through which the commands for postural motor responses pass. The commands originate somewhat lower in the nervous system than do volitional commands, but the pathway is the same. The latency of response is shorter because the site at which the responses are generated is below the cortex of the hemisphere. The *pyramidal tract* is the pathway through which the motor commands must pass in order to get to the muscles of the limb and the trunk. Muscle contractions are then generated in the form of ankle, hip, and step strategies. If there is a lesion in the pyramidal pathways anywhere from the point at which the origin of the response is generated, up through the point at which it must be carried forth, you will have disruption of the postural strategy mediated by the limb that is being supplied by that pyramidal pathway. These areas include the subcortical areas of each hemisphere, the internal capsule, the pyramidal tract in the brainstem, or the corticospinal tract in the spinal cord.

What are these disruptions? Depending on the degree of impairment of the pyramidal tract, the force of the response or the latency of the response, or both, may be significantly affected. The number of motor units, the amplitude of motor units, the time at which the first motor unit contracts, and the time over which all of the motor units are able to act may all be distorted. In other words, the response may be delayed in onset, too weak, and the generation of force may be spread over such a long period of time that the postural response is ineffective.

The demands on the pyramidal system for automatic postural responses far exceed those associated with volitional movements. When testing strength, the pyramidal system is evaluated in the functional setting by asking patients to generate volitional, tonic contractions of their muscles. Hundreds of milliseconds are allowed to recruit as many of the motor units as possible. In order to determine whether the pyramidal system function is sufficient for postural responses, it must be realized that the response occurs in only 100 milliseconds, most of the response must be applied over another 50 or 60 milliseconds thereafter, and the force must be quite high. Standard muscle testing does not evaluate whether the pyramidal system is impaired in a way that disrupts postural motor responses. In practical terms, many patients who have hemiparesis but recover volitional strength will still present with significant impairments of postural motor responses in the involved extremity. This impairment manifests itself as instability in the joint control of the limb. Postural sway will be increased because the force at the ankle is applied too late and spread over too much time. Therefore, patients with pyramidal lesions can have excessive sway and demonstrable dyssynergy in the limb due to muscle weakness, a disruption in the timing of automatic postural responses, or a combination of these impairments. Evaluation must attempt to delineate the problems in order to properly form a treatment plan.

Cerebellar System Lesions

The cerebellum (Figure 9.3) modulates postural responses much in the same way it does for volitional movements (25,26). It is not a generator of movement. It matches the amplitude of the response to the ampli-

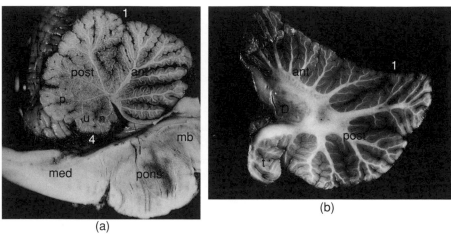

Figure 9.3 *Sections through the cerebellum: (a) in the midline, showing division of cerebellar vermis; (b) oblique, passing through the dentate nucleus. ant = anterior lobe; D = dentate nucleus; l = lingula; mb = midbrain; med = medulla; n = nodulus; p = pyramis; post = posterior lobe; t = tonsil; u = uvula; 1 = primary fissure; 4 = fourth ventricle. (Reprinted from Esiri MM, Oppenheimer DR. Diagnostic neuropathology: a practical manual. Oxford: Blackwell Scientific, 1989:38.)*

tude of the stimulus. If there is a perturbation of a medium amplitude, the muscle forces must be of a similar amplitude to stabilize the center of gravity in a coordinated manner. If too much force is applied to the muscle, the center of gravity sway will not only be counteracted but will be driven beyond the initial position, and the body will be thrown back beyond the initial position. If too little force is applied, the sway will not be counteracted and the fall in the direction of the perturbation will not be avoided. Patients with cerebellar lesions tend to have an overshooting of the intended response (*hypermetric responses*). This sets up a "to and fro" oscillation of center of gravity movement, leading to overshooting in each direction. The response is ineffective because of the uncoordinated amplitude. This is most noticeable at the knee and is observed as an excessive flexion–extension oscillation. The knee appears weak or unstable.

Basal Ganglia Lesions

The basal ganglia control the sequencing of balance strategies (27,28). Severe basal ganglia pathology, such as Parkinson's disease, is thought to cause a simultaneous firing of both the ankle and hip strategies. Each individual strategy has the proper force and timing; however, they are generated simultaneously. Thus, the muscles on the anterior and posterior aspects of the hip, knee, and ankle joints contract at the same time, essentially freezing the joints and producing a rigid posture. Patients with basal ganglia lesions retain some ability to control postural sway about the ankles; therefore, these patients can remain balanced if they are not significantly perturbed. When there is a significant perturbation, an abrupt fall usually occurs with the appearance that no balance strategy has been generated. In reality, however, both hip and ankle strategies have been simultaneously produced.

Thalamic Lesions

If they are small enough, thalamic lesions will involve only the ascending vestibular pathways (29,30). Patients will be posturally biased

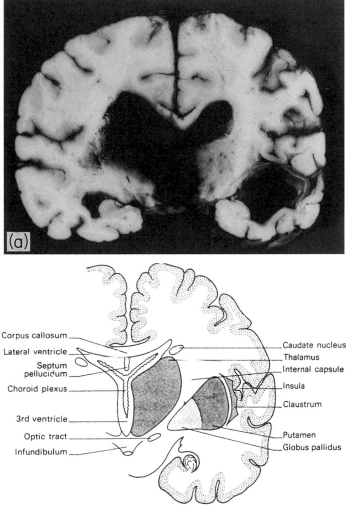

(b)

Figure 9.4   (a) Cerebral hemorrhages in a hypertensive, 61-year-old woman. The lesion involves the *right* thalamus, causing a postural bias to the *left* side. (Reprinted from Esiri MM, Oppenheimer DR. Diagnostic neuropathology: a practical manual. Oxford: Blackwell Scientific, 1989:103.) (b) The thalamus and 3rd ventricle in coronal section. (Reprinted from Ellis H. Clinical anatomy, 9th ed. Oxford: Blackwell Science, 1997:373.)

toward the contralateral side. With extensive lesions, patients have a significant hemisensory loss and demonstrate marked incoordination of postural motor responses on the contralateral side (Figure 9.4). Postural bias occurs to the contralateral side, perhaps onto a limb that is uncoordinated because of poor sensory mapping.

Parietal Lesions

Parietal lesions will affect the nervous system's sensory map. As discussed earlier, vestibular pathways terminate in this region of the brain (13,18). With a right parietal lesion, the patient will be biased to the left and will have poor sensory mapping of the left limbs. All motor activity planned with a poor sensory map will be uncoordinated.

CLINICAL EXAMPLES

The following examples will provide information regarding clinical findings with lesions in two different areas of brain involving vestibular pathways. Table 9.1 provides a summary of the comparison of the examples.

Lateral Medullary Infarct

A lesion in the lateral medulla can involve two neurologic structures that will directly affect postural control: the cerebellar connections and vestibular inputs (Figure 9.5). This lesion causes a sudden loss of vestibular inputs unilaterally to one side of the nervous system. Slowly, the brain adjusts by using visual and proprioceptive information to

Table 9.1. Comparison of Left Lateral Medullary and Paramedian Pontine Lesions

	Lateral Medullary (Brainstem)	Paramedian Pons-Midbrain (Midbrain)
Critical structures	Left unilateral vestibular pathways Left unilateral cerebellar pathways	Right unilateral vestibular pathways Bilateral cerebellar pathways Right pyramidal tract
Postural bias	Left	Right
Other clinical signs	Abnormal perception of upright Sensory organization deficit	Abnormal perception of upright Sensory organization deficit

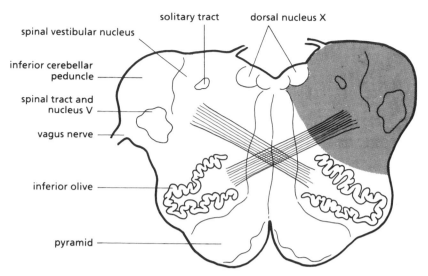

spinal vestibular nucleus

solitary tract

dorsal nucleus X

inferior cerebellar peduncle

spinal tract and nucleus V

vagus nerve

inferior olive

pyramid

Figure 9.5 *Area of the medulla commonly supplied by the posterior inferior cerebellar artery (stippled). Structures involved in the lateral medullary syndrome include the inferior cerebellar peduncle, containing the dorsal spinocerebellar tract and olivocerebellar fibers from the opposite side; the spinal (descending) vestibular tract and nucleus; emerging and entering fibers of the vagus nerve; the spinal (descending) trigeminal tract and nucleus; and a mixture of ascending and descending pathways, continuous with the anterolateral columns of the cervical cord, including the spinothalamic and spinoreticular (sensory) pathways and the upper sympathetic fibers running from the hypothalamus to the intermediolateral columns of the spinal cord. Damage to the cerebellar and vestibular connections affects postural control.* (Reprinted from Esiri MM, Oppenheimer DR. Diagnostic neuropathology: a practical manual. Oxford: Blackwell Scientific, 1989:376.)

relearn that the earth's vertical (and the world) is not tipped to the side of the lesion. A patient who has a left brainstem infarct will perceive the world as being tipped to the left. Consequently, this person stands with a bias to the left, and all postural responses are generated relative to this new perception of the center of gravity and the limits of stability. The result is that this patient will weight-shift too far to the left without preventing a fall, but will generate premature postural responses with right-sided weight shifts.

The patient with a lateral medullary lesion is unable to differentiate between accurate and inaccurate proprioceptive and visual inputs, leading to sensory selection problems and use of incorrect strategies. In addition, because of loss of accurate vestibular input, this patient will not perform hip strategies when nearing a loss of balance.

Cerebellar involvement affects the coordination of motor responses in the arm and leg. With a lesion on the left, postural motor synergies on the left side will be inappropriately mediated, resulting in overshooting of limb movement in all directions. Consequently, this patient presents with major problems of knee control when trying to maintain postural stability. Patients with this clinical profile are perversely tipped toward the side of their lesion and bear weight primarily on the pathologically involved lower extremity. However, this limb is not able to generate effective postural motor responses. A patient with pure motor hemiparesis or any other brain injury that does not involve vestibular pathways will have a postural bias toward the uninvolved side, rather than the involved side. The prognosis for improvement of balance disorders associated with a lateral medullary infarct is good. The incoordination and abnormal segmental control impairments also improve, but to a variable degree.

Paramedian Pons-Midbrain Infarct

Traveling through the medulla, the vestibular pathways cross (decussate) and proceed to the medial brainstem. Vascular lesions often occur in the paramedian pons or midbrain secondary to the rich vascularity of this brain region (Figure 9.6). The critical structures for balance in this area are the ascending vestibular pathways, the decussating cerebellar pathways, and the pyramidal tract. A patient with a paramedian pons or midbrain lesion will also manifest a postural bias. In this case, the bias occurs to the opposite side of the lesion, but again, toward the impaired extremity. A patient with a left paramedian infarct is biased to the right, since the vestibular information is coming from the right inner ear prior to the crossing of the fibers. Since there is right pyramidal tract involvement, many of these patients are described as

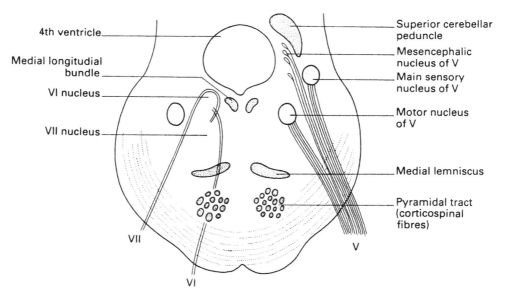

Figure 9.6 The pons—level of the right 4th nerve nucleus and the intrapontine course of the facial nerve and, on the left, of the nuclei of V. (Reprinted from Ellis H. Clinical anatomy, 9th ed. Oxford: Blackwell Science, 1997:369.)

having pure motor hemiparesis. The common classification for this patient is ataxic hemiparesis or hemiataxia. Postural responses on the right are uncoordinated because of pyramidal and cerebellar pathway involvement. Treatment for these patients should also consider the mild incoordination on the contralateral side. This is due to the fact that the cerebellar pathways are decussating in this region.

These patients are more difficult to rehabilitate than patients with a lateral medullary lesion. The recovery process is often longer than in the lateral medullary lesion, and the prognosis is often underestimated because the treating clinician relates the decreased limb coordination to pyramidal effects rather than to the cerebellar insult. With involvement of the cerebellar pathways, the clinician must recognize that until natural recovery begins the patient will not shift weight onto the unaffected side. This limitation can significantly impair the patient's early performance in therapy.

CLINICAL EVALUATION

Preparation/Chart review

The clinician's assessment must begin before meeting the patient by reviewing his or her medical record. It is important to look in the history for initial or persistent symptoms of vertigo, nausea, vomiting, double vision, or swallowing problems, as these symptoms are indicative of vestibular, brainstem, or cerebellar dysfunction. Acute neuroimaging studies combined with the neurologist's assessment will help determine the location and size of the lesion. It is essential to know the location of the lesion. The fact that initial neuroimaging studies are negative may not be conclusive. Lesions, especially small ones within the cerebellum, midbrain, pons, and brainstem, are often not detected by brain CT scans. Therefore, the clinical assessment and later MRI reports are important in determining whether a patient has had damage in any of these areas. If available, results of specific vestibular testing can localize lesions to the vestibular system, helping to determine the patient's prognosis. Examples of vestibular tests include electronystagmography, calorics, brainstem auditory responses, sinusoidal rotary chair, and dynamic posturography.

ASSESSMENT

Balance involves cognitive, perceptual, musculoskeletal, neuromuscular, vestibulo-ocular, and vestibulospinal components. Most of the guidelines presented here are focused on understanding the balance impairments that are produced by vestibular dysfunction, or those which cannot be accounted for on the basis of cognitive, musculoskeletal, tonal, or sensorimotor deficits. If the latter areas are involved, it is assumed that they will be evaluated and treated in conjunction with the vestibular deficits.

There are a number of assessment tools in the literature (31–35). Table 9.2 is an example of a balance evaluation. The Appendix to this chapter provides the detailed guidelines for performing and documenting the evaluation. The evaluation is separated into four parts. The emphasis is on standing balance. However, Parts I–III can be applied to sitting balance, if needed, depending on the functional level of the patient. The evaluation should be performed without upper extremity support.

When the evaluation is complete, the clinician should develop an impression of the specific reason the patient has a balance impairment. If there is more than one reason, the clinician must try to discern the relative contribution and prognosis of each factor. Only then can sound plans be made for the type, timing, and progression of treatment for the balance impairment.

PRINCIPLES OF TREATMENT

There are many variables to be considered in planning treatment for patients with balance impairment. Answering the question of why the patient is not producing effective balance reactions becomes a primary precursor to treatment. The clinician should identify the areas of the nervous system involved and relate the pathology to which impairments are likely to spontaneously resolve, which are irreversible, and which can be remedied by therapy. For example, in a 70-year-old male who suffers a stroke resulting in disruption of balance control who has a history of macular degeneration and peripheral neuropathy, it becomes obvious that the irreversible elements of his history (macular degeneration and peripheral neuropathy) will hinder CNS compensation for his deficits through use of vision and proprioception. A person with the same primary diagnosis with normal vision and proprioception could use these systems to provide compensatory input for balance control.

The treatment variables to be considered and manipulated when designing treatment plans include the sensory environment, the type of movements or tasks required of the patient, the base of support, and the difficulty of, or multiplicity of, the tasks. Treatment plans should be creative and designed to place demands on each of the variables involved. The parameters of balance addressed in treatment are the same as those initially assessed. This section will provide more specifics

Table 9.2. *Balance Evaluation*

Section I Static Balance—Limits of Stability

POSITION	ASSISTANCE	SWAY	POSTURE	COMMENTS
Sit-static				
Sit-L.O.S. (Lateral)				
Sit-L.O.S. (A-P)				
Stand-static				
Stand-L.O.S. (Lateral)				
Stand-L.O.S. (A-P)				

Perception of Midline:	

Section II Automatic Postural Responses

POSITION	1	2	3	ASSUME	STRATEGY	SWAY	COMMENTS
Preferred B.O.S. ( )							
Narrow B.O.S. ( )							
Tandem							
Beam-Lateral							
Beam-A-P							
Unilateral-L							
Unilateral-R							
Eyes Closed							
Foam							
Foam, eyes closed							
Induced hip strategy							

Section III

FUNCTIONAL BALANCE		ASSISTANCE	COMMENTS
SIT/STAND			
REACHING 1	1 (<25% LOS)		
	2 (25–75% LOS)		
	3 (75–100% LOS)		
Sit → stand			
Stand → sit			
Stand → floor			
Floor → stand			

Table 9.2 (continued)

Section IV *GAIT EVALUATION*

Specific patient complaints: _____

Deviations: _____

Specific observations (circle items below)

Initiation of gait	normal	mildly decreased	significantly decreased	
Rate of gait: (time per 50 ft)	fast (<20)	normal (20–25)	slow (50)	very slow (75) (seconds)
Step length symmetry:	normal	short bilateral	short left	short right
Degree:	N/A	mild	moderate	severe
Stance phase duration:		symmetrical	long left	long right
Accuracy of foot placement	Left:	normal	mildly decreased	significantly decreased
	Right:	normal	mildly decreased	significantly decreased
Base of support	wide	normal	narrow	
Postural bias:	none	left	right	Anterior Posterior
Postural bias rating:	none N/A	mild left stance	moderate right stance	severe both
Phase of loss of balance:				
Direction of loss of balance:	N/A Left/Ant.	Left Left/Post.	Right Right/Post.	Anterior, Posterior Right/Ant.

GAIT ENDURANCE: Normal

	Level 1:	More than 500 feet causes decreased quality, but patient can safely continue
	Level 2:	More than 500 feet causes decreased quality and patient must rest.
	Level 3:	Tolerates 200 to less than 500 feet.
	Level 4:	Tolerates 51 to 199 feet.
	Level 5:	Tolerates 5–50 feet.
	Level 6:	Unable to ambulate > 4 feet.

Level of Assistance	I	Cues	S	CG
	Min	Mod	Max	D

Table 9.2 (continued)

AMBULATION	TIME	ASSISTANCE	LOSS OF BALANCE	LINE OF PROGRESSION	COMMENTS
Forward 50 ft.					
Head turns 50 ft.					
Eyes closed 25 ft.					

FUNCTIONAL GAIT	ASSISTANCE	COMMENTS
Tandem		
Beam-lateral		
Beam A-P		
Pivot quickly		
Sudden stop		
Uneven surface		
Step-over		
Backwards		
Narrow area		
Carrying a glass		
Stairs		

ADVANCED GROSS MOTOR ACTIVITIES

	ASSISTANCE	#REPS/TIME	COMMENTS
Jumping Jacks			
Hopping L/R			
Split Jacks			
Running 50 ft.			

FUNCTIONAL GAIT CATEGORY (circle one)

Non-ambulatory
Therapeutic ambulator
Assisted household ambulator
Limited household ambulator (independent)
Household ambulator (independent)

Limited community ambulator (independent)
Community ambulator (independent)
Unlimited ambulator (including sports/fitness activities)

regarding treatment guidelines and suggestions for progressive treatment activities.

Center of Gravity Control

The combination of maintaining one's center of gravity in midline with correct postural alignment is the precursor to all progress in treatment. There are three primary areas to be addressed when treating center of gravity control problems. These areas are postural alignment, center of gravity alignment, and limits of stability.

Corrections of poor postural alignment incorporate any activities that will improve segmental alignment, which, in turn, will affect center of gravity alignment. Stretching and strengthening exercises are important for normalizing postural alignment. For some patients, abnormal center of gravity control is related to postural alignment deficits caused by abnormal tone, decreased active movement, or biomechanical constraints. In other cases, patients have an abnormal perception of center of gravity alignment. These individuals perceive their center of gravity as being in midline, when it is actually shifted (biased) to one side. As discussed, this is common in the hemiataxic patient with unilateral cerebellar or unilateral central vestibular damage who presents with a bias toward the involved side. In either case, the goal of treatment is to teach the patient to maintain the center of gravity in midline over the given base of support and with as normal a center of gravity as possible.

Retraining perception of center of gravity alignment requires the patient to be able to follow instructions so that he or she can learn how to use available normal sensory inputs to correct the postural bias. In situations where patients are unable to follow instructions, the therapist may manually assist the patient to perform treatment activities and experience more normal alignment of the center of gravity. Retraining the perception of center of gravity alignment starts with the patient's gaining an understanding of the concept of center of gravity. Patient education centers around increasing the patient's awareness of how to use feedback from varied senses to detect midline. For example, a patient can use the sensation of pressure under his feet to detect midline center of gravity. For the patient who presents with a rightward bias, learning that midline is realized when he feels more pressure under his *left* foot is essential prior to further instruction. This involves a degree of trust as well as the provision of visual feedback to reinforce midline. The most effective feedback is that which coincides with the center of gravity alignment, as opposed to just postural alignment.

Another key concept the patient must understand about center of gravity control is that in order to successfully internalize normal center of gravity alignment, he has to move his posture to midline through use of volitional movements. Patients who fail to do this will not change their postural bias. For the patient with a rightward bias, failure to truly internalize center of gravity alignment may result in lateral trunk flexion to the left, but with a majority of weight still shifted to the right. It is vital that a patient develop a sense of normal center of gravity alignment because problems in this area will cause problems in all areas from static stance, dynamic stance, and walking. Table 9.3 provides treatment guidelines and suggestions for center of gravity control problems, including the components of postural alignment, center of gravity alignment, and limits of stability.

Sensory Organization

Varying the sensory environments during the patient's evaluation and subsequent therapy sessions permits the therapist to identify sensory organization problems. Treatment plans begin with patient education and retraining the perception of center of gravity alignment. Patients will learn how to use available sensory information, starting with the maximum use of proprioceptive and visual feedback. Treatment progresses by applying activities commensurate with each patient's sensory dependency. Table 9.4 outlines treatment concepts and suggestions to consider for patients with visual and/or support surface dependency.

Table 9.3. Treatment Suggestions for Patients with Center of Gravity Control Problems

Treatment Goal	Treatment Suggestions
Postural Alignment	
Normalize muscle length/joint range of motion, and segmental alignment.	Stretching/strengthening exercises focusing on cervical, trunk and lower extremity muscles Neuromuscular techniques
COG Alignment	
Retrain midline	Midline stance using maximum feedback. Stand in front of mirror, stance in front of grid scale representative of sway area, or on computerized force plate system
Retrain lateral limits of stability	Midline stance, weight shift lateral limits of stability to 50% Attach flashlight to belt and weight shift between two targets on the wall
Retrain anterior-posterior limits of stability	Midline stance, weight shift anterior-posterior limits of stability to 50%
Increase speed of movements	Increase speed of weight shifts using an auditory pacing device
Vary BOS	Narrow BOS, one-legged stance
Vary visual or proprioceptive inputs	Midline stance with eyes closed or on compliant surface
Progress by:	Increasing target distance Increasing speed of weight shifts Decreasing visual and proprioceptive cues

Table 9.4. Treatment Suggestions for Patients with Visual and/or Support Surface Dependency

Treatment Goal	Treatment Suggestions
Visually Dependent	
Provide maximum, accurate proprioceptive inputs	Stand on firm support surface
Reduce the availability of accurate visual orientation inputs	Eyes open, look at target/no target Eyes closed, intermittently at first
Gradually increase the availability and complexity of visual inputs for postural orientation	Standing weight shifts while looking at checkerboard or striped background
As patient progresses, slowly decrease available proprioceptive inputs	Weight shifting, marching with movement occurring in visual environment Any of above activities while standing on a compliant surface
Support Surface Dependent	
Provide maximum accurate visual inputs	Stand in stable environment with fixed visual targets
Reduce the availability of accurate proprioceptive inputs	Narrow base of support
As patient progresses, slowly decrease the available visual inputs	March in place Stand on foam/compliant surface Walk on uneven terrain Incorporate head turns and body turns to above activities Add eye closure and more complex visual environments

For patients with a combination of visual and support surface dependency, conflicts occur when they are asked to rely on vestibular inputs alone. The critical clinical decision is to determine which area is more involved, vision or proprioception. Based on this assessment, the goal is to decide how and when to maximally challenge each sensory dependency. The treatment suggestions listed in Table 9.4 can be combined to increase patient reliance on vestibular inputs.

Automatic Postural Reactions

The therapist must attempt to identify the specific abnormalities in automatic postural response: for example, onset, latency, amplitude, coordination, or selection of the response. Treatment activities (Table 9.5) are designed to facilitate each strategy by utilizing context-specific techniques. Remember to consider what is appropriate for each patient given his or her age and living situation. For instance, a young healthy person should rely primarily on an ankle strategy when standing on a balance beam. Conversely, an elderly person with decreased ankle strength and range of motion should utilize more of a hip strategy in this same situation.

Table 9.5.   Treatment Suggestions for Patients with Automatic Postural Reaction Abnormalities

Treatment Goals	Treatment Suggestions
Ankle Strategy	
Maximize proprioceptive input from the support surface for orientation	Lateral weight shifts Anterior-posterior weight shifts
Maximize external feedback, including vision	Reaching, head and/or trunk turns
Facilitate forces at the ankles, without movement at the hips and knees	
Incorporate into functional activities	
Hip Strategy	
Reduce ability to exert ankle torque to the support surface	Tandem stance and walking External perturbations
Facilitate reciprocal hip movements	Balance beam activity Activities involving movement of center of gravity to outer edges of BOS Unilateral stance Standing on foam Kicking a ball Stand on tilt/rocker board
Stepping Strategy	
Final strategy essential in preventing a fall when limits of stability are exceeded	Activities involving movement of center of gravity outside of BOS Large external perturbations to produce a step Unweight the "stepping leg"

Balance Training in Ambulation

The principles outlined in Table 9.5 also should be utilized during gait balance training. The goals are the same for gait as they are for retraining standing balance. Specifically, they are to train normal perception and control of center of gravity during the gait cycle, to enhance the patient's ability to maintain center of gravity control within altered sensory environments, and to facilitate automatic postural responses appropriate to the environment. The following is a sample of activities that go beyond the basic forward progression gait training.

- Walking with head turns
- Variations in speed
- Sudden stops
- Carrying objects
- Reading a book
- Narrowed base of stability
- Random turns
- Backwards/sideways
- Consistently altered environment
- Random altered environment

CASE EXAMPLE

A 68-year-old woman presents with a chief complaint of progressive unsteadiness and bouts of dizziness over 4 years. She is a diabetic with associated retinopathy and peripheral neuropathy and with known multi-infarct disease. She reports a good deal of low-back pain and pain in the right leg and thigh. She describes a tendency to experience dizziness, which is largely confined to times when she rises rapidly or quickly changes position from supine to standing. This resolves in minutes. The patient has had many falls that she attributes to her unsteadiness and not to dizzy spells. She reports no spontaneous dizziness. She has mild, insidiously progressive hearing loss but no tinnitus.

The patient lives with her husband who is able to physically assist her. She is independent in all activities of daily living in sitting and standing positions. She walks in the home independently but generally uses the furniture and walls for support. She does not walk in the house at night alone and requires her husband's arm for support whenever walking outside. She reports she has not walked outside alone for about 1 year and during that time the most she would walk at any one time is 4 to 5 minutes. She does light meal preparation but no other housework.

An MRI of the brain performed 1 year ago disclosed moderate cortical atrophy and small focal lesions in the periventricular areas, left caudate, and globus pallidus and in the brainstem. A repeat MRI 1 month prior to evaluation revealed additional, widespread periventricular small vessel disease in the right caudate, putamen and thalamic regions, central pons, and left paramedian pons.

The current neurology examination revealed normal auditory canals and tympanic membranes with functional hearing. There is one-half to three quarters of the normal range of motion in the neck with no complaints of pain. Visual acuity is 20/25 in the left eye and essentially absent (blind) in the right eye. There is no spontaneous or gaze nystagmus but post head shaking there is a brief burst of left beating horizontal nystagmus behind Fresnel glasses. Positional testing discloses a low intensity but persistent static second degree left beating nystagmus behind Fresnel glasses most evident with the right ear down.

Sensory exam discloses dulling of vibration at the ankles symmetrically and moderate loss of proprioception at the toes bilaterally. There is dulling of superficial sensations in a stocking distribution symmetrically. Joint range of motion is functional except for $-10°$ from neutral in the left ankle and $-15°$ degrees in the right ankle. Muscle tone is normal. Stretch receptor reflexes are 1+ in the upper extremities and absent in the lower extremities. Muscle flexibility is mild to moderately diminished in the lumbar extensors, quadriceps, hamstrings, and gastrosoleus bilaterally, somewhat greater on the left. There is no focal weakness in the legs; however strength is generally 4/5 on the right and 4+/5 on the left. Limb coordination is mildly decreased in the right leg on heel-to-shin testing.

The patient is able to rise from sitting but with decreased forward flexion to initiate, and she requires upper extremity support. She is able to stand with a 3-inch base of support (BOS) on a flat, stable support surface, but there is increased postural sway, a clear right bias, and a slight anterior bias given her preferred posture which is with 10° to 15° of hip, knee, and ankle flexion bilaterally. When attempts are made to correct her posture volitionally, there is a moderate posterior bias of center of gravity. The patient's attempt to control postural sway involves poorly coordinated ankle strategies manifested by out of phase oscillations of low amplitude and high frequency at the knees and ankles, right greater than left. The remainder of the body is held rigidly. The patient is unable to maintain her balance with eye closure in the 3-inch base of support on a compliant piece of foam, falling backward and to the right without evidence of balance reactions. She is unable to stand on one foot or tandem walk along a 3-inch-wide beam. She produces no hip strategies, but there are ineffective lateral step strategies stimulated in these tasks. Volitional weight shifts are within 40% to 50% of the normal range to the left and 65% to the right.

Unassisted, the patient's walking discloses a staggering, ataxic gait. Specific deviations include minimally decreased initiation; increased base of support; moderately, but right greater than left, shortened stride length; right postural bias and decreased weight shift to the left; and inaccuracy of right foot placement. She generally requires minimal assistance to walk 25 feet. Line of progression is slightly right but overall staggering. She falls when asked to perform head turns, eye closure, or full turns.

Computerized vestibular function testing discloses an asymmetry of vestibulo-ocular reflex responses at high peak velocity stimulus (300 degrees per second). This finding documents a unilateral lesion involving vestibulo-ocular pathways, likely on the right. Visuo-ocular/vestibulo-ocular integration testing was abnormal, with a failure of fixation suppression documenting a central locus of vestibular pathology involving those pathways.

The sensory organization portion of the dynamic posturography provided no localizing information in that the patient was only able to sustain balance when provided with maximal visual and support surface cues. She fell to the right and posterior with any changes in vision or support surface cues. Electromyographic monitoring of long latency automatic postural responses produced by upward rotations of the platform, demonstrated significant prolongation of latency of onset and severe delay in time to peak of response. These findings indicate that the peripheral neuropathy in this patient is contributing significantly to the impairment in postural responses mediated by the lower extremities.

It is well documented that the patient has multisystem pathology largely as a consequence of her diabetes. The assessment has confirmed this and added more specific localization and correlation with her functional impairments. Specifically, the patient does indeed have vestibular system involvement from her brainstem small vessel disease, which correlates with the documented infarct in the right paramedian pons. This central vestibular lesion is almost certainly responsible for the patient's motion/position induced dizziness and is a significant component of her gait ataxia. Her clear postural bias to the right is a common manifestation of lesions at this site. It is well documented that the patient has peripheral neuropathy, and the postural electromyographic results signify that this is contributing to her disequilibrium out of proportion to that expected from her afferent (sensory) loss as seen on physical exam alone. The patient's marked visual and support surface dependence is due to the combination of her peripheral neuropathy and her central vestibular lesion. The patient's lower extremity dyssynergy of postural automatic responses is on the basis of both peripheral neuropathy and mild cerebellar pathway involvement in the brainstem. The patient's visual disturbances also contribute to her balance impairment, but it is difficult to know the actual degree. It is clear that none of this pathology is reversible.

Given these findings, the potential for functional improvement in gait is very guarded. However, the patient does not have a degree of weakness and is able to participate and understand the rationale for treatment. Additionally, she has family available to assist her in carrying out a home program. Consistent, daily performance of exercises and cueing as to the appropriate execution of balance retraining tasks is imperative. Given her lack of activity over the past year, she will also benefit from the conditioning aspects of a physical therapy program. It will be clearer after 2 or 3 weeks of aggressive balance retraining whether she has the potential to achieve independent ambulation within the home and endurance for ambulatory distances that will allow her to functionally access the community with a minimum of assistance.

The primary goals of therapy are to determine if the patient can learn to attain midline center of gravity alignment and control volitional weight shifts symmetrically in all planes to at least 65%. Treatment should also focus on providing the patient with the most suitable assistance and assistive devices. Of course, initial treatment goals would also include increasing range of motion and strength, improving bed mobility, sitting, sit to stand, and static standing activities.

If the patient does attain the initial balance goals, progression should be aggressive and include altering visual input to maximize the use of available proprioceptive input. Initially the patient should be allowed to have a wide, stable base of support. However, varied stance positions and widths should be introduced as soon as possible. Treatment principles should be extended to gait as early as possible. It is important to have the patient feel safe but work without actual physical assistance during practice sessions. Teaching the family to provide this type of "guarding" is extremely beneficial so she can have frequent exposure to "feeling" her own balance. During daily activities, she should be given physical assistance for safety.

It is unlikely that this patient will regain functional hip strategies due to the multiplicity of her deficits. Treatment should, however, include some work in this area with the goal of improving her overall balance reactions.

CONCLUSION

Balance is a complex neurobehavioral function that can be disrupted by a number of neuropathologies. The neurologic rehabilitation model insists on accurate diagnosis of handicapping conditions produced by the underlying lesions. Treatment planning then unfolds based on a realistic assessment of what can be remediated, what can be compensated for, and, finally, what should either spontaneously improve or be accepted as irreversible.

References

1. Nashner LM, McCollum G. The organization of human postural movements: a formal basis and experimental synthesis. Behav Brain Sci 1985;8:135–172.
2. Shumway-Cook A, Horak FB. Vestibular rehabilitation: an exercise approach to managing symptoms of vestibular dysfunction. Semin Hear 1989;10:196–209.
3. Hayes KC. Biomechanics of postural control. Exerc Sport Sci Rev 1982;10:363–391.
4. Moore SP, Horak FB, Nashner LM. The effect of prior leaning on human postural responses. Gait Posture 1993;1:203–210.
5. Murray MP, Seireg A, Scholz RC. Center of gravity, center of pressure and supportive forces during human activities. J Appl Physiol 1967;26:831–838.
6. Palmer CE. Studies of the center of gravity in the human body. Child Dev 1944;15:99–179.
7. Webb P. Bioastronautics data book. NASA SP-3006. Washington, DC, 1964.

8. Balance master system operator manual, version 2.10. Clackamas, OR: Neurocom International, Inc., 1989.

9. McCollum GM, Leen TK. Form and exploration of mechanical stability limits in erect stance. J Motor Behav 1989;21:225–244.

10. Horak FB, Nashner LM. Central programming of postural movements. Adaptations to altered support surface conditions. J Neurophysiol 1986;55:1369–1381.

11. Nashner LM. Fixed patterns of rapid postural responses among leg muscles during stance. Exp Brain Res 1977;30:13–24.

12. Amblard B, Assainanle J, Cremieux J, Marchand AR. From posture to gait: which sensory input for which function? In: Brandt TH, Paulus W, Bies W, et al, eds. Disorders of posture and gait. New York: Elsevier Science, 1990:168–176.

13. Baloh RW, Honrubia V. The central vestibular system. In: Clinical neurophysiology of the vestibular system. Philadelphia: FA Davis, 1979: 47–100.

14. Quoniam C, Roll JP, Deat A, Massian J. Proprioceptive induced interactions between segmental and whole body posture. In: Brandt TH, Paulus W, Bies W, et al, eds. Disorders of posture and gait. New York: Elsevier Science, 1990:194–197.

15. Kotaka S, Croll GA, Bles W. Somatosensory ataxia. In: Brandt TH, Paulus W, Bies W, et al, eds. Disorders of posture and gait. New York: Elsevier Science, 1990:177–183.

16. Nashner LM, Black FO, Wall C. Adaptation to altered support and visual conditions during stance. Patients with vestibular deficits. J Neurol Sci 1982;5:536–543.

17. Nashner LM, Woollacott M, Tuma G. Organization of rapid responses to postural and locomotor-like perturbations of standing man. Exp Brain Res 1979;36:463–476.

18. Baloh RW, Honrubia V. Clinical neurophysiology of the vestibular system. Philadelphia: FA Davis, 1979.

19. Black FO, Shupert CL, Horak FB, Nashner LM. Abnormal postural control associated with peripheral vestibular disorders. In: Pompeiano O, Allum JHJ, eds. Progression in brain research. New York: Elsevier Science, 1988:263–275.

20. Horak F, Nashner LM, Diener HC. Postural strategies associated with somatosensory and vestibular loss. Exp Brain Res 1990;82:167–177.

21. Brandt TH, Paulus W, Straube A. Vision and posture. In: Brandt TH, Paulus W, Bies W, et al, eds. Disorders of posture and gait. New York: Elsevier Science, 1990:157–175.

22. Forssberg H, Nashner LM. Ontogenetic development of postural control in man: adaptation to altered support and visual conditions during stance. J Neuro Sci 1982;5:545–552.

23. Equitest System, version 4.0. Data Interpretation Manual. Clackamas, OR: Neurocom International, Inc., 1991.

24. Nashner LM, Cordo PJ. Relation of automatic postural responses and reaction-time. Voluntary movements of human leg muscles. Exp Brain Res 1981;43:395–405.

25. Dichgans J, Diener HC. Different forms of postural ataxia in patients with cerebellar diseases. In: Brandt TH, Paulus W, Bies W, et al, eds. Disorders of posture and gait. New York: Elsevier Science, 1990:207–215.

26. Horak FB, Diener HC. Cerebellar control of postural scaling and central set in stance. J Neurophysiol 1994;72:479–493.

27. Knutsson E, Martensson A. Posture and gait in Parkinson's patients. In: Brandt TH, Paulus W, Bies W, et al, eds. Disorders of posture and gait. New York: Elsevier Science, 1990:217–229.
28. Nutt J, Horak F, Frank J. Scaling of postural responses in Parkinson's disease. In: Woolacott M, Horak F, eds. Posture and gait: control mechanisms, vol. II. Eugene, OR: University of Oregon, 1992:4–7.
29. Masdeu JC, Gorclick PB. Thalamic astasia: inability to stand after unilateral thalamic lesions. Ann Neurol 1988;23:596–603.
30. Dieterich M, Brandt T. Which thalamic infarctions cause postural imbalance? In: Woolacott M, Horak F, eds. Posture and gait: control mechanisms, vol. II. Eugene, OR: University of Oregon, 1992:51–54.
31. Berg KO, Wood-Dauphinee S, Williams IJ, Maki B. Measuring balance in the elderly: validation of an instrument. Can J Public Health 1992;83(suppl):57–61.
32. Shumway-Cook A, Horak FB. Assessing the influence of sensory interaction on balance. Phys Ther 1986;66:1548–1550.
33. Tinetti ME. Performance-oriented assessment of mobility problems in elderly patients. J Am Geriatric Soc 1986;34(2):119–126.
34. Shumway-Cook A, Horak FB. Rehabilitation strategies for patients with vestibular deficits. Neurol Clin 1990;8:441–457.
35. Herdman SJ. Assessment and treatment of balance disorders in the vestibular deficient patient. In: Duncan P, ed. Balance proceedings of the APTA forum. Nashville, TN, 1990:87–94.

APPENDIX: GUIDELINES FOR BALANCE EVALUATION

Documentation Definitions

Assistance: I = Independent; Cues = Needs cues but no physical help;
S = Supervision; Min = Minimal; Mod = Moderate; Max = Maximal;
D = Dependent

Sway: Amount of postural sway = none, min, mod, severe

Posture: Describe any deviations

Comments: Comment on any of the following that apply:
Body alignment (trunk, extremities)
Segmental control
COG alignment ("postural bias")
Direction of LOB
Latency of automatic postural response
Presence and effectiveness of automatic postural response
Is assistance needed to maintain balance once patient assumes the position?

If patient "free-falls," note either:
   a) unaware of fall/LOB
   b) aware of LOB, but unable to correct
Presence of dizziness (vertigo, lightheadedness, and/or spatial disorientation)
Presence of compensation techniques such as increasing BOS or using arms
Finally, note any modification of the test position

PART I. STATIC BALANCE AND LIMITS OF STABILITY

Specific Tests

Sit: Static

Test: Sit straight with both feet on the floor, hands folded across chest, with midline COG

Normal response: No postural sway, midline COG alignment, neck neutral, thoracic extension with neutral pelvic tilt. Accurate perception of location of COG.

Sit: LOS (Lateral)

Test: Shift your weight as far to the right as possible without losing your balance. Then return to midline. Repeat to left. Return to midline.

Normal response: Weight shift initiated at pelvis with trunk elongation to the weight bearing side. Symmetrical left/right weight shifts while maintaining neutral trunk extension. Minimal to no postural sway. LOS: 75–100% depending on age. Accurate perceived limits of stability (PLOS).

Sit: LOS (Anterior-Posterior)

Test: Shift your weight as far anteriorly as possible without losing your balance. Then return to midline. Repeat posteriorly. Return to midline.

Normal response: Anterior weight shift with relatively straight spine, shoulders ending up over knees while maintaining an anterior pelvic tilt with forward movement of the pelvis over the femur. Posterior weight shift–posterior pelvic tilt combined with an increase in lumbar and thoracic flexion. Minimal to no postural sway. LOS: 75–100% depending on age. Accurate PLOS.

Stand: Static

Test: Stand straight with arms at your side, feet hips width with midline COG.

Normal response: No visible sway with normal standing alignment and midline COG. Accurate perception of location of COG.

Stand: LOS (Lateral)

Test: Shift your weight as far to the right as possible without losing your balance. Return to midline. Repeat to left. Return to midline.

Normal response: Weight shift initiated at ankles while maintaining proximal joint stability of the trunk, hip, and knee joints. (COG is shifted by moving the body about the ankle joints.) Minimal to no postural sway. LOS: 75–100% depending on age. Accurate PLOS.

Stand: LOS (Anterior-Posterior)

Test: Shift your weight as far anteriorly as possible without losing your balance. Return to midline. Repeat posteriorly. Return to midline.

Normal response: Weight shift initiated at ankles while maintaining proximal joint stability at trunk, hip, and knee joints. Minimal to no postural sway. LOS 75–100% depending upon age. Accurate PLOS.

Perception of Midline

State whether your patient has an accurate perception of midline.

Documentation   Intact or abnormal? If abnormal, note: Direction of postural bias (left, right, anterior, posterior)

Severity of postural bias (minimal, moderate, severe)

PART II. AUTOMATIC POSTURAL RESPONSES

The purpose of this part of the evaluation is to assess the presence and effectiveness of automatic postural responses (APRs). For any of the standing tests beyond preferred BOS there can be a wide variation in the APRs (i.e., type of strategy, amount of sway) especially when attempting to assume the position. This variation is seen in the general population as well as the elderly. However, a patient's inability to assume or maintain any of these positions has functional significance.

Documentation Definitions

Time (1, 2, 3):   The goal is 20 seconds, 3 repetitions should be performed

Assume: The level of assistance needed to assume the test position

Strategy: Ankle, hip, step, mixed strategies, suspensory "Free-fall" = no strategy, requires full assistance to prevent a "fall"

Specific Tests

Preferred BOS

Test position: Standing with arms by side, feet hips width apart with midline COG. Measure BOS (distance between medial malleoli).

Normal response: No visible sway. Maintain with ankle strategy with normal standing alignment and midline COG.

Narrow BOS

Test position: Standing with feet together. Modification—If patient is unable to do this, ask patient to stand with feet 1–2 inches apart and document.

Normal response: Minimal sway. Maintain with ankle strategy with normal standing alignment and midline COG.

Tandem

Test position: Place one heel directly in front of the opposite toes. Both feet facing forward. Then reverse foot position. Modification—Place one heel next to the medial arch of the opposite foot. Both feet facing forward. Then reverse foot position.

Normal response: To assume the position initially requires a mix of hip and ankle strategy with minimal to moderate sway. Once the patient assumes the position, the patient should maintain with an ankle strategy with minimal sway.

Beam: Lateral

Test position: A 3–4 inch balance beam is positioned a few inches off the floor. Stand in tandem position on the beam. Modification—same position with the beam on the floor.

Normal response: Often requires 1–3 initial attempts to assume and/or excessive hip and upper body movements to gain balance. By then patient should maintain with ankle strategy with minimal sway.

Beam: Anterior-Posterior

Test position: Beam off the floor. Stand with the middle of foot across the beam. Feet hips width apart. Modification—same position with beam on the floor.

Normal response: To assume, initially requires a mix of ankle and hip strategy with minimal to moderate sway. Once patient assumes the position, patient should be able to maintain with an ankle strategy with minimal sway.

Unilateral Stance

Test position: Stand on one foot. The other foot should be 4–5 inches off the floor and should not touch the weight-bearing lower extremity.

Normal response: Initially, it may require l–3 attempts to assume this position. Once patient assumes the position, patient should be able to maintain with an ankle strategy with minimal sway and increased muscle activity about the foot and ankle. Normal knee alignment varies from 5° flexed to mild hyperextension.

Eyes Closed

Test position: Stand with arms by side, feet hips width apart, midline COG with eyes closed.

Normal response: Minimal to no sway. Maintain with ankle strategy with normal standing alignment and midline COG.

Foam

Test position: Standing on foam (compliant enough so that the patient does not sink all the way to the floor), with feet hips width apart.

Normal response: To assume, initially requires a mix of ankle and hip strategy. Once patient assumes the position, patient should maintain with ankle strategy with minimal sway and increased muscle activity about the foot and ankle, midline COG.

Foam, Eyes Closed

Test position: Standing on foam with feet hips width apart. Allow the patient to stabilize and then close eyes.

Normal response: It is normal to observe a mild increase in sway compared to foam alone and eyes closed alone. However, patient should be able to maintain with an ankle strategy with increased muscle activity about the foot and ankle with midline COG.

Induced Hip Strategy

There are two general types of patients who up to this point have not produced a hip strategy.

1. Patients who were able to maintain their COG within the BOS and did not require a hip strategy
2. Patients who were unable to produce a hip strategy when needed and exhibited an early step strategy, free-fall, or an excessive ankle strategy

If this is the case, the following are ideas to further assess the presence of a hip strategy.

1. Passively move patients beyond their biomechanical LOS and cue them not to take a step. This can be done on the beam, foam, or level surface.
2. Cue patients to actively weight shift beyond their biomechanical LOS. This can be done on beam, foam, or level surface.
3. External perturbations by therapist.

PART III. FUNCTIONAL BALANCE

The purpose of this section of the evaluation is to assess your patient's ability to integrate maintenance of balance while performing a functional activity. For any of these tests, there can be a wide variation of responses. This variation is seen in the general population as well as the elderly.

Specific Tests

For reaching tests, circle which test position is used, either Sitting or Standing depending on level of function.

Reaching: Level I

Test: Evaluate your patient's ability to carry out a reaching activity which consists of:

1. Minimal to no movement of COG over BOS (<25% LOS)
2. Manipulate an object weighing up to 1 pound

Examples: Grooming activities, setting a table, light meal preparation, removing clothes from a bureau or closet

Reaching: Level 2

Test: Evaluate your patient's ability to carry out a
                   reaching activity that consists of:

                   1. Minimal to moderate movement of COG over
                      BOS (25–75% LOS)
                   2. Manipulate an object weighing up to 10
                      pounds

Examples: Grocery shopping, cooking activities, yard work,
                   housecleaning activities

Reaching: Level 3

Test: Evaluate your patient's ability to carry out a
                   reaching activity which consists of:

                   1. Maximum movement of COG over BOS (75%
                      to >100% LOS) and/or the ability to quickly
                      change your BOS when needed while
                      performing a bending, reaching, or lifting
                      activity
                   2. May include an unstable or uneven support
                      surface

Examples: Any activity related to fitness/sports, leisure, or
                   employment

Sit → Stand

Test: Without the use of upper extremities, from a non-
                   fixed chair of average height (approximately 17
                   inches). Patient begins seated at the edge of a
                   chair and assumes a standing position.

Stand → Sit

Test: Patient begins in standing and assumes a sitting
                   position in the chair without the use of the
                   upper extremities.

Stand → Floor

Test: Patient begins in standing and assumes a prone,
                   supine or sidelying position on the floor.

Floor → stand

Test: Patient begins on the floor and assumes a standing position.

PART IV. GAIT EVALUATION

This evaluation is to be done without an assistive device whenever possible. Note if the evaluation is done with an assistive device and/or orthotic.

Documentation Definitions

Specific patient complaints: Obtained through patient interview.

Deviations: Document standardized gait deviations seen during swing and stance phase.

Specific observations: Circle the appropriate description for each category.

AMBULATION

The purpose of this section of the evaluation is to further assess the presence of a postural bias, frequency of LOB and your patient's ability to safely ambulate with head turns and with decreased visual input.

Documentation Definitions

Loss of balance: Note frequency of loss of balance (LOB).
   Loss of balance = excessive postural sway to the degree which patient

a. Needed to stop to regain balance
b. Needed to take a deviant step to prevent a fall
c. Required physical assistance to prevent a fall

   Line of progression = straight, left, or right.
      If abnormal, note severity: min, mod, severe (or obtain specific measurements), and direction.

Specific Tests

Forward 50 Feet

Test: Walk 50 feet straight ahead.

Normal response: 20–25 seconds, no LOB, straight progression, normal gait pattern.

Head Turns 50 Feet

Test: Walk 50 feet straight ahead turning your head to the left and right every other second.

Normal response: 25–30 seconds, no LOB, straight progression, normal gait pattern.

Eyes closed 25 Feet

Test: Walk straight ahead 25 feet with eyes closed.

Normal response: 10–20 seconds, verbal cues for reassurance, no LOB, mild veering to either side, mild ↑ BOS, mild ↑ stance time bilaterally, mild ↓ step length bilaterally.

FUNCTIONAL GAIT

The purpose of this section of the evaluation is to assess your patient's ability to maintain balance during various functional activities.

Documentation Definitions

Comments: Presence and direction of postural sway and/or LOB
Strategy (APR) used in response to LOB
Awareness of LOB, perception of stability
Postural alignment abnormalities
Changes in gait pattern
Onset of dizziness, vertigo, or spatial disorientation

Specific Tests

Tandem

Test: Perform tandem walking 15–25 feet (heel-toe gait).

Normal response: Maintain balance with minimal to moderate postural sway and mix of ankle > hip strategy.

Beam: Lateral

Test: Stand across a 3-inch beam, arches over the beam. Perform sidestepping to left and then right on the beam (beam off floor if possible).

Normal response: Initially, may require 1–3 attempts with excessive upper body motion needed to maintain balance. Then patient should perform the activity with minimal postural sway and a mixture of ankle and hip strategy.

Beam: Anterior-Posterior

Test: Perform tandem gait on beam (beam off floor if possible).

Normal response: Initially, may require 1–3 attempts with excessive upper body motion needed to maintain balance. Then patient should perform the activity with minimal to moderate postural sway and mixture of ankle and hip strategy.

For the remaining tests, there is a wide variation in the normal response of the general population as well as the elderly. The main question is whether the patient can perform the task. Also consider whether he/she uses compensatory strategies effectively and whether he/she approaches the task safely.

Pivot Quickly

Test: Walk straight ahead at a brisk pace and stop and pivot quickly on left foot. Repeat with right foot.

Sudden Stop

Test: Walk straight ahead at a brisk pace and stop quickly.

Uneven Surface

Test: Walk straight ahead on a mat or outdoors on an uneven surface.

Step-Over

Test: Walk straight ahead and step over a small object.

Backwards

Test: Walk 15–25 feet backwards.

Narrow Area

Test: Walk through an area/passageway smaller than hip/shoulder width.

Carrying a Glass

Test: Walk forward carrying a glass/cup $^4/_5$ full of water.

Stairs

Test: Walk up and down 8 stairs, without a railing, step-over-step.

ADVANCED GROSS MOTOR ACTIVITIES

Documentation Definitions

Assistance: If the patient is unable to perform with minimal assistance or less, do not continue.

Reps/time: For a 10 second period, count the number of repetitions.

Comment: Quality of movement pattern, coordination, postural alignment abnormalities, presence and direction of LOB strategy (APR) used in response to LOB.

Specific Tests

Jumping Jacks (Bilateral Symmetrical Activity)

Test: Perform jumping jacks for 10 seconds.
Normal response: 10–12 reps/10 seconds.

Hopping

Test: Hop on one foot for 10 seconds.
Normal response: 19–23 reps/10 seconds.

Split Jacks (Bilateral Asymmetrical Activity)

Test: Perform split jacks for 10 seconds. (For split jacks, patient is positioned with one foot forward to the other, opposite arm forward to the other arm. The patient jumps, reversing position of the arms and legs.)
Normal response: 10–12 reps/20 seconds.

Running 50 Feet

Test: Run 50 feet straight ahead.
Normal response: Pace is variable depending on age. Smooth, coordinated motion.

FUNCTIONAL GAIT CATEGORY (CIRCLE ONE)

0. Nonambulatory
1. Therapeutic ambulator
2. Assisted household ambulator
3. Limited household ambulator (independent)
4. Household ambulator (independent)
5. Limited community ambulator (independent)
6. Community ambulator (independent)
7. Unlimited ambulator (including sports/fitness activities)

Use of the Neurologic Rehabilitation Model in the Assessment and Treatment of Patients with Functional Memory and Daily Planning Problems

Ann Gillespie and Jeffrey S. Kixmiller

Memory impairments are not only the most commonly reported cognitive problem following brain injury (1,2), but also one of its most disabling (3–5). When these patients are augmented by those who have "memory-like" impairments due to attentional-organizational deficits seen with frontal systems dysfunction (6–8), the number of rehabilitation patients who present with memory and organizational complaints becomes staggering. Consequently, rehabilitation clinicians must be prepared to address memory deficits in all post-acute settings. This chapter reviews how the neurologic model of rehabilitation assists with developing and implementing the use of organizational and memory systems in those settings. Its application generally follows the same logic as that in the acute rehabilitation setting. However, most patients come to post-acute rehabilitation when the biologic component of their underlying neurologic disorder is becoming fixed, and further improvement due to the natural history of recovery is not expected. Nonetheless, a thorough understanding of a patient's neurologic profile in post-acute rehabilitation continues to affect the delivery of rehabilitation services by assisting rehabilitation therapists with the following:

1. *Problem identification*—targeting cognitive and functional domains that need to be assessed given certain types of neurological damage
2. *Selecting appropriate interventions*—assisting the clinician with planning, developing, and implementing specific treatment approaches given the neurologic profile
3. *Setting realistic outcome goals*—maintaining a focused treatment regimen that is aimed at attaining functional goals that are reasonable in scope and probability of success given a patient's specific residual deficits
4. *Maintaining realistic expectation*—assisting with setting and sustaining a course of treatment that is clearly attainable.

A commonly used rehabilitative intervention for such disturbances is the application of external memory and organizational systems aimed at cueing patients to organize and recall information more effectively. Thus, the introduction of memory logs and organizational planners are used to assist neurologically impaired patients with recalling and organizing information in such a way as to help alleviate the functional deficits that exist in everyday life. Such strategies have been shown to be quite successful in many instances (9–11).

There are many types of externally applied memory and organizational systems available to address rehabilitation patients' functional deficits in memory and organization, but they generally fall into two types. *Memory logs* are those external devices that are used to help cue or remind a patient to remember information. Examples of memory logs include diaries, calendars, reminder lists, and categorized memory workbooks. *Organizational systems* are external rehabilitation aids that assist patients with planning and organizing their time more efficiently; these include daily or weekly time planners, organizational folders, itineraries, beeper systems, computer/phone cueing systems, checklists, posted signs, and symbols. Memory logs and organizational systems are often used in conjunction with one another, and it is the responsibility of the rehabilitation clinicians to choose the optimal combination of external aids to assist patients with their functional memory and organizational problems.

TRADITIONAL USE OF EXTERNAL MEMORY AND ORGANIZATIONAL AIDS IN POST-ACUTE REHABILITATION

The decision to use external memory and organizational aids in treatment is generally made by the team when the patient's deficits in these areas are sufficiently severe that that they cannot learn more internally motivated strategies. The traditional approach for the team in determining and choosing external memory and organizational aids for the patient's treatment is to:

1. Determine that a patient's memory and/or organizational deficits are disrupting their ability to function in everyday life
2. Design an external memory/organizational system to address the functional deficit(s)
3. Teach the use of the external aid to the patient
4. Assist the patient to extend the use of the external memory aid into the everyday environment.

There are some common problems with this traditional approach. Organizational and memory systems often prove to be only partially effective, or fail entirely, because the team fails to recognize that a patient's neurologic deficits precluded the successful use of the external memory or organizational aid. Oftentimes this is due to assessments in which a patient's unique memory profile was characterized unitarily as a "bad memory." As a result, the subsequent planning, teaching, and institution of the aids are not sufficiently tailored so that the patient could learn and use the memory aids optimally. Some rehabilitation programs purchase mass quantities of identical memory books and organizational systems and attempt to use the same aids and systems with every patient who presents with memory or organizational deficits. Another common mistake is that therapists devise highly complex systems and fail to recognize that utilizing such systems is beyond the cognitive capacities of the patient. The application of either generic or complex aids without addressing how each patient's neurologic deficits will interact with the external aids will be ineffective or will only moderately improve the patient's ability to function in the real world.

THE NEUROLOGIC MODEL APPLIED TO THE USE OF MEMORY/ORGANIZATIONAL AIDS IN POST-ACUTE REHABILITATION

The neurologic model of rehabilitation incorporates each patient's neurologic and neuropsychological strengths and weaknesses within every aspect of rehabilitation programming. In this way, the initial evaluation, choice of rehabilitation goals, teaching styles used, and selection of interventions are all framed according to what is reasonable based on the patient's neurologic profile of strengths and weaknesses (Table 10.1).

ASSESSMENT

Using memory impairments as an example, the first step in the assessment of memory problems includes an analysis of functional memory

Table 10.1. *Steps Involved in Establishing Memory/Organizational Systems Using the Neurologic Rehabilitation Model*

Assessment
1. Determine that a patient's memory/organizational deficits are disrupting his/her ability to function in everyday life.
2. Conduct an in-depth evaluation of the patient's memory or organization as it relates to each of the "stages," processes, or components of that system.
3. Identify the specific areas in which the patient is having significant difficulties, as well as those areas of memory or organization that are intact.
4. Incorporate other neurologic and neuropsychological information about a patient with his/her memory and/or organizational functioning to determine the level of assistance that is needed, as well as specific areas of deficits that need to be targeted.

Design, Teaching, and Use of Memory Aids
5. Determine if the patient is capable of learning self-motivated, self-cueing organizational or memory cues that would not require using external systems. If not,
6. Design an external memory/organizational system that can address the functional memory deficits but that is also within the cognitive capacity of the patient to learn and use effectively.
7. Choose specific teaching strategies that are directed at, and use, the patient's cognitive strengths.
8. Assist the patient to extend and incorporate the external memory aid into his/her everyday environment.

Generalization and Evaluation
9. Assist the patient to extend and generalize his/her use of the external memory or organizational aid into his/her everyday environment.
10. Assess whether the intervention is being used properly and generalized for the purpose it was intended.
11. Evaluate the overall effectiveness over a specified period of time.

deficits. It is important to determine, for instance, that either self-reported memory complaints or memory deficits detected by neuropsychological tests represent real world obstacles to daily functioning. A functional assessment ensures that patients' memory ability in their natural environment is actually problematic for day-to-day activities. Suggested areas of day-to-day functional activities that should be assessed are patients' abilities to: 1) access their community's resources, 2) shop, 3) access public transportation, 4) plan their time and follow their own schedule, 5) manage their money, 6) engage in leisure activities, 7) use the telephone effectively for communication, 8) maintain their self-care and safety, and 9) access emergency procedures.

The next step consists of breaking down the functional activities that are problematic to the patient into their component parts. Most real-world tasks represent the end result of multiple routines and tasks that relate to various cognitive processes that can be differentially affected following neurologic illness. It is therefore crucial for clinicians to analyze the precise areas of memory difficulties that a patient is experiencing and determine which memory processes are relatively intact in order to formulate realistic and attainable treatment plans.

Review of Memory Stages and Processes

Impairments of memory have often been observed as sequelae of brain damage, following head trauma, strokes, encephalitis, progressive dementing illnesses, and long-term substance abuse. However, there has been a tendency to treat memory disturbances as a unitary deficit despite the fact that there is a considerable amount of heterogeneity in patients' clinical presentation of memory problems. Thus, too often, rehabilitation clinicians have approached "memory" as a single entity. Behavioral neurology and neuropsychology have shown, however, that memory is actually comprised of a number of multidimensional "systems" or "processes" that can be differentially disrupted following various types of neurologic damage. Hence, in order to more appropriately assess and develop interventions for memory disorders in rehabilitation, information regarding the specific nature of each patient's memory disturbance is crucial.

Research in memory has posited the existence of multiple, distinct memory systems or processes that work in conjunction to form the complex process commonly referred to as "memory." There continues to be a great deal of research devoted to determining ways in which memory can be differentially affected by neurologic insult. Several proposed components of memory have generally become accepted and regarded as unique memory "subsystems." These components tend to be based on temporal processing differences (e.g., short-term vs. long-term memory) or are based on the type of information that is processed by each memory sub-system (e.g., memory for playing a piano versus recalling what *chair* means). Some of the most agreed on memory systems are discussed below.

Short-Term, Long-Term, and Remote Memory

One of the most clinically used, and often misused, memory systems defines memory as occurring in "stages." From this perspective, short-term memory is a stage that processes information for several seconds prior to "consolidating" memories into long-term memory. Long-term memory is a subsequent stage of memory processing that stores information in a more "permanent" fashion, such that memories can be recalled minutes, hours, and even years after being transferred from short-term memory. Remote memory, on the other hand, refers to those events and information that have been consolidated from the distant past (i.e., years or even decades), and refers to such recalled events as childhood memories and old news events. In general, research has demonstrated that each of these "subsystems" can be differentially affected following brain damage, and thus each stage needs to be assessed separately in order to determine which memory components are contributing to observed "memory" impairments.

Explicit Memory and Implicit Memory Systems

Explicit and implicit memory systems represent two major "types" of memory that differ according to whether memories can be accessed consciously or not. *Explicit memory* (also known as *declarative memory*) represents those events, episodes, and facts that can be recalled consciously through explicit, or effortful, retrieval (i.e., trying to remember something). These memories are typically further partitioned into two subdivisions: episodic and semantic memories. *Episodic memory* processes information that corresponds to our personal experiences of events or episodes, and contains information about the surrounding context of these memories. For example, when asked to recall what you did on your birthday last year, you will most likely remember what you did, as well as who you were with and where you were at the time. In other words, episodic memories are believed to be intimately connected to the environmental and temporal context in which the events and episodes occurred. *Semantic memory*, on the other hand, is the memorial process that represents our knowledge of facts, rules, and principles. Recollection of semantic memories, unlike episodic memory, is not dependent on the temporal context in which information is learned. This is presumably because such information, through time, has lost its connections to specific contextual and temporal episodes, leaving semantic knowledge as something "you just know" (oftentimes without knowing where you learned the information or when). Thus, for example, your knowledge of what a "birthday" means is semantic in nature, since it is unlikely that your recollection of such knowledge requires that you also recall the specific episode in which you learned this concept.

Implicit memory (also known as *procedural memory*) represents our knowledge of the world that is not available through conscious awareness. Instead, implicit memories include our stored repertoire of knowledge that can be performed virtually without our conscious recollection. Therefore, implicit memories represent our unconscious knowledge of information such as skill learning (e.g., how to ride a bike and play a musical instrument), as well as "holding" more automatic mental knowledge and procedures (e.g., how to read and add numbers together).

Knowing the distinction between explicit and implicit memory is important in that brain damage can differentially affect these memory systems. It is possible to find patients who have memory profiles characterized by severe explicit memory deficits within the context of intact implicit memory. Further, neurologic patients can often have relatively intact memory of semantic information and yet demonstrate relatively severe episodic memory impairments.

Anterograde and Retrograde Memory Problems

Another distinction in memory is based on the period of time for which patients have their memory deficits. *Anterograde memory* deficits refer to the impaired ability to form and "consolidate" new memories from the time since the neurologic insult. In such cases, patients are not readily able to learn new information since the onset of their neurologic damage. Conversely, *retrograde memory* impairments refer to difficulties in retrieving memories that were formed prior to the brain injury. This can include instances of "post-traumatic amnesia," in which patients cannot recall events leading up to the point of brain damage for minutes, hours, or even months prior to injury. In addition, episodes of retrograde amnesia can exist for years or even decades following neurologic insults that are a result of severe, global amnesia.

Prospective Memory

A final memory process that has become increasingly investigated is the degree to which patients can "remember to remember something"; this process of recognizing the need to recall something else in the future is referred to as *prospective memory*. This concept is especially pertinent to providers of rehabilitation services because if memory-disordered patients are unable to remember to use external memory aids that are designed to assist these patients to recall important information, then these external memory aids will not be used by patients at all.

Other Functional Brain Systems

It is important to remember that the memory processes reviewed here are interrelated with multiple other functional brain systems. Damage to the brain in one system will often affect other brain processes. For example, prospective memory deficits will often result in impairments in executing complex, organized behavioral plans, because the ability to do so typically requires remembering what actions need to be carried out at the appropriate time in the future (i.e., remembering to remember). As a result, multiple systems can be adversely affected by damage to one functional system.

This concept also applies to memory, where impairments in other brain systems can adversely affect memory abilities. One of the most common examples of this is seen with impaired attentional processes. When attentional capacities are impaired by some neurologic insult (e.g., acute confusional states following acquired brain trauma, metabolic encephalopathies) disturbances are noted in simple attention, vigilance, and inability to maintain coherent thoughts. As a result, information is not easily attended to or encoded into memory; this often leads to misdiagnosed "memory deficits" that are actually attentional disturbances. Again, proper assessment of which systems are impaired does influence rehabilitation goals. In the case of attentional deficits, for example, providing repetition and drilling and allowing a patient to write information down with a pencil and paper can often improve the ability to get information into memory.

Summary: Memory Stages and Processes

The memory processeses described above are by no means exhaustive of all the possible types of memory systems that exist. It does, however, represent a brief review of many of the most clinically encountered "memory" systems that are discussed by neurologists and neuropsychologists. Such distinctions are vital, not merely pedantic dissociations, because in each case, brain-damaged patients have been found who show differential impairments across these memory processes. The proper use of the term *amnesia*, for example, is for instances in which patients have 1) generally intact short-term memory, 2) severe anterograde amnesia for both episodic and semantic information, 3) variable levels of retrograde amnesia that is especially pronounced for episodic information, but 4) intact implicit/procedural memory. Conversely, patients who are described to have evidence of *dementia* often have 1) impaired short-term memory and diminished consolidation of memories, 2) impaired long-term memory that includes 3) the loss of anterograde and retrograde memory, as well as 4) the loss of episodic and semantic knowledge. Thus, as will be seen, information regarding the nature and type of memory that is affected and preserved in neurologically impaired patients can assist rehabilitation practitioners with developing a better characterization of each patient's memory profile, as well as incorporating such information into treatment planning and services.

The final stages of the assessment process consist of integrating observed memory deficits within the context of other cognitive-neurologic functions. A rehabilitation clinician needs to know if additional areas of cognitive functioning are impaired (e.g., aphasia, apraxia, and executive-frontal lobe deficits), as well as what cognitive functions appear intact. It is also important to determine whether the memory impairments are the result of, or interact with, other cognitive deficits. For example, it is possible that a patient's memory impairments are really due to poor attentional capacities that prevent a patient from encoding new information rather than to memory impairments per se. Similarly, existent memory deficits could be complicated by the fact that a patient has significant executive deficits that hamper a patient's ability to retrieve information from memory, yet with suffi-

Table 10.2. Neurologic Rehabilitation Factors Related to Assessment and Treatment

Neurologic Factors
- Psychiatric history
- Substance use history
- Premorbid medical and neurologic history
- Injury severity indices (e.g., Glasgow Coma Scale scores, length of post-traumatic amnesia)
- Neuroimaging data
- Neurologic syndrome presentation
- Natural recovery course
- Prognosis

Neuropsychological Factors
- Intelligence (verbal, performance)
- Attention (attention span, concentration, sustained, divided)
- New learning (encoding capacity, learning capacity)
- Memory (immediate, short-term, long-term, retrieval)
- Visual-spatial/visual-motor functioning (e.g., drawing ability)
- Level of insight and awareness
- Executive functioning (e.g., planning, organization, impulsivity)
- Emotional functioning (pseudobulbar affect, depression, anxiety)
- Behavioral/psychosocial issues (e.g., compulsions, social behavior)

cient retrieval cues, these same patients would be capable of recalling learned information. Finally, it is important to integrate knowledge about the specific memory difficulties with other neurologic factors, such as whether the patient has undergone all of the natural recovery that can be expected and determining what sorts of factors could be impinging on prognosis (e.g., history of alcohol abuse). Examples of neurologic factors to consider are given in Table 10.2.

DESIGN, TEACHING, AND USE OF MEMORY AIDS

When patients' memory disturbances are deemed to be functionally significant and of a severity that these patients would be incapable of learning and using internally motivated memory strategies, it is time to design and teach the use of external memory aids. In designing such systems, there must always be a balance between the level of need for external assistance and what a patient is capable of actually learning and using. For instance, if a patient's memory deficits are noted to be particularly severe for anterograde memories, then interventions may need to focus on intact procedural skills in order to teach an external memory system.

In addition to teaching to the relative strengths of a patient, the design and teaching of external memory systems must also conform to, or work around, each patient's neurologic deficits. In other words, it is imperative that components of any external memory system are within the patient's neurologic capacities to learn and use. As mentioned, rehabilitation clinicians often develop generic memory systems that they apply to numerous patients' memory difficulties. Yet, this practice ignores important neurologic factors that could be used to tailor the use of a memory aid in much more specific and reasonable ways. Thus, for example, existing attention deficits often make learning a new memory system very difficult. The design of any external memory aid therefore must include adaptations to cue a person's attention to use his or her memory system. In teaching a memory system to an attentionally impaired patient, interventions for poor attention may be necessary. Examples of such teaching adaptations are using frequent but short teaching sessions, teaching the system in a graduated way that breaks down complex tasks into easier subparts, using a relatively distraction-free area for teaching the memory system, and giving the patient frequent rest breaks during the learning process to avoid depleting attentional reserves. Thus, neurologic factors need to be addressed in both the design and teaching of external memory aids in order to expect that a patient can realistically learn and use the system successfully.

GENERALIZATION OF MEMORY AND ORGANIZATIONAL AIDS

Generalization of patients' ability to use memory and organizational aids from a controlled rehabilitation environment to their daily lives has become one of the most important challenges confronting therapists in post acute rehabilitation. There seems to be some common causes that underlie patients' failure to generalize skills learned in rehabilitation to their own living environment. Too often, rehabilitation treatment plans are based on outcome goals and assessments that were not clearly defined from the onset. As a result, rehabilitation interventions are aimed at deficit areas that may not be the most needy areas for assisting the patient with making functional changes in their daily lives. For instance, a patient and her family may have indicated that a memory problem was the most difficult deficit they noticed within the patient's daily functioning. Yet, a more defined functional assessment may show that what appears to be memory disturbance, as reported by the family and patient, is actually due to executive dysfunction that is hampering a patient's daily functioning. If interventions are instituted without verifying the functional validity of the complaints, a considerable amount of time and effort can be wasted by the clinical team.

It is important to consider how the patient will function independently away from the supportive rehabilitative environment. Many neurologically impaired patients can learn and use extensive external memory and organizational aids with the assistance of the structure, routine, and feedback that naturally occurs within the rehabilitative treatment regimen, yet be completely unable to maintain the use of these interventions in the real world due to its lack of structure and routine.

Some memory and organizational aids may be inappropriately introduced during the evolving course of natural recovery of a memory disorder. Whereas a memory system devised may have been comprehensive and fitting to the memory disorder at a particular time in the patient's recovery, the system can often become less pertinent and applicable to the patients' lives as their memory impairments improve.

The final reason aids falter following post-acute rehabilitation is that there is little follow-up concerning how well the aids are working in the patient's daily life. It is usually the rule, and not the exception, that unexpected difficulties with memory and organizational aids will arise that could never have been anticipated during the design and teaching of the system during post-acute rehabilitation. Consequently, it is essential that clinicians follow up with patients and monitor their outcomes so that accommodations can be made as problems arise.

CASE STUDIES

The following case studies illustrate the use of the neurologic rehabilitation model as it relates to the teaching three patients with unique profiles of neurologic impairments to use memory and organizational aids. Table 10.3 presents an overview of these case examples.

Traumatic Brain Injury: Patient G.L.

Assessment

G.L. is a 36-year-old right-handed female and single parent who, prior to her injury, was working part time as a waitress. She was active in her community and had many friends. G.L. was involved in a motor vehicle accident and sustained a traumatic brain injury with severe diffuse axonal injury (DAI) and focal injury. Her initial Glasgow Coma Scale score was 4 to 5 and she had a 4-week coma and $3^1/_2$ month posttraumatic amnesia. Her head CT scan showed a left temporal contusion and scattered petechial hemorrhages. Following her 4-month inpatient rehabilitation program, she had some insight into her memory impairments and showed good progress in her cognitive functioning. Her neurologist anticipated that G.L. would have permanent memory deficits due to the severity of her DAI and nature of her focal brain injury. Consistent with this prognosis, neuropsychological testing conducted at 1 year post injury indicated that G.L. was completely amnesic for verbal and visual information that had been previously encoded 30 minutes earlier. As a result, her prospective memory was very poor. Procedural/skill learning was average, and she had good attention and long-term memory. Executive-frontal processes were generally intact as well. G.L. was frustrated with her memory deficits and showed some reactive depression.

She enrolled into a post-acute rehabilitation program after being referred by her physician. The severity of her amnesia suggested that memory deficits would be the largest obstacle to her independent daily functioning and the predominant focus of the program. G.L. was motivated to address these issues given that she had some insight into her memory deficits.

The speech evaluation performed in the post-acute program noted that G.L.'s spoken and written language and comprehension were intact for all her functional needs in the community. The functional evaluation, conducted in the patient's home, indicated that while G.L. was familiar with various community resources, she was not utilizing them. She was overwhelmed when asked to carry out multistep plans. She could not accurately dictate a short message given over the phone or remember the information on her own. She was frequently unable

Table 10.3. Overview of Three Case Illustrations

	GL	SB	TL
Diagnosis	TBI	Anoxia	Stroke
Cognitive problems	Severe verbal and visual memory impairments	Mild attention and concentration problems	Prospective memory poor
	Anterograde and prospective memory problems	Slow new learning	Mild concentration problems
	Good insight into memory problems	Severe anterograde amnesia	Poor insight into deficits
	Mild/mod. problems in concentration	Reduced insight into memory deficits	Poor executive functioning
	Mild learning impairments	Moderate executive dysfunction	Compulsions, utilization behavior, orality
	Good executive functions	Decreased problem solving	Inappropriate social behavior
	Easily frustrated	Reactive depression	Good ability to learn and remember information
	Decreased problem solving skills	Using drugs and alcohol	
Daily functional problems	Could not outline a daily schedule	Difficulty accessing emergency numbers	Initiation decreased for daily activities
	Inability to take phone messages	Could not take a phone message	Could not self-monitor behaviors
	Forgot to pay bills	Failed to record in time planner or note financial transactions	Unable to take a phone message reliably
	Scattered memory system	Unable to use community resources	Inability to organize or structure time
	Could not remember daily activities and social exchanges	Forgot social functions and appointments	Unable to function in the community independently
Goals	Teach GL to establish a function time planner system	Develop a more appropriate memory log system to assist with daily functioning	Be able to use a time planner on a daily basis to organize time
	Proceduralize its use in daily activities	Be able to use the system with some degree of independence	Participate in daily structured activities
	Learn system to accurately record information to be used daily	Be accurate in recording events/activities	Use system to better regulate behavior
Methods	Establish a small memory book	Replace current monthly planner with small weekly book	Establish use of monthly pocket calendar designed by staff and patient
	Use a weekly system within the book	Add small pad for separate memory log	Beeper system instituted to cue to look at book
	Repetitive practice and prompting to promote proceduralized learning	Slowly, concretely teach steps of memory system	Written cues in colorful cards in book for behavioral cueing
	Taught in graduated steps	Taught 1 to 1 in distraction-free environment	Use of felt tip pen for all recordings to deal with utilization behavior and orality
	Consistent note-taking system established	Promoted encoding (put teaching in his own words)	
	Maximal cueing to record (then fade prompts)	Resource and emergency numbers in separate section with an "issue resolution" section	
	Easy labeling system	Colorful index card system for cues for system	
	Emergency directory		

to recall the gist of a detailed message that was given to her verbally. She required moderate verbal cues and modeling to outline a daily schedule and accommodate new appointments. She could not manage her financial affairs, failing to remember when bills were to be paid and on several occasions paying a bill twice. G.L. needed almost constant reminders and prompts to engage in any kind of leisure activity. Prior rehabilitation attempts to institute a note-keeping system to compensate for her memory deficits had been unsuccessful. Notes were scattered all over the house and in her pocketbook, and it appeared that her memory aids were confusing her more than assisting her. Finally, observations of G.L. in the community indicated that she was unable to recall what she had ordered in a restaurant for lunch or how much money she had brought to spend. She required a loan to pay the bill.

To institute an external memory system, we analyzed G.L.'s existing neurologic deficits to determine those that might hamper the teaching and use of a memory aid system:

1. While G.L.'s basic undivided attention was intact, she was susceptible to distraction.
2. Initial learning of new information was slow, and G.L. rapidly forgot information after a delay; therefore, she would likely require a great deal of practice and prompting to use a new memory aid effectively.
3. While G.L. had little executive (frontal) dysfunction, she did exhibit some problem-solving difficulties. There was concern that she might become easily confused attempting to use a memory system in novel situations.

There were, however, a number of cognitive strengths to support the attempted use of a memory aid with G.L. Her intellectual capacity was well within the average range, suggesting that she should not have difficulty understanding the purpose and rationale of the aid. Her basic attention was good, suggesting that if the memory aid could be taught in a relatively distraction-free environment and for short intervals, she would likely be able to attend to the teaching.

Design, Teaching, and Use of a Memory Aid

G.L.'s stated goals were to be more independent in all aspects of her life, including driving, cooking, managing her finances, and caring for her daughter. The rehabilitation team wanted to teach G.L. to establish and proceduralize the use of a time planner on a daily basis to cope with her memory deficits. G.L. was already utilizing scraps of paper and several books as a memory system. The team wanted her to use one memory book to reduce the complexity of the system that she was using. This would assist G.L. with regaining a sense of control over her daily functioning.

With assistance, G.L. purchased a new 3×6 log book in which all of her to-be-remembered information would be recorded and stored in her pocketbook. G.L. had previously used a monthly system that was too complex. We converted her to a weekly calendar. A cued-procedural learning approach was used. The goal was spontaneous use of the memory log without explicit recall of the treatment plan. Teaching sessions consisted of recording information in the log repetitively, prompted as needed when she could not recall previous learning of the memory system. Because of her limited concentration and slow encoding, the system was introduced in graduated steps across multiple sessions. Her frustration level was monitored so that she did not become too upset during the teaching of the system. Because the functional evaluation had previously shown that G.L. had difficulty both recording to-be-remembered information (e.g., taking a message) and understanding later what she had written, a very clear and easily comprehensible note-taking system was devised. G.L. consistently recorded the topic, as well as key words, to assist her in recalling the event (e.g., what, when, and where the occurrence occurred). Cues to record messages in this fashion were affixed to each page of her memory log. Finally, to address the memory and initiation difficulties that were noted in the functional evaluation, we promoted the use of the system with maximal cueing immediately following any occurrence that was to be recorded. We then began to fade the amount of assistance that was provided. In this way, G.L. was able to learn the system without experiencing too many failures and setbacks. All areas of the book were labeled as simply as possible to assist with problem solving and organizational issues. A directory of emergency numbers, most commonly used phone contacts, and resources were listed in the book as well.

Generalization and Evaluation

At 1 month, G.L. was using her time planner reliably enough that she could make and keep track of her appointments independently, with only a few mistakes. A modification had been instituted to her memory system after several weeks, however, in order to address G.L.'s continued need for frequent prompts to take her time planner out of her pocketbook. It eventually surfaced that at least a portion of this reluctance was psychologically motivated in that she did not want to rely on this external device to remember information. However, with continued encouragement to use her system, and after experiencing several negative social consequences of missing appointments that were not recorded in her book, her use of the log improved considerably. By the second month of post-acute treatment, she was recording important information in her time planner and was requiring only minimal assistance from staff to check her work for accuracy. There was an unexpected and beneficial generalization. Prior to her injury, G.L. had read many novels. She spontaneously discovered that use of the memory book faciliated reading because she could record information such as the general story line or where she had left off reading.

Final Outcome and Reassessment

At the end of 20 weeks of treatment in post-acute rehabilitation, G.L. was consistently logging her daily activities independently without cues and was using this information to guide her interactions with others. A 6-month follow-up documented that she was still recording information consistently and was functioning more independently.

Anoxic Brain Injury: Patient S.B.

Assessment

S.B. is a 42-year-old single male construction worker who developed cognitive impairments following three cardiac arrests, the latest of which resulted in a lengthy resuscitation before he was able to breathe independently. A toxicology screen further indicated the presence of cocaine. During his early recovery, a 2 to 3 week post-traumatic amnesia (PTA) was noted, and later it was observed that his learning and remembering new information were severely impaired after his PTA cleared. Following discharge to home, S.B. became frustrated, depressed, and socially withdrawn, and he began drinking alcohol excessively. A neurologist's reevaluation at 1 month post brain injury indicated that S.B. continued to exhibit significant anterograde and retrograde amnesia. These difficulties were exacerbated by executive deficits as well, evidenced by poor initiation, diminished insight, and impairment of abstraction abilities. In response to strong encouragement by the neurologist, S.B. enrolled in a post-acute rehabilitation program to become more independent, monitor compliance with drug and alcohol treatment programs, and develop recreational interests. S.B.'s prognosis was guarded concerning his ability to return to his former occupation, although there was hope that he could work in a routinized job or volunteer position.

As part of an evaluation to assess S.B.'s appropriateness for participation in a post-acute rehabilitation program, a neuropsychological evaluation was conducted. S.B. reported that his typical day was consumed "sitting in the house being depressed and bored." He admitted to "some memory problems," but insight into the ramifications of his deficits remained quite limited. He denied any current or recent use of alcohol or drugs. S.B. had forgotten two prior appointments for the evaluation, even when he was contacted by telephone on the day of each appointment several hours in advance. Results of neuropsychological testing indicated that attention and concentration were moderately impaired. Verbal and visual recall was severely impaired as well, and S.B. retained only a small amount of previously encoded information over a long delay. Executive problems in strategy planning, setshifting, and problem solving were seen. Finally, S.B. was experiencing significant depression, which was related to frustration and diminished functional independence.

A time planner was proposed as a major rehabilitation goal in order to compensate for S.B.'s attentional, executive, and memory deficits. Observations from a functional evaluation in S.B.'s home supported the need for this intervention. For instance, while S.B. could readily identify community resources, he was not independently utilizing them. He could not consistently access information that was important for emergencies. Moderate to maximum assistance was required before he could accurately dictate a message over the telephone. S.B. indicated that he had already instituted a time planner system, yet team observation showed that he required maximal assistance to interpret and follow through with his own written plans. He frequently forgot to put important information into his time planner and to forget to review his book to determine whether there were any appointments or messages. His financial records demonstrated organizational problems as well in that he repeatedly failed to record banking transactions. S.B.'s memory deficits were adversely affecting his social relationships: his friends were frustrated about his frequent instances of forgetting arrangements and meeting times.

The rehabilitation team and S.B. decided to set a goal to develop a more appropriate memory log system that would help him to plan, schedule, and remember his daily activities. The critical issues addressed were the following:

1. Recovery had plateaued, and dramatic spontaneous improvement in memory and executive functioning was not expected.
2. S.B.'s neuropsychological profile did not support dementia. His syndrome was consistent with focal amnesia, although mild to moderate attention and executive deficits were also present. In addition, thinking style was concrete, which would make him especially vulnerable to feeling overwhelmed with tasks and activities that required abstract problem solving and novelsolution generation. Further, because his organization was impaired, explicit assistance with organizing information was needed.

3. S.B had some awareness of his memory deficits; therefore, he was motivated to learn and use a time planner to maximize independence and control over his life.

Design, Teaching, and Use of Memory/Time Planner

S.B.'s own appointment book, although appropriately convenient and small, was a monthly planner with printed time segments provided. The team replaced it with a weekly planner without time slots so that it was less distracting and visually complex. The teaching approach consisted of multiple, interspersed, short teaching sessions aimed at slowly and concretely introducing the steps of the time planner. As S.B. became familiar with the information, additional steps were introduced in a clear and concise manner that avoided overburdening his slow information processing. Because S.B.'s attention deficits left him highly susceptible to interference and distractibility, teaching was performed one-on-one in the most distraction-free environment available. Encoding of information was assessed repeatedly by asking S.B. to repeat the information in his own words. Frequently utilized resources and emergency numbers were written on the front cover of the book. A logging system was developed to record issues that had been resolved or achieved successfully, addressing S.B.'s tendency to perseverate on problems or appointments that had already been completed or kept. This procedure provided S.B. the opportunity to recall earlier resolutions of problems (e.g., recorded that bills had been paid or that he had discussed an important issue with his mother).

After 1 month of intensive, repetitive teaching sessions and practice, S.B. was able to use his memory log with moderate independence. He also used a small, pocket-sized time planner, in addition to a memory log that was attached to the time planner. The decision to use both a separate time planner and memory log was based on S.B.'s tendency to become confused regarding whether recorded information was an appointment or information that he would need to recall for more than a single instance.

At the end of 10 weeks of treatment, S.B. was able to merge his time planner and memory log into a single system. He continued to carry the time planner consistently and was finally using a strategy of including to-be-recalled items into his memory book. S.B. was consistently recording at least one key piece of information in the planner with one or no verbal cue 75% of the time. Difficulties, however, were noted in carrying over this system to his home without staff reminders.

Refinement of the Design, Teaching, and Use of Memory/Time Planner

To promote better generalization of his memory log and time planner at home, the staff set up a system in which S.B. was reminded twice a day to review his planner for upcoming appointments and accuracy of verbalizations (e.g., report on what he had done the previous evening). A sample entry was provided in the book as a guide. Also, the staff attached an index card to his planner to alert him to look in the book for certain information. The card was colorful and captured his attention. Its placement on the cover of the book instructed S.B. to look in his planner. It was found that this visual cue assisted him with initiating the use of the book in the community and home setting.

Generalization and Outcome

At the end of 20 weeks of treatment, S.B. was able to check his entries for accuracy on a daily basis. The visual cue of the index cards was helping him to carry over the use of the memory system to his home environment. S.B. was volunteering 4 days per week and recently asked his supervisor for more hours. He was scheduling and following through with all of his own transportation, substance abuse treatment, medical appointments, and recreational activities. At 6 months post treatment, the time planner was still being used consistently and was self-reportedly his "life-line," without which he could not manage.

Stroke: Patient T.L.

Assessment

T.L. is a 46-year-old, left-handed male who suffered an aneurysm rupture and repair of his anterior communicating artery (ACoA) resulting in bilateral frontal lobe lesions. He was a corporate executive who was married with three young children and active in community activities. During both inpatient and outpatient rehabilitation, T.L. exhibited problems with executive functions such as poor initiation, inappropriate social behavior, irritability, impulsivity, poor judgment, perseveration, and obsessive compulsive behavior. T.L. and his family were interested in enrolling him in a post-acute rehabilitation program because he "wanted to return to normal." T.L. was dissatisfied with his current sedentary lifestyle in which he reportedly "ate, read the paper, watched TV, ate, watched TV, ate, and went to sleep." His family was having difficulty adjusting to T.L.'s pronounced personality changes.

A neurologic evaluation revealed that T.L. had significant bifrontal damage confirmed by CT, MRI, and SPECT imaging. Prognosis for further recovery was limited. Neuropsychological testing revealed that T.L.'s intellectual capacity remained within the high average range and that short-term memory, concentration, and encoding of new information was very good. T.L.'s memory was generally intact, with only mild decrements in delayed recall. Memory for day-to-day events was good.

However, prospective memory was impaired: T.L. often forgot to complete prearranged activities on time, such as transmitting messages and following through on responsibilities. Poor insight into deficits was noted in that T.L. would deny inadequacies and maintain denial in the face of failures. He was incapable of comprehending how deficits were affecting his functional behavior and relationships. He exhibited compulsions, utilization behavior, orality, and inappropriate social comportment.

Findings from a speech evaluation revealed the problem areas in T.L.'s self-initiation, self-monitoring, and body language communication (e.g., flat affect, poor eye contact). Community evaluation findings indicated that while T.L. was readily able to identify community resources, he was not using them. This was at least partially related to the fact that T.L. and his family felt that his inappropriate social behaviors were embarrassing the family. T.L. was unable to take a message over the phone or present a message to another person. While he was able to identify many leisure activities, he did not participate independently in any because of his innappropriate social behaviors and impulsivity. T.L.'s ability to organize his time was impaired, and he would sit on the couch for hours unless cued to move. While T.L. was pleasant and cooperative, he did not interact with others spontaneously. The family indicated that they were devastated by his personality, behavior, and cognitive changes.

Factors that were considered especially important in devising the organizational system were the following:

1. The frontal syndrome exhibited by T.L. was extensive and would be a significant obstacle to implementation of the external aid. Yet, if the organizational system could be taught successfully, it could potentially improve his independence; thus, the attempt was clinically justifiable.
2. T.L. had previously begun to use an appointment planner, but he was using it inconsistently and failing to schedule and follow through with most important appointments and activities.
3. T.L. had premorbidly relied on a secretary to maintain his work and social schedules; therefore, there was no preexisting proceduralized knowledge to assist us with teaching him the organizational system.
4. Teaching efforts would need to take into account T.L.'s poor insight; otherwise, it was unlikely that he would be sufficiently invested in learning the organizational system or to use it consistently.
5. T.L.'s initiation would be a problem because he needed cues to follow through with nearly all intentional behaviors and plans.
6. Compulsive behaviors could be problematic because once T.L. began certain repetitive rituals (e.g., switching lights on and off), he did not stop until cued.

7. Many of T.L.'s executive/frontal deficits were seen in intrusions, perseverations, disorganization, and planning impairments. All of these difficulties would influence the actual use of the organizational/time planner (e.g., diminish regular use or accuracy) and would need to be anticipated.

It was decided that the best way to approach T.L.'s organizational and time management impairments was to establish a structured schedule to increase his independent functioning. In this case, T.L.'s time planner would operate as an organizational aid rather than a memory aid. The goal was to have T.L. use a time planner on a daily basis so that he could attain a greater amount of independence in daily functioning and establish a more interesting daily schedule of events.

Design, Teaching, and Use of Organizational/Time Planner

The teaching of the organizational system was conducted in a slow and organized manner. Consistent with neuropsychological findings, T.L. was able to learn and remember the system quite well when the information was presented in a concrete and organized manner. To promote consistency and familiarity, T.L.'s time planner was adopted for use in post-acute rehabilitation. It consisted of a monthly calendar that could fit into his pocket. He had already demonstrated that he rarely forgot to bring his time planner with him to therapy, and since we adopted a system that T.L. had designed himself, he was much less resistant in using it for an organizational system. The defensiveness that normally accompanied any attempts to address his deficits was avoided. His time planner was modified in the following ways. First, a beeper system was used to cue him to look at his schedule each hour. Given that T.L. rarely consulted his time planner without cueing, the team decided that a consistent reminder was preferable, whether staff was present or not. The second modification was aimed at reducing T.L.'s repetitive behaviors that interfered with his ability to utilize the time planner. A behavioral cueing system was instituted in which written cues were provided on colorful cards and attached to his time planner. When the beeper signaled for T.L. to take out his time planner, the written cues instructed him to refrain, or cease, from engaging in certain inappropriate behaviors (e.g., "do not switch the light switch"). Surprisingly, these simple cues were sufficient to interrupt his compulsive behaviors in most instances.

Generalization and Outcome

At the end of the first month, T.L. was using the time planner well, with the combined aid of the beeper, written cues, and, occasionally, verbal cues. Unfortunately, frequent instances occurred in which the information recorded was inaccurate. In addition, several of T.L.'s "frontal" behaviors were beginning to escalate in severity and centered around the use of the time planner. For example, T.L. was adamant that he did not want anyone to see what he had written and would shield his time planner from staff. Also, his utilization behavior was more pronounced. For example, he chewed the erasers off his pencils. To address these issues, a "check-in" time was agreed on in which T.L. would allow staff to review his time planner. His pencils were substituted with a felt-tip pen. At the end of 10 weeks of treatment, T.L. had made progress in using his time planner with cues, but it remained partially inaccurate. At the end of 14 weeks of treatment, the time planner intervention was discontinued when he decided that he did not want to rely on any external aids and would rather "just remember things" on his own. It was decided that his frontal behaviors were of a nature and type that prevented him from successfully utilizing the organizational aid. In the end, a more conservative approach was used in which T.L.'s wife maintained responsibility for his schedule and appointments. Eventually, T.L.'s family was unable to manage him at home due to his behaviors and he was placed in a long-term care setting where he now resides.

ACKNOWLEDGMENT

The work reported in this chapter was funded in part by NINDS grant NS 26985 to the Boston University School of Medicine. The authors express their appreciation to Yvette McMullen and Ellen Spiegel for editorial comments.

References

1. O'Connor M, Verfaellie M, Cermak LS. Clinical differentiation of amnesic subtypes. In: Baddeley AD, Wilson BA, Watts FN, eds. Handbook of memory disorders. Chichester, England: Wiley, 1995:53–80.
2. Sunderland A, Harris JE, Baddeley AD. Do laboratory tests predict everyday memory? A neuropsychological study. J Verbal Learning Verbal Behav 1983;22:341–357.
3. Brooks N, ed. Closed head injury: psychological, social, and family consequences. Oxford: Oxford University Press, 1984.
4. Lewinsohn PM, Graf M. A follow-up study of persons referred for vocational rehabilitation who have suffered brain damage. J Commun Psychol 1973;1:57–62.

5. Mateer CA, Sohlberg MM, Crinean J. Focus on clinical research: perceptions of memory function in individuals with closed-head injury. J Head Trauma Rehabil 1987;2:74–84.

6. Schacter DL. Memory, amnesia, and frontal lobe dysfunction. Psychobiology 1987;15:21–36.

7. Stuss DT, Benson DF. The frontal lobes. New York: Raven Press, 1986.

8. Wood RL. Disorders of attention: their effect on behaviour, cognition, and rehabilitation. In: Wilson BA, Moffal N, eds. Clinical management of memory problems. San Diego: Singular Publishing Group, 1992:213–239.

9. Kurlychek RT. Use of a digital alarm chronograph as a memory aid in early dementia. Clin Gerontolog 1983;1:93–94.

10. Lawson MJ, Rice DN. Effects of training in use of executive strategies on a verbal memory problem resulting from closed head injury. J Clin Exp Neuropsychol 1989;11:842–854.

11. Zencius A, Wesolowski M, Burke L. The use of a visual cue to reduce profanity in a brain injured adult. Behav Residential Treatment 1990;5:143–147.

Table 11.3. Psychiatric
Complications Following Traumatic Brain Injury

Amnestic Disorder

Anxiety Disorder

Delirium

Dementia

Impulse Control Disorder

Mood Disorder
* Depressive
* Bipolar

Personality Change

Psychotic Disorder

Sleep Disorder

Somatoform Disorder

Table 11.4. Medications with Potential to Cause Regression in Cognitive Function

Antibiotic	**Antiparkinson**	**Sedative-hypnotic**
Acyclovir	Amantadine	Barbiturates
Amphotericin B	Benztropine	Benzodiazepines
Cephalexin	Biperiden	Glutethimide
Chloroquine	Carbidopa	**Sympathomimetic**
Isoniazid	Levodopa	Amphetamines
Metronidazole	**Analgesic**	Disulfiram
Rifampin	Opiates	Metrizamide
Anticholinergic	Salicylates	Phenylephrine
Atropine	Synthetic narcotics	Phenylpropanolamine
Belladonna alkaloids	**Cardiac**	Propylthiouracil
Phenothiazines	β-blockers	Quinacrine
Scopolamine	Clonidine	Theophylline
Tricyclic antidepressants	Digitalis	**Over-the-counter**
Anticonvulsant	Disopyramide	Compoz
Phenobarbital	Lidocaine	Excedrin PM
Phenytoin	Mexiletine	Sleep-Eze
Antiemetics	Quinidine	Sominex
Promethazine	Procainamide	**Miscellaneous**
Antihistamine	**Drug withdrawal**	Aminophylline
Cimetidine	Alcohol	Bromides
Promethazine	Barbiturates	Chlorpropamide
Anti-inflammatory	Benzodiazepines	Lithium
Corticosteroids		
NSAIIs		
Phenylbutazone		

SOURCE: Modified from (9).

adverse central nervous system (CNS) effects. The development of adult respiratory distress syndrome is another secondary medical complication that can produce unanticipated clinical deterioration and worsen outcome. The management of these difficulties is beyond the

Problem Patients: Outliers in Rehabilitation

John W. Cassidy

To the inexperienced clinician, all patients with neurologic problems may appear unique and as such become viewed as outliers. However, the underlying premise of this text is that most properly diagnosed patients presenting to a neurorehabilitation program will have a predictable course of recovery over a discernible period of time. Yet, even under the best of circumstances, there are occasions when the statistically expected fails to materialize in a particular case. Such patients are by definition "outliers"; that is, their courses of improvement do not conform to the expected and their outcomes are markedly different from others with the same diagnosis. Thus, outliers can occur at every point in the continuum of recovery.

Those who have a more rapid and complete recovery than expected may humble our sense of clinical omniscience, but they and their families are rarely displeased by their outcomes. On the other hand, those that do worse than expected can test the mettle of any rehabilitative team and the forbearance of even the healthiest of families. These outliers tend to plateau at lower levels of functioning than anticipated and as such, their outcomes are poor and they often require ongoing, specialized care. Providing this care is problematic for families, expensive for financial sponsors, and impractical for standard rehabilitation programs. Nonetheless, an extension of the neurologic model can aid in the diagnosis and management of even these difficult patients.

Nowhere is the outlier problem more acute than in patients who have sustained traumatic brain injury (TBI). These young, impulsive, predominantly male individuals present challenges throughout their rehabilitation, problems that more easily diagnosable, older patient populations, such as those who have had a stroke, do not. For this reason, the final chapter of *Neurologic Rehabilitation* will focus on this group of individuals.

As noted in Chapter 4, TBI occurs along a continuum of severity, from mild to severe. Interestingly, outliers present at both ends of this spectrum. As emphasized throughout this text, incomplete or improper diagnosis is a major contributor to the variability of outcome found amongst a group of patients felt to be "phenotypically" similar in presentation. However, even correctly diagnosed cases may exhibit deviation from the anticipated. For example, at the mild end of the continuum in acceleration-deceleration injuries, diffuse axonal damage forms the substratum of the expected neuropathology. It is also known that despite the widespread nature of this neuropathology, it has a certain predilection for disrupting frontal systems functioning. Therefore, we should anticipate that this diffuse axonal injury may produce some attentional problems that commonly lead patients to complain of "memory difficulties," especially during the first 3 months following the concussive event. However, every experienced clinician has seen individuals with this diagnosis who exhibit amnesia dense enough to preclude recognition of their own children and recall of personal information, such as birth date and age. Under such circumstances, these individuals are correctly categorized as outliers. However, since we know that such presentations are impossible with mild acceleration-deceleration injuries, differential diagnosis becomes paramount in understanding what, if anything, is wrong with these individuals. The extension of the neurologic model of rehabilitation to these patients requires a concomitant understanding of neuropsychiatry. While seemingly a daunting leap of faith, such a development is little more than the logical evolution of the constructs already developed in this text and are explicated in the sections that follow.

ASSESSMENT

When a patient with a TBI falls off the expected recovery curve, the first response of the treatment team must be to look for evolving secondary complications, be they medical, neurologic, or psychiatric. This task routinely falls to the attending physicians and nursing staff. However, given that other team members spend a great deal of time with these patients, it is incumbent upon each treating clinician to notice and report all deviations from the expected to the appropriate "case-manager." Tables 11.1, 11.2, and 11.3 list the important diagnostic considerations in each specialty area.

Table 11.1. Medical Complications

Pulmonary
Acute cardiac failure
Adult respiratory distress
  syndrome (ARDS)
Airway obstruction
Apnea
Atelectasis
Chest wall injuries
Diaphragm paralysis/rupture
Embolism
Cardiovascular
Cardiac dysrhythmias
Deep venous thrombosis
Pulmonary embolism
Disseminated intravascular
  coagulation
Fluid—Electrolytes
Hyponatremia
Hypernatremia
Diabetes insipidus
Nutrition
Malnutrition

Hemothorax
Hypo/hyperventilation
Neurogenic pulmonary edema
Neurogenic ventilation/perfusion defect
Pre-existing pulmonary disease
Pneumonia
Pneumothorax
Pulmonary contusion/edema

Table 11.2. Neurologic Complications

Depressed sensorium—Drug reactions
                    Metabolic Disorders
                    Infection
                    Primary brain complications—Hematoma or
                                                hygroma
                                              Seizures
                                              Hydrocephalus
                                              CSF leak
                                              New trauma
                                              Traumatic aneurysm
Spasticity
Unrecognized spinal cord injury
Pain syndromes

Secondary medical complications occur more frequently than one might expect. Vigilant nursing and expectant medical care are the appropriate antidotes for many of these difficulties. Although the issue of drug side effects has been reviewed *ad nauseam*, a full medication review is warranted in any patient whose condition unexpectedly deteriorates. Table 11.4 lists some common medications and their potential

Table 11.3. Psychiatric
Complications Following Traumatic Brain Injury

Amnestic Disorder

Anxiety Disorder

Delirium

Dementia

Impulse Control Disorder

Mood Disorder
• Depressive
• Bipolar

Personality Change

Psychotic Disorder

Sleep Disorder

Somatoform Disorder

Table 11.4. Medications with Potential to Cause Regression in Cognitive Function

Antibiotic	**Antiparkinson**	**Sedative-hypnotic**
Acyclovir	Amantadine	Barbiturates
Amphotericin B	Benztropine	Benzodiazepines
Cephalexin	Biperiden	Glutethimide
Chloroquine	Carbidopa	**Sympathomimetic**
Isoniazid	Levodopa	Amphetamines
Metronidazole	**Analgesic**	Disulfiram
Rifampin	Opiates	Metrizamide
Anticholinergic	Salicylates	Phenylephrine
Atropine	Synthetic narcotics	Phenylpropanolamine
Belladonna alkaloids	**Cardiac**	Propylthiouracil
Phenothiazines	β-blockers	Quinacrine
Scopolamine	Clonidine	Theophylline
Tricyclic antidepressants	Digitalis	**Over-the-counter**
Anticonvulsant	Disopyramide	Compoz
Phenobarbital	Lidocaine	Excedrin PM
Phenytoin	Mexiletine	Sleep-Eze
Antiemetics	Quinidine	Sominex
Promethazine	Procainamide	**Miscellaneous**
Antihistamine	**Drug withdrawal**	Aminophylline
Cimetidine	Alcohol	Bromides
Promethazine	Barbiturates	Chlorpropamide
Anti-inflammatory	Benzodiazepines	Lithium
Corticosteroids		
NSAIIs		
Phenylbutazone		

SOURCE: Modified from (9).

adverse central nervous system (CNS) effects. The development of
adult respiratory distress syndrome is another secondary medical complication that can produce unanticipated clinical deterioration and
worsen outcome. The management of these difficulties is beyond the

scope of this text, but can be found in a number of comprehensive texts and reviews (1,2).

Neurologic complications can eventuate into neurosurgical emergencies. The slowly expanding subdural hematoma or the insidious evolution of obstructive hydrocephalus can lead to unexpected regression in functioning that if not immediately reversed can result in death. Seizures are another late neurologic complication that can produce deviation from an expected trajectory of recovery. Although perhaps less common than once believed, these disorders are now far more treatable than ever before given the recent introduction of several new anticonvulsant medications.

Reassessment of the patient's initial injury characteristics must also be undertaken when salient hallmarks of recovery are not met within the expected time frames. Although repeated neuroimaging studies may be undertaken, far more revealing are the initial emergency medical service and emergency department records. Very often, the contribution of diffuse hypoxemic-ischemic injury to the overall picture is underestimated. The clinical hallmarks of this condition are outlined in Chapter 4, but to recapitulate briefly they are cardiopulmonary or pulmonary arrest, profound hypotension, and significantly increased intracranial pressure. These patients plateau early and have worse outcomes than those with diffuse axonal injury alone. Unrecognized focal contusional injury, especially that occurring in the frontal or anterior temporal cortices, is another harbinger of a nondiffuse axonal injury recovery curve. Rather than following a 12 to 18 month trajectory to social and vocational reentry, these patients plateau at 4 to 6 months and are left with substantial executive dysfunction.

Acute psychiatric problems also lead to humbling reassessments of the trajectory of recovery and outcome. A number of behavioral disorders can occur early in the course of rehabilitation. These are conceptualized as falling into one of three rubrics (see Figure 11.1). Not surprisingly, most rehabilitative clinicians have been reluctant to use psychiatric diagnostic strategies; however, the extension of the neurologic model requires that we do so. Historically, as has been the case with the physical expressions of neurologic disability, clinicians have focused on the surface manifestations of the behavioral problems that present in these patient populations. Subjective clinical impressions or rating scales, such as the Katz Adjustment Scale (KAS) or the Overt

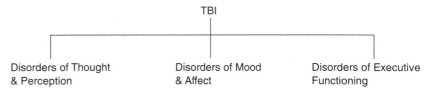

Figure 11.1   *Categories of Neuropsychiatric Disorders Following TBI.*

Aggression Scale (OAS), have been used in these circumstances. Thus, when describing behavioral disorders, the extant rehabilitation literature is replete with considerations of aggression, agitation, disorders of conduct, disorders of will, and disinhibition. However, these characterizations are no more helpful to a treating clinician using the neurologic model of rehabilitation than is the broad diagnosis of "traumatic brain injury." Although not yet traceable to a distinct neuropathology, a formal diagnostic inquiry can lead to the diagnosis of a well-described neuropsychiatric syndrome that has treatment designed to decrease handicap.

During the acute phase of rehabilitation, many of these behavioral difficulties pass with the clearing of post-traumatic amnesia and require little more than temporary environmental modification. However, if behavioral disabilities persist, they are often the problems that prevent full participation in rehabilitation and delay discharge. This is the group of patients that generally become outliers.

Persistent aggression is one such problem. Although we all seem to know conceptually what aggression is, it has been a difficult construct to define operationally. In some settings, agitation is the descriptor of choice, in others irritability. For the purposes of this chapter, the phrase *destructive behavior* will be used to subsume all of the terms listed above. Destructive behavior is defined as behavior that results in partial or complete injury to the physical or psychological integrity of a person or object. However, neither destructive behavior nor aggression is a diagnosis, but rather a sign or a behavioral manifestation that serves to indicate the presence of malfunction or disease. This sign is a component of many neurobehavioral syndromes and therefore always has a differential diagnosis. The diagnostic process begins where it always does, with taking a history and examining the patient.

EVALUATION OF THE PATIENT

Ideally, one should carefully evaluate the premorbid functioning of the patient, the characteristics of the injury, concomitant complications, and the current learning environment. In reality, this type of evaluation can only be performed when the patient is no longer in acute crisis.

A structured interview with the family focusing on previous neuromedical or neuropsychiatric disorders will begin to elucidate premorbid functioning. In addition, external validators such as education, military, and vocational histories should be requested when possible. These adjunctive sources can help balance retrospective falsification that may occur following injury. Previous substance abuse or criminal history must be explicitly sought, for they are rarely spontaneously disclosed. A detailed family history may identify specific familial neuropsychiatric diatheses that may aid both diagnosis and treatment. Another important aspect of the history involves gathering information about the injury characteristics. This area is completely reviewed in Chapter 4.

The evaluation of destructive behavior in relationship to the learning environment is vital. Issues central to any behavioral analysis should be considered: antecedent behaviors noted by the staff, particular precipitating environmental stimuli, and the consequences already occurring in the treatment environment when the behavior is seen. Diurnal variation is common and may be related to an underlying neuropsychiatric syndrome, a cyclic reinforcer in the milieu, such as morning activities of daily living, shift changes for the nursing staff, or fatigue.

The next step in the analysis is the clinical examination. It should incorporate elements of naturalistic behavioral observation, a psychiatric mental status, and an extended neurologic examination. Behavioral observation should test hypotheses already gleaned from the history. Whenever possible, direct observation of antecedent environmental factors as well as the problematic behavior is necessary. In particular, inferences regarding premeditation, volition, confusion, and psychosis should be evaluated. Episodic behaviors will require examination of the patient during the expression of the targeted behavior. At times, manifestations of the syndrome noted in the latter circumstance will not be evident when the patient is in behavioral control.

Following behavioral observation, one begins the extended neuropsychiatric examination, which ideally includes a structured evaluation of cortical functioning. A model that incorporates elements from Strub and Black (3), Taylor (4), and Folstein (5) fulfills these criteria. Special attention should be directed toward the patient's arousal and attention, orientation, speech, perception, affect, and memory. This approach helps refine the focus of possible neuroanatomic abnormalities that may have pharmacologic implications (6). It also establishes a clinical baseline of cognitive functioning, which can be easily followed over time to monitor both beneficial and deleterious effects of any prescribed medication.

Next, the clinician should proceed to a comprehensive neurologic examination. This examination may allow for further anatomic localization, as well as identifying concomitant conditions that may affect medication selection. As an example, a patient with prominent parkinsonian features secondary to hypoxemic-ischemic injury to the basal ganglia would be a poor candidate for high-potency neuroleptics, even if psychosis were evident. This evaluation allows the clinician to assess the language and motor effects seen with certain classes of medication in relationship to a preestablished baseline. Correlation of this information with the results of neuroimaging, electroencephalographic, and neuropsychological testing will often suggest underlying path physiologic processes involved in the expression of the maladaptive behavior.

Management

Outliers are difficult to manage in traditional rehabilitation settings. Their management varies depending on the acuity of the presentation and the degree of threat they pose to themselves or others. In the acute phases of recovery, management tends to focus on environmental prosthesis and neuropharmacologic interventions. The latter have a celebrated history. In the late 1960s through the mid-1970s, pharmacologically induced behavioral control was essentially associated with the reintroduction of coma. The backlash from such interventions was inevitable, and from the late 1970s through the late 1980s all psychotropics were summarily banished from the rehabilitation pharmacopoeia. Instead, patients were essentially permitted to express any type of behavior as long as they were trailed by 1 : 1 or 2 : 1 staff supervision or banished to the hinterlands of "behaviorally" based postacute treatment programs. Obviously, either approach missed the point: patients must regain behavioral control so they can perform necessary rehabilitation tasks designed to reduce their level of handicap as efficiently as possible. Thus, a more contemporary approach to these patients incorporates the positive elements of both philosophies into a coherent treatment program. In addition, psychosocial interventions are of benefit if they are appropriately directed toward those with some capacity for reflection and retention associated with the return of continuous, episodic memory.

SYNDROMES ASSOCIATED WITH DESTRUCTIVE BEHAVIOR

Delirium

Delirium is a syndrome that affects arousal, attention, orientation, perception (e.g., visual and auditory illusions or hallucinations), motor activity (generally increased), mood, and memory. Many patients show diurnal variation in symptoms as well as disturbed sleep cycles. It is one of the more common syndromes associated with destructive behavior seen early in the course of rehabilitation, often occurring as the patient emerges from coma. The problematic behavior can range from periods of uncontrollable restlessness (where wandering and the disconnection of intravenous lines can occur) to florid episodes of uncontrollably destructive behavior.

Although delirium can be a consequence of the injury itself, other etiologic factors need to be ruled out. Independent of brain injury, delirium represents a potentially life-threatening syndrome with mortality rates at 1 year reported by some centers as high as 35% (7). A full review of this topic is beyond the scope of this chapter and interested readers are referred to Strub and Black (3) and Lipowski (8) for further details. However, all medications should be carefully reviewed since many, including commonly prescribed agents such as phenytoin and analgesics, have been implicated in inducing this condition.

The Management of Delirium

There are no controlled treatment studies with idiopathic, delirious TBI or similar patients (9). Rather there are series or case reports that currently guide the clinical management of these patients (8,10). Given that this condition is principally biologically mediated, neuropharmacologic agents and environmental manipulations become the treatments of choice.

Generally, most pharmacologic interventions for delirium are directed at containment and tranquilization. Intravenous haloperidol is considered the drug of choice, administered either as a bolus (10) or as a continuous drip (11). Given its relative specificity for dopamine receptors, it produces little hypotension, has few if any anticholinergic effects, and does not suppress the respiratory drive (9). Sos and Casem (12) and Tesar and colleagues (13) have used this agent extensively in idiopathic, agitated deliriums with good result and little morbidity. Interestingly, when this medication is given intravenously it produces fewer extrapyramidal side effects than when administered orally (14). Following TBI, the lowest possible effective doses should be employed. Thus, 2 mg may be administered every 30 minutes until reasonable control has been achieved or a maximum of 15 mg per 24 hours. Acceptable results have also been obtained when low dose benzodiazepines are combined with neuroleptics (15). Lorazepam (1 to 2 mg) administered intravenously or intramuscularly may reduce the dose of haloperidol needed to produce the desired clinical outcome. Delirium is usually time limited and begins to end with the clearing of the posttraumatic amnesia (16). Thus, these interventions need to be carefully reviewed on a daily basis. Once the patient has stabilized, the haloperidol should be gradually reduced over a period of 3 to 5 days rather than abruptly discontinued (9). Clinical experience suggests that a prolonged delirium following TBI can evolve into a number of neuropsychiatric syndromes as the patient's consciousness clears. These include secondary psychoses, amnestic disorder, and dementia.

Management also focuses on environmental prosthesis. To that end it attempts to reduce the handicapping conditions of the patient and provide for the safety of all concerned. First, the environment must be

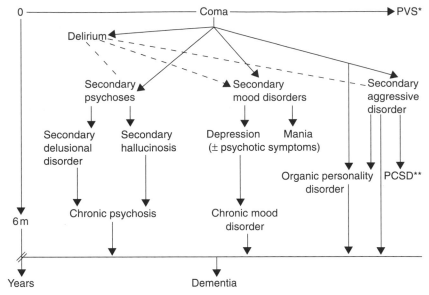

* Persistent vegetative state. ** Partial complex seizure disorder

Figure 11.2 *Secondary Psychiatric Syndromes.*

controlled and quiet. The notion that a stimulating environment helps a damaged CNS recover is absurd. Therefore, all non-essential personnel should be excluded from the treatment milieu. The environment must be as clear of obstacles as possible, overhead paging systems eliminated, and, when necessary, 1 : 1 staffing provided. Diurnal variation in lighting and activity should be continued. Focus must be maintained on providing respiratory support, intravenous and enteric access to sustain life. Thus, restraints may become necessary if the patient consistently compromises the integrity of these supports. When such measures are employed, the staff must be prepared to explain the rationale behind their use to the patient's family. The so-called Craig bed cannot provide this level of support to the patient and its use should be avoided under most circumstances. Behavioral and psychosocial strategies are less effective at this point in time.

As delirium clears, a patient can be handicapped by a number of psychiatric disorders best conceptualized (at least at first) as secondary to the underlying neuropathology. These difficulties fall into three broad categories: disorders of thought or perception, mood disorders, and disorders principally characterized by frontal system deficits (personality disorders). They may evolve into a number of more specific diagnoses (Figure 11.2).

Secondary Disorders of Thought or Perception

In other patients with TBI, their initial recovery is complicated primarily by the presence of perceptual distortions or delusional thinking (referred to as secondary psychotic disorders) (17,18,19). Frequently these sensory and cognitive difficulties are accompanied by destructive behavior that can be unpredictable. These symptoms are transient and will abate spontaneously with the clearing of consciousness. Under these circumstances, no pharmacologic intervention is warranted. In the acute stages of rehabilitation, several circumstances can alter this recommendation. First, the disturbances continue beyond several days. Second, the hallucinations or delusions become "commanding" in nature (i.e., the individual is "told to do" certain life-threatening things, like harm himself or others). Third, the accompanying destructive behavior cannot be contained within the treatment milieu.

There are no controlled studies to guide the pharmacologic therapy of the TBI patient with a secondary psychotic disorder. However, there are numerous controlled studies of the use of these agents in patients with idiopathic psychotic disorders and some case reports in the TBI literature (20,21). Selection of an appropriate agent is determined more by the wish to avoid certain side effects than by drug specificity. The recent introduction of risperidone and olanzapine has simplified this process, as both medications are relatively free of the motor, cardiovascular, and anticholinergic side effects that plagued older antipsychotic agents. The older antipsychotic agents cluster into two categories. First, low-dose, high-potency agents such as pimozide, haloperidol, thiothixene, or fluphenazine lack anticholinergic and autonomic effects. However, they are more likely to cause pseudoparkinsonian side effects such as tremor, gait disturbance, and akathisia. Second, high-dose, low-potency drugs such as chlorpromazine and thioridazine are less likely to produce motor side effects but are more sedating and produce both anticholinergic and autonomic side effects. Both groups are now reserved for treatment refractory patients who fail to respond to either risperidone or olanzapine.

Clozapine, another atypical antipsychotic, has an important, but limited role to play in those with TBI and chronic psychoses. It is the most effective antipsychotic agent currently available in the United States. Like risperidone and olanzapine, clozapine produces few if any extrapyramidal effects and has not been implicated in causing tardive dyskinesia (22). In fact, it may improve dyskinetic movements in patients who already manifest this disorder. However, it is epileptogenic, profoundly sedating, and can produce agranulocytosis. Thus, it should be used cautiously in patients with a high risk of seizures or in those being treated with carbamazepine or other agents likely to suppress bone marrow functioning. Clozapine may be used in conjunction with sodium valproate for patients with seizure disorders for whom no other neuroleptic alternatives exist. In addition, the Food and Drug Administration (FDA) requires that patients receiving this medication have weekly blood counts before their 7-day supply of medication can be released from a pharmacy. Hypotension, tachycardia, and hyperptyalism also need to be carefully monitored. Michals and colleagues (23) reported their experience in using clozapine with nine TBI patients in 1992. All were in the very late phases of post-acute rehabilitation. Approximately 33% of these patients had a positive response to this medication. However, two of the nine had its use precluded by the onset of seizures.

Secondary Mood Disorders

Mania

Disorders primarily involving mood and its accompanying neurovegetative signs may also present early in the course of rehabilitation in association with destructive behavior. Secondary mood disorder, manic type, is generally seen toward the end of post-traumatic amnesia (PTA). If this condition occurs later, a second pathophysiologic process—such as development of a subdural hematoma, seizure disorder, or intracerebral infection—should be sought. These patients will present with pressured speech, flight of ideas (often grandiose in nature), motor hyperactivity, and insomnia. Their sensorium is usually clear, but they may become confused as their condition worsens.

No controlled studies have been done with destructive TBI patients with a secondary mania. The neuropsychiatric literature includes controlled studies of the agents discussed below, used with patients who suffer from idiopathic mania. Rare case reports have included TBI patients.

If psychosis accompanies symptoms of mania (see section "Secondary Disorders of Thought or Perception"), a brief trial of a neuroleptic is indicated by clinical experience. However, if psychosis is not present and the difficulties persist beyond 7 to 10 days, lithium should be considered, as its efficacy has been conclusively demonstrated in controlled studies. Some clinicians have been concerned about the epileptogenic potential of lithium, yet Erwin and colleagues (25) reported a 36% reduction in the number of seizures seen in 17 lithium-treated, epileptic patients. Close blood monitoring (twice per week) is suggested, especially early after its initiation until steady-state conditions are reached.

During the past two decades, anticonvulsants have demonstrated efficacy in the treatment of both primary and secondary mania. Ballenger and Post (26) were the first to study systematically the use of carbamazepine in controlled trials for this indication. It may be used as a single agent or in combination with lithium. Although reports of neurotoxicity have appeared when these two agents have been used in combination, they are rare (27). An adequate therapeutic response is often obtained with blood levels in the 8 to 10 ng/dL range (28,29). In uncontrolled trials, McElroy and colleagues (30) and McElroy and Pope (31) have used sodium valproate for these syndromes. This group reported two patients with secondary mania caused by TBI who responded to valproate (32). Of particular interest was the fact that neither had responded to other more standard treatments before the valproate trial. Freeman and colleagues (33) in a controlled study, noted that valproate may be of greater benefit than lithium to individuals with "mixed mania," which is often associated with destructive behavior. Blood levels need to be monitored and should be maintained between 55 and 100 ng/dL, although most investigators have found the higher end of the therapeutic range to be optimal (34).

Secondary Depression

Depression should always be considered in the differential diagnosis of destructive behavior. This is especially true if a patient, who has been otherwise stable, begins to deteriorate behaviorally.

No controlled studies with TBI patients who sustained moderate or severe injuries have been reported. However, the controlled studies of non-TBI patients (especially those with post stroke depression) are relatively abundant in the neuromedical literature and support the efficacy of antidepressants in treating such conditions. Varney and colleagues (35) reported an uncontrolled series of 51 patients with TBI who responded positively to thymoleptic therapy. The author (36) reported a series of nine patients with severe TBI treated with the newer selective serotonin reuptake inhibitor (SSRI), fluoxetine. In an uncontrolled open trial, over 60% of these individuals benefited from treatment with few side effects. Thus, depressed patients with TBI manifesting destructive behavior should be tried on an antidepressant. Newer agents such as the SSRIs (fluoxetine, fluvoxamine, paroxetine, or sertraline) should be considered the drugs of choice. However, depression and destructive behavior associated with psychosis will require treatment with both an antidepressant and an antipsychotic medication. This has been demonstrated in controlled studies in the psychiatric literature (37), and clinical experience with TBI patients concurs.

Partial Complex Epilepsy

Late-onset, partial complex epilepsy also may be rarely associated with episodic, nondirected destructive behavior. Historically, patients with intermittent explosive disorder have been considered a subset of this group, and limbically active anticonvulsants, such as carbamazepine and sodium valproate, are therefore the drugs of choice (38). Accompanying, so-called interictal personality disturbances are rarely responsive to anticonvulsants alone. Paranoid delusions may develop, even years after the onset of seizures, which require concomitant management with neuroleptics. This is also true of associated mood disturbances that require treatment with appropriate thymoleptics (39).

Frontal System Disorders

Secondary Aggressive Disorder

Another syndrome that may be seen after the patient with TBI has emerged from coma is organic aggressive disorder described by Silver and colleagues (40). In this disorder, destructive behavior is observed, while difficulties with orientation are less pronounced than in delirium. Abnormalities in thought content or perception do not predominate, and a change in personality is not a requirement of diagnosis. Quasi-controlled studies exist in the TBI literature. Numerous case reports exist in both the non-TBI and TBI neurobehavioral literature.

Rao and colleagues (41) (in a quasi-controlled study) have treated this group of patients successfully with oral haloperidol with doses in the 2–15 mg/day range. They reported no significant differences in rehabilitative outcome between the treated and control groups. Nevertheless, the period of post-traumatic amnesia was significantly longer in the treated group. However, this difference may be attributable to increased severity of neurologic impairment in the treated group. Theoretical challenges to this study have been partially based on an earlier study by Feeney and colleagues (42), who reported that haloperidol impaired motor recovery following brain injury in animal models, presumably by disrupting dopaminergic transmission. Although the applicability of these findings to humans is unknown at this time, they stimulated the search for other agents with which to treat these patients.

Trials with various antidepressants have been one response to this dilemma. Jackson and colleagues (43) were the first to report the use of amitriptyline for aggression in 1985. In that report, they discussed a patient who responded to 50 mg of amitriptyline administered orally at bedtime. Their group (44) did a follow-up study involving 20 patients with secondary aggression. Dosages of this agent ranged up to a maximum of 150 mg/day. However, like the Rao study, only 50% of the treatment group cleared post-traumatic amnesia. Again, the non-treated group was not a true control group since they had already had a return of continuous memory and did not exhibit behavioral difficulties significant enough to warrant entry into the treatment group. A few case reports of organically impaired (but not head-injured) patients with aggression have shown a good response to the serotonergically active antidepressant trazodone. The mean dose of trazodone has been 200 mg, but some clinicians have used up to 600 mg/day in divided doses.

A non-benzodiazepine anxiolytic, buspirone, may also come to play a role in the treatment of these patients (45). At low doses, it is a direct 5-HT1A agonist (46). Levine (47) presented a case report using buspirone in a patient with TBI and organic aggressive syndrome. Sustained improvement occurred at 10 mg given three times per day. In general, the side effects of buspirone are few and mainly confined to mild sedation. However, a few scattered reports have been found that suggest it may produce akathisia and tinnitus (48).

Psychostimulants such as dextroamphetamine and methylphenidate have also been tried in case reports of TBI patients with secondary aggression (49). Results have been mixed, and some patients developed what appeared to be tolerance to these medications. Amantadine, a direct and indirect dopamine agonist, has been used with some success in these patients. Chandler and colleagues (50) reported on two patients with relatively acute aggressive disorder, secondary to TBI, who responded satisfactorily to amantadine following failure of other medications. Amantadine had a favorable toxicity profile and was not epileptogenic. Other direct-acting dopamine agonists such as bromocriptine, pergolide, and low-dose apomorphine may also benefit certain individuals who do not respond to amantadine or the indirect-acting psychostimulants.

Although not well studied in patients with acute secondary aggressive disorder, adrenergically active agents have been considered as second-line drugs by experienced clinicians. The author prefers to use a transdermal clonidine patch (0.3–0.6 mg/day/week) for these patients. This agent is discussed in detail below.

Secondary Personality Disorder

More chronic destructive disorders occurring with personality changes, independently of major mood or perceptual abnormalities, may be seen after the sensorium has cleared. They are usually episodic in nature and often related to persistent frontal system deficits or disconnection syndromes. Various labels have been given to the former condition, ranging from "frontal aggression" to "organic personality disorder, explosive type." Few controlled studies exist in the TBI and neuromedical literature, although there are abundant case reports.

Elliott (51) first reported on the use of propranolol, a beta-adrenergic receptor blocker, in patients with organic difficulties and agitation. All of the patients in this open study improved with doses ranging between 60 and 1600 mg/day. A number of similar studies followed Elliott's report, demonstrating improvement in 86% of the over 200 patients treated with this agent (52,53). However, Greendyke and colleagues (54) reviewed the use of propranolol in a double-blind crossover study, and although they found a statistical reduction in the number of assaults in the treatment group, the absolute number was not markedly decreased. Silver and colleagues (40) offer guidelines for the use of this agent.

With increased use of propranolol, the initial enthusiasm regarding its role in secondary personality disorder has waned. This has occurred for several reasons. First, it takes considerable time to gradually titrate the dose upward toward the recommended target dose of 640 mg/day. Second, the drug must be withheld due to clinically significant postural hypotension that occurs on a regular basis in this patient population. Third, it can take many weeks after reaching a relatively high dose to know whether the medication will be effective and such time is not generally available for most "managed care" patients.

Therefore, other alpha- and beta-blockers have been evaluated. In case reports, nadolol has been reported to be efficacious in doses between 40 and 160 mg/day. The utility of this agent suggests that peripheral as well as central mechanisms may be important in the usefulness of this class of drugs (55). Greendyke and Kanter (56) reported their use of pindolol (up to 60 mg/day) in similar patients. This agent appears to have an advantage over propranolol in that it produces less hypotension, apparently due to its intrinsic sympathomimetic activity.

Clonidine, an α_2-adrenergic agonist, has been shown to benefit some of these patients. It acts primarily on the presynaptic α_2-adrenergic autoreceptor, effectively inhibiting noradrenergic activity throughout the CNS. Side effects include sedation and postural hypotension. There is a significant "first pass" effect on blood pressure, so the initial dose is preferably small and given at bedtime. Then, the amount is gradually titrated up to approximately 0.6 mg/day (57). A transdermal preparation of this agent is available providing sustained release of up to 0.3 mg/day over a week.

Lithium carbonate has also been prescribed under these circumstances and is associated with a comparatively large literature in the head-injured population. Lithium has been used in the treatment of syndromes associated with destructive behavior with or without associated head injury (58,59). Hale and Donaldson (60) reported its use in five patients broadly diagnosed as having organic brain syndrome. Three of the five individuals in this study, however, had major head trauma. Each of the patients demonstrated improvement on lithium with blood levels between 0.6 and 0.8 mEq/L. None of the patients in this group had evidence of a primary affective disorder. Three of the subjects reported improved cognitive functioning while being treated with this agent; however, this has not been a consistent finding throughout all studies. Haas and Cope (49) reported a single case of aggression that was unresponsive to benzodiazepines, neuroleptics, propranolol, and methylphenidate. Lithium was significantly helpful. The response to lithium occurred within several days. Lithium levels ranged up to 0.8 mEq/L. Williams and Goldstein (61) reported on its effectiveness in a number of patients with organic brain syndromes, including one case associated with cerebrovascular accident. Again, none of the patients had a clear-cut mood disorder and agitation was severe in most. Glenn and colleagues (62) reported on the use of lithium in ten TBI patients described as aggressive or affectively unstable. Six of these patients had a positive response to this intervention, although one "regressed" after the seventh week of the study. Adverse neurologic effects were noted in three of these patients; however, only one was being treated with lithium alone.

Serotonergically active agents that reduce most forms of destructive behavior have also been used in secondary personality disorders. Ratey and colleagues (63) reported using buspirone to treat agitation and maladaptive behavior in two patients with acquired brain injuries. Low doses in the range of 10–15 mg/day were found effective for these patients. Generally, the response to buspirone is rapid. Therefore, Gualtieri (64) recommends discontinuing buspirone if it is not effective within several days following its initiation.

Direct and indirect dopamine agonists have also been used in this syndrome. In particular, psychostimulants—primarily dextroamphetamine and methylphenidate—have been used in treating destructive patients when they are inattentive and underaroused. Lipper and Tuchman (65) reported the first case where dextroamphetamine was tried. The patient was described as agitated and depressed, in addition to having memory and cognitive problems. He was apparently unresponsive to amitriptyline or a perphenazine-amitriptyline combination. Dextroamphetamine was successfully employed with gradually increasing doses up to 15 mg twice a day. The medication was briefly discontinued; however, its reinstitution did not lead to another positive response. Since that report, a number of clinical investigators have reported the effectiveness of methylphenidate and pemoline in similar situations (64,66).

Mooney and Haas (67) reported a controlled study where methylphenidate was used to treat "anger" in post-acute TBI patients who sustained severe injuries. A randomized, pretest, posttest, placebo control group, single blind design was employed to evaluate the effectiveness of methylphenidate. Several interesting findings were reported: short-term treatment with the active agent significantly reduced anger in this patient population. Patients with higher pretreatment anger scores responded better to methylphenidate than those with lower pretreatment anger scores. Further, this drug reduced the level of general psychopathology in the treatment group without producing significant adverse effects. However, attention, as measured by a variety of neuropsychological tests, unexpectedly did not improve with treatment.

Speech and colleagues (68) came to the opposite conclusion regarding dysregulated behavior in a double-blind, placebo-controlled randomized study of methylphenidate using a crossover design. The contradictory results are particularly problematic since these two studies are among the best in the pharmacologic treatment of behavioral disturbances following TBI. However, the two study designs are not equivalent in several important ways. First, the length of treatment in the Speech study was significantly shorter, 1 week compared to 6 weeks in the Mooney study. Second, over half of the patients in the Speech study were women, while Mooney studied men exclusively. Third, Speech grouped moderate and severe TBI patients together; Mooney and Haas restricted their study to those with severe injuries only. Finally, different outcome measures were used to determine the effects of methylphenidate.

Clinical experience suggests the usefulness of methylphenidate despite the conflicting reports. Furthermore, given its relatively benign side-effect profile and potentially rapid onset, it remains the initial drug of choice for this disorder. Adrenergically active agents run a close second.

Dementia

In later stages of rehabilitation and community reentry, other syndromes associated with destructive behavior begin to emerge. For some patients, the global CNS dysfunction of delirium will evolve into the more permanent problem of dementia. In other patients, dementia appears to be the final common pathway to which other secondary psychiatric disorders devolve.

Controlled treatment studies do not exist for this syndrome, nor are there any clearly defined TBI case reports. Thus, treatment is guided by non-TBI case reports, clinical experience, and attempts to treat potentially treatable subsyndromes of this condition.

When evaluating patients with dementia, it is vital to consider the "pseudodementia" of depression in the differential diagnosis. Many clinicians have suggested at least a 6-week trial of an antidepressant in this subgroup of patients, since the prognosis for those with frank dementia is so poor. Neuroleptics have been used in this population with varying degrees of success (69). However, given the chronicity of this condition, newer agents that do not produce tardive dyskinesia are the drugs of choice. Occasionally, benzodiazepines have been successfully used in those who have agitation associated with dementia. For this indication, oxazepam is the most frequently used agent from this class of medications (70). More recently, buspirone has been used successfully to manage destructive behavior occurring with dementia (71). Given its benign side-effect profile, buspirone should be considered the drug of choice in this subgroup of patients. Theoretically, other serotonergically active agents should be effective as well. Thus, a trial of fluoxetine, fluvoxamine, sertraline, or paroxetine may be warranted if buspirone fails to improve the agitation associated with dementia.

BEYOND PSYCHOPHARMACOLOGY

As much as any of us might wish for a magic elixir that transforms maladaptive, dysregulated behavior into appropriate and controlled conduct, such an agent does not yet exist and likely never will. Therefore, other nonpharmacologic strategies must be employed to help improve these patients' outcomes. These approaches center on the use of environmental prosthesis, behavioral programming, and psychotherapeutic techniques. A full discussion of each is beyond the scope of this text and the interested reader is referred to a number of texts that focus exclusively on these strategies (72,73). However, a few comments are warranted.

First, although we wish to believe that most treatment programs are comprehensive enough to care for even the worst of TBI outliers, the fact of the matter is that they are not, nor should they be. The attempt to be all things to all patient populations produces inescapable mediocrity for the whole. Very few programs see enough outliers to become expert in their management. Therefore, clinicians in general programs should recognize the need to refer these patients to specialized settings where the major focus of treatment centers on these handicapping conditions.

Second, environmental prosthesis must occur in even the most basic of neurorehabilitation settings. As noted above, such prosthesis centers on creating a quiet, secure, and safe treatment milieu. Such an environment is the antithesis of most acute rehabilitation hospital settings. However, it can be created if the will to do so exists both clinically and administratively. The constant background din of television sets, overhead paging systems, and modern cleaning equipment is not conducive to healing a damaged central nervous system, when inattentiveness and slowed processing speed must be overcome for learning to occur.

Third, inconsistently applied and ill-conceived, "cookbook" behavioral programming is worse than none at all. It rapidly devolves into a draconian punishment system that demoralizes both patients and staff. Therefore, most general programs are well advised to confine their behavioral interventions to "time out" and praise. Disruptive behavior is best dealt with by brief periods of "time out" in a "quiet-room." Generally, within 5 minutes, the calmer patient is quietly encouraged to reenter the treatment milieu and retry the activity or interaction that precipitated his or her dysregulated response. Praise, for even the smallest successes, goes a long way toward providing the only positive reinforcement most of us, including our brain-injured patients, need to continue to persevere at tasks that must be accomplished despite reluctance to believe that such mastery can be achieved.

Fourth, psychotherapy is not a technique to be practiced just because a patient and a clinician can both talk. It is rarely indicated for those with significant cognitive impairment or major psychiatric sequelae.

Standard practice must be modified to a more active, coaching technique that focuses on practical day-to-day problem solving and acceptance of those deficits that are unlikely to improve with time. Although improvement of self-awareness is a noble goal of psychotherapy, it is rarely achieved in those with true anosognosia. Finally, an hour's worth of psychotherapy once a week is no substitute for repeated encouragement from a caring staff, genuinely interested in the welfare of its patients.

Case Study

At the time of his work-related injury, W.D. was 21 years old. He was struck by an automobile while riding his bicycle and immediately rendered unconscious. Emergency medical service (EMS) records indicated that he had an initial Glasgow Coma Scale (GCS) score of 3. He was in respiratory distress and intubated at the scene. Upon arrival at the emergency department, his post-resuscitation GCS score had risen to 6. His initial brain CT revealed diffuse petechial hemorrhages and bilateral intraventricular bleeding. A ventriculostomy was placed for 2 weeks to control increased intracranial pressure. True coma lasted for 5 days, but he remained mute for over a month. He remained confused throughout his acute hospitalization. Subsequent brain CT scans revealed the following: left orbital frontal and inferior opercular contusions, right thalamic infarcts, and bilateral posterior and periventricular encephalomalacia.

At 2 months post injury, he was transferred to an acute rehabilitation hospital. In that setting, the patient remained confused and extremely agitated. He spent the majority of his days restrained in a chair bolted to the floor. When released from restraints, he would unpredictably strike out at staff and on one occasion assaulted a staff member, breaking her jaw. His treating physician tried a number of medications in an attempt to improve his behavior. These included pindolol, amantadine, and lorazepam. He did not benefit from these interventions. A repeat brain CT revealed a 3×3 cm left orbital and frontal polar contusion and moderate diffuse cerebral atrophy.

At 6 months post injury, he remained confused and agitated with a Galveston Orientation and Amnesia Test (GOAT) score of 40. During a phase of increased agitation, the amantadine was discontinued and his GOAT score decreased to 17. Subsequent trials on buspirone and carbamazepine were not particularly helpful. Buspirone was discontinued, and doxepin was begun along with low-dose haloperidol. The dosage of pindolol was increased and lithium was added to his medication regimen. On these agents, his aggression persisted; he required eight staff members to complete activities of daily living (ADLs) and ten to restrain him when he became violent. He was subsequently referred to a behavioral rehabilitation program at 5 months post admission.

At the time of admission to the behavioral rehabilitation program, he was confused, with a GOAT in the mid-30s, acutely agitated, extremely perseverative, and aphasic. Admission medications included haloperidol (2 mg IM three times/day), lithium carbonate (600 mg PO twice/day and 900 mg PO at bedtime), and lorazepam (2 mg IM every 4 hours) as needed for agitation. The manifestation of his destructive behavior showed no discernible pattern and was extremely unpredictable. His mental status examination revealed significant suspiciousness in thought content and hypervigilance. General physical examination was essentially unremarkable. Neurologic examination revealed profound parkinsonism, bilateral hyperreflexia, and frontal release signs on the right. Repeat brain CT revealed left frontal and right parietal infarcts and the aforementioned hydrocephalus ex-vacuo. An EEG demonstrated left frontal slowing, but no electrographic seizures.

All of the patient's medications were discontinued, and he was observed for 2 weeks free of medication. During this time, it was noted that his disorder of thought content worsened; he exhibited frank paranoia and appeared to be responding to internal stimuli. Although his parkinsonism improved off the haloperidol, it did not completely abate. He did not clear post-traumatic amnesia. At the end of 14 days, he was begun on clozapine and restarted on amantadine. His environment was simplified, and no staff members other than those trained in the management of aggressive behavior were permitted to interact with him. On 300 mg/day of clozapine and amantadine, he exhibited considerable improvement in his thought disorder and, subsequently, in his destructive behavior. At day 14 the restraints were discontinued and he was permitted to ambulate with assistance in the treatment milieu.

Subsequently it was noted that his destructive behavior would reemerge when he became frustrated performing tasks that he felt were "beneath" his abilities. Therefore, clonidine and labetalol were added to his medications. With the addition of these medications, he began to respond to behavioral cues and was able to perform all ADLs with only stand-by assistance. At 6 months post entry into the behavioral rehabilitation program, he was able to make the transition to a community-based residential facility.

This patient's course emphasizes the effects of focal contusional and diffuse hypoxemic injury on outcome. These neuropathological substrates produced fixed deficits that were unresponsive to standard remediative therapies. Furthermore, it became clear that the secondary delusional disorder producing abnormalities in his thought content had been unresponsive to haloperidol and that other medications "generically" prescribed to improve "phenotypic" agitation were unsuccessful in altering the course of his condition. Using the extension of the neurorehabilitation model, it became clear that both newer antipsychotic agents and medications designed to aid secondary personality disorder were necessary to improve his condition. Implementation of these more specific therapies reduced his level of disability and permitted his transfer to a less restrictive and less costly treatment environment.

OUTLIERS AND MINOR BRAIN INJURY

At the other end of the TBI continuum, a significant minority of patients with concussive events remain handicapped long after the predicted 3 months needed to restore most healthy patients to their baseline. In this circumstance, an adage from Johann Wolfgang von Goethe (1749–1832) seems appropriate: "We see what we look for. We look for what we know." Such is the case with minor brain injury (MBI), for if we do not clearly understand the syndrome, we have no hope of managing its outcome.

From its inception as a diagnosis in the mid-1800s, MBI has been a subject shrouded in controversy. It has been variably conceptualized, first as a "functional compensation neurosis" and then as "organic disorder" on par with "stroke." During the last decade, those who favored an organic explanation had their position bolstered by increasingly sophisticated basic research that described the pathophysiology of minor, diffuse axonal injury as a process mediated unequivocally by "biomechanical perturbations." However, in recent years, the acceptance of MBI's organic etiology has tended to obfuscate its nonorganic manifestations and confused its causality with patient outcome. These constructs are best understood in the context of the case presentation that follows.

Case Study

Leigh, a nurse-case manager for a large national case-management firm, called the author's office concerned about a client of hers with a presumed MBI, who had been inexplicably deteriorating over the past several months. S.L., a 26-year-old "roustabout" with no prior history of neurologic disorder, was now nearly 2 years post injury. At the time of the call, he was in treatment at a brain injury rehabilitation day program some distance from his home. The program employed a multidisciplinary treatment team and was run by a neuropsychologist. The patient was complaining of severe amnesia and the inability to read or write. Numerous treatment strategies had been employed, but none produced lasting benefit. Recently, his speech and language pathologist began using the program "Hooked on Phonics," which his wife had ordered for their 4-year-old daughter. Although the patient said that he liked this program and religiously used it twice a day, he remained unable to sign his name or to read. He was becoming more miserable by the day and had recently threatened to assault his wife and one of his therapists. Both the treatment team and his family were exasperated with him. It was in this context that the call was made to request a "second opinion."

S.L. arrived, unaccompanied, for evaluation nearly 1 month after that first phone call. He was tall and somewhat unkempt, with long, unwashed black hair pulled tightly back into a ponytail, but generally cooperative as he signed his admission paperwork with a witnessed X. He was tired from his early morning flight and elected to "turn in" for the day. Staff assisted him with unpacking, and he proudly placed his "Hooked on Phonics" tapes on his dresser. He produced a business card from his wallet that was inscribed with the following: "I'm sorry I'm so slow and can't read, but I had a brain injury last year and I'm still trying to recover. Please bear with me. Thanks." He said that he gave the card out several times a day and just wanted the staff to have one for his chart so the entire team would understand his limitations.

The next morning he outlined his history for me during morning work rounds. He could recall, in exquisite detail, how he slipped on the top metal step of the oil rig platform he'd been assigned to repair, fell down ten stairs "head over heels," and landed on his "butt." He could not recall if he lost consciousness, but remembered two coworkers coming to assist him after "they heard all the commotion." He had several abrasions that were treated and shortly thereafter a helicopter arrived to transport him to a mainland medical center. He complained of headache, but his evaluation was unremarkable; thus, he was released to return home with a recommendation to see his family physician the next day.

Despite this admonition, it was a full week before he saw his doctor. Complaints of headache, dizziness, and memory problems were paramount. He was started on Fiorinal (butalbital, aspirin, caffeine) with codeine, Naprosyn (naproxyn sodium), and Flexeril (cyclobenzaprine) and told to remain off work for the next 2 weeks. At the next visit, S.L. told his doctor that he felt worse than he had at the first appointment. New medicines were ordered and a course of physical therapy was prescribed.

Weeks passed, then months. Five physicians with specialties ranging from otolaryngology to orthopedics were consulted, and neuropsychological testing was ordered. Each physician listed "concussion" as one of his impressions (in addition to a host of other problems), and the neuropsychological testing "confirmed the presence of a traumatic brain injury with severe neurocognitive deficits." Each clinician recommended a different treatment plan, but the patient's condition continued to worsen and soon his lawyer recommended that he apply for Social Security disability benefits to supplement his income from workers' compensation. He was deemed to be totally and permanently disabled and, of course, unemployable. Finally, as a "last ditch effort," his treating physician referred him for intensive, outpatient rehabilitation with a special emphasis on "cognitive retraining" and speech therapy. Twenty weeks into the program, he was nearly amnestic and could neither read nor write.

What can be learned from this case? First, refocusing this patient's complaints in the context of his diagnosis and its natural history permits a broader understanding of his situation and suggests strategies for its management. The first step using this paradigm is to understand clearly his injury characteristics. As previously noted, this information is best obtained from the early vocational and medical records, such as the "employer's first report of injury or illness" or a police citation. Documentation of witnessed alteration of awareness or confusion, not loss of consciousness, is the critical factor. Without alteration of awareness, there is, by definition, no diffuse brain injury. There may have been a head injury, but not a brain injury. This distinction is critical in predicting the expected sequelae from the accident. If the patient can recall the injury—remember how it occurred, who was at fault, the sequence of events that injured his head—and explain what happened following it—the likelihood that this event produced a brain injury is remote. First responder reports often include such information and can be used to corroborate or refute the patient's recollection when the history is elicited later. Ambulance reports should always be consulted, as emergency medical technicians are adept at recording which areas of the body have been injured as well as the individual's mental status. GCS scores are routinely noted in most cases where injury has occurred to the head or can be reconstructed from the records. Confusion is generally noted, but its length is not easily established. However, a comparison of the EMS notes with the mental status recorded at the time of arrival to the emergency department can provide a rough estimate of its duration.

At the emergency department, the medical record becomes more focused. In this setting, the triage nursing notes are helpful because they often record the history verbatim from the patient. The neurologic and mental status examinations provide another point of reference in understanding the extent and degree of the patient's confusion. Furthermore, the patient's complaints generally center on typical concussive symptoms, such as headache, dizziness, and nausea. Initial neuroimaging studies, if indicated and performed, can clarify the presentation of focal injury. In the case of true MBI, they are always normal.

In S.L.'s case his initial injury characteristics were somewhat confusing. First, the event itself was unwitnessed. Second, the first responders did not record their impressions. Third, he has a good recollection of the accident, no retrograde amnesia, questionable loss of consciousness, possible confusion, and little, if any, post-traumatic amnesia. The EMS report recorded a GCS score of 15 and noted that he was "alert and oriented." However, the record revealed that they received the call for assistance 30 minutes before their arrival at the scene, and therefore his confusion could have cleared while they were en route. The emergency department noted complaints of generalized pain and headache and a small abrasion to his left supraorbital region, but no abnormalities in either his elemental neurologic or basic mental status examinations. A CT study of his brain was normal. Using the neurologic model, the patient's diagnosis was "possible minor head and brain injury, characterized by diffuse axonal injury."

Now that we know the diagnosis, we can predict the natural history of this disorder as well as the anticipated outcome at various points in time. It has become clear that the vast majority of these patients, up to 95%, gets better as time progresses. Since S.L. has gotten worse, he is, without a doubt, an outlier. These outliers may have persistent concussive disorder (PCS), but other syndromes must be considered as well. The next question to be answered was the correspondence of his presentation with that of other patients with PCS. The most commonly documented symptoms of this disorder include headache, dizziness, fatigue, and attentional problems that produce some problems with episodic memory and emotional lability. S.L.'s complaints far exceeded those seen in patients with true PCS, and, as such, he could not have this syndrome.

If not PCS, then what? Rather than add dense amnesia, alexia, and agraphia to the list of symptoms seen in this patient population, it is far more prudent to use our model to suggest a number of currently recognized syndromes for differential diagnosis. With the use of neuropsychiatric constructs, the somatoform disorders need to be considered in the differential diagnostic process in addition to malingering and factitious disorders.

Somatoform disorders are defined by the American Psychiatric Association's Diagnostic and Statistical Manual, IV edition (DSM-IV) (74) as a group of disorders characterized by the presence of physical symptoms that suggest a physical disorder, but cannot be fully explained by it. The symptoms must cause clinically significant distress or impairment in social or occupational functioning. In contrast to malingering and factitious disorders, the production of the physical symptoms is not intentional. They include somatization disorder, conversion disorder, pain disorder, hypochondriasis, and body dysmorphic disorder. Diagnostic criteria for each of these conditions are listed in Table 11.5.

Malingering is defined as the intentional production of false or grossly exaggerated physical or psychological symptoms, motivated by secondary gain generally for financial compensation. Factitious disorders are characterized by physical or psychological symptoms that are intentionally produced or feigned in order to assume and maintain the "sick role."

With these differential diagnoses in mind, a plan for evaluation evolved. First, direct staff observation noted inconsistencies in the patient's degree of disability. At times, he would converse with them as

Table 11.5. *Diagnostic Criteria for Somatoform Disorders*

Somatization disorder

A. A history of many physical complaints beginning before age 30, occurring over a period of several years resulting in treatment being sought or significant impairment in social, occupational, or other important areas of functioning.
B. Each of the following criteria must have been met, with individual symptoms occurring at any time during the course of the disturbance.
   (1) four pain symptoms
   (2) two gastrointestinal symptoms
   (3) one sexual symptom
   (4) one pseudoneurological symptom
C. Either:
   (1) after appropriate investigation, each of the symptoms in Criterion B cannot be fully explained by a known general medical condition or the direct effects of a substance
   or
   (2) when there is a related general medical condition, the physical complaints or resulting social or occupational impairment are in excess of what would be expected from the history, physical examination, or laboratory findings.
D. The symptoms *are not* intentionally produced or feigned.

Conversion disorder

A. One or more symptoms or deficits affecting voluntary motor or sensory function that suggest a neurological or other general medical condition.
B. Psychological factors are judged to be associated with the symptom or deficit because the initiation or exacerbation of the symptom or deficit is preceded by conflicts or other stressors.
C. The symptom or deficit is not intentionally produced or feigned
D. The symptom or deficit cannot, after appropriate investigation, be fully explained by a general medical condition, or by the direct effects of a substance, or as a culturally sanctioned behavior or experience.
E. The symptom or deficit causes clinically significant distress or impairment in social, occupational, or other important areas of functioning or warrants medical evaluation.
F. The symptom or deficit is not limited to pain or sexual dysfunction, does not occur exclusively during the course of Somatization Disorder, and is not better accounted for by another mental disorder.

Pain disorder

A. Pain in one or more anatomical sites is the predominant focus of the clinical presentation and is of sufficient severity to warrant clinical attention.
B. The pain causes clinically significant distress or impairment in social, occupational, or other important areas of functioning.
C. Psychological factors are judged to have an important role in the onset, severity, exacerbation, or maintenance of the pain.
D. The symptom or deficit is not intentionally produced or feigned.
E. The pain is not better accounted for by a Mood, Anxiety, or Psychotic Disorder and does not meet criteria for Dyspareunia.

Hypochondriasis

A. A preoccupation with fears of having, or the idea that one has, a serious disease based on the person's misinterpretation of bodily symptoms.
B. The preoccupation persists despite appropriate medical evaluation and reassurance.
C. The belief in Criterion A is not of delusional intensity and is not restricted to a circumscribed concern about appearance.
D. The preoccupation causes clinically significant distress or impairment in social, occupational, or other important areas of functioning.
E. The duration of the disturbance is at least six months.

Table 11.5. *Continued*

F. The preoccupation is not better accounted for by Generalized Anxiety Disorder, Obsessive-Compulsive Disorder, Panic Disorder, a Major Depressive Episode, Separation Anxiety or other Somatoform Disorder.

Body dysmorphic disorder
A. Preoccupation with an imagined defect in appearance. If a slight physical anomaly is present, the person's concern is markedly excessive.
B. The preoccupation causes clinically significant distress or impairment in social, occupational, or other important areas of functioning.
C. The preoccupation is not better accounted for by another mental disorder.

SOURCE: (74).

if he were entirely free of cognitive dysfunction, and, while on community outings, he managed to find personal hygiene items without assistance or random searching. At other times, he complained bitterly that he could remember nothing and had no hope of returning to a normal life. His premorbid history became clearer as school and work records arrived for evaluation. It was learned that he was a below-average student who left school after failing his junior year of high school. He never sat for the GED and had no specialized job training. His work history was spotty, with numerous job changes and no steady income. He had been employed less than a month at the job where he was injured. Finally, forced-choice neuropsychological tests and the Rey 15 item test suggested exaggeration of symptoms, if not outright malingering.

Given that the diagnosis of malingering is best confirmed by the individual's eventual admission to dissimulation, a drug-assisted interview was undertaken. Following the induction of significant sedation with intravenous diazepam, S.L. was interviewed by his attending physician and the procedure recorded on videotape. During this interview it was learned that he had indeed feigned his symptoms at the "suggestion" of his lawyer, for "with brain injury cases you always have to add at least one zero when it comes to settlement." He stated that he felt trapped by his symptoms and did not know how to "get out of this situation." The following day he was shown the tape during an extended consultation with his physician. During that visit, he openly admitted that he had "faked" his problems and wondered what he should do next. A dialogue was opened with his case manager and she facilitated closing the case and referred final disposition to the company's legal department.

Other patients, while not intentionally feigning their disabilities, have complaints that exceed their underlying neuropathology. Under these circumstances, the somatoform and mood disorders must be systematically considered. Criteria for major depressive disorder are listed in Table 11.6. Patients presenting with memory complaints and depression often respond to questions with "I don't know" rather than incorrect answers. Treatment of the depression with medications leads to a

Table 11.6.   *Diagnostic Criteria for Major Depressive Disorder*

A. Five or more of the following symptoms have been present during the same 2-week period and represent a change from previous functioning; at least one of the symptoms is either (1) or (2).
   (1) depressed mood most of the day, nearly every day, as indicated by either subjective report or observation made by others.
   (2) markedly diminished interest or pleasure in all, or almost all, activities most of the day, nearly every day.
   (3) significant weight loss when not dieting or weight gain or decrease or increase in appetite nearly every day.
   (4) insomnia or hypersomnia nearly every day.
   (5) psychomotor agitation or retardation nearly every day.
   (6) fatigue or loss of energy nearly every day.
   (7) feelings of worthlessness or excessive or inappropriate guilt (which may be delusional) nearly every day.
   (8) diminished ability to think or concentrate, or indecisiveness, nearly every day.
   (9) recurrent thoughts of death, recurrent suicidal ideation without a specific plan, or a suicide attempt or a specific plan or committing suicide.
B. The symptoms cause clinically significant distress or impairment in social, occupational, or other important areas of functioning.
C. The symptoms are not due to the direct physiological effects of a substance or general medical condition.

SOURCE: (74).

remission of their memory difficulties. Those with conversion disorder or hypochondriasis are more difficult to treat and are best managed by clinicians who have considerable experience managing patients with somatoform disorders.

CONCLUSION

We have now come full circle, and it should be clear that outliers occur at each end of the spectrum of severity. Variation from the expected is the defining quality of their presentation. However, proper extension of the principles of the neurologic model of rehabilitation provides for appropriate diagnosis and management of these challenging patients.

References

1. Cooper PJ, ed. Head injury. 3rd ed. Baltimore: Williams & Wilkins, 1993.
2. Rosenthal M, Griffith ER, Bond MR, Miller JD. Rehabilitation of the adult and child with traumatic brain injury. Philadelphia: F.A. Davis, 1990.

3. Strub RL, Black FW. Neurobehavioral disorders: a clinical approach. Philadelphia: F.A. Davis, 1988.
4. Taylor MA. The neuropsychiatric mental status examination. New York: S.P. Medical and Scientific Books, 1981.
5. Folstein MF, Folstein SE, McHugh PR. Mini-mental state. A practical method for grading the cognitive state of patients for the clinician. J Psychiatr Res 1975;12:189–195.
6. Flor-Henry P. Cerebral basis of psychopathology. Boston: J. Wright, 1983.
7. Rabins PV, Folstein MF. Delirium and dementia. Br J Psychiatry 1982; 140:149.
8. Lipowski ZJ. Delirium: acute confusional states. New York: Oxford University Press, 1990.
9. Wise MG, Brandt GT. Delirium. In: Hales RE, Yudofsky SC, eds. Textbook of neuropsychiatry. Washington, DC: American Psychiatric Press, 1987:89–106.
10. Lipowski ZJ. Delirium updated. Compr Psychiatry 1980;21:190–196.
11. Fernandez F, Holmes V, Adams F, Kavanaugh J. Treatment of severe, refractory agitation with a haloperidol drip. J Clin Psychiatry 1988;49:239–241.
12. Sos J, Cassem NH. Managing postoperative agitation. Drug Ther 1980;10:103–106.
13. Tesar GE, Murray GB, Cassem NH. Use of high-dose intravenous haloperidol in the treatment of agitated cardiac patients. J Clin Psychopharmacol 1985;5:344–347.
14. Menza M, Murray G, Holmes V, Rafuls WA. Decreased extrapyramidal symptoms with intravenous haloperidol. J Clin Psychiatry 1987;48:278–280.
15. Adams F. Neuropsychiatric evaluation and treatment of delirium in the critically ill cancer patient. Cancer Bull 1984;36:156–160.
16. Brooke MM, Questad KA, Patterson DR, Bashak KJ. Agitation and restlessness after closed head injury: a prospective study of 100 consecutive admissions. Arch Phys Med Rehabil 1992;73:320–322.
17. Achte KA, Hillbom E, Aalberg V. Psychosis following war brain injuries. Acta Psychiatr Scand 1969;45:1–18.
18. Davison K, Bagley CR. Schizophrenia-like psychosis associated with organic disorders of the central nervous system. Br J Psychiatry 1969;4:113–184.
19. Shapiro LB. Schizophrenia-like psychosis following head injuries. IMJ 1939;10:150–254.
20. Donaldson SR, Gelenberg AJ, Baldessarini RJ. The pharmacologic treatment of schizophrenia: a progress report. Schizophr Bull 1983:504–527.
21. Janicak PG, Davis JM, Preskorn SH, Ayd FJ, eds. Principles and practice of psychopharmacolotherapy. Baltimore: Williams & Wilkins, 1993: 93–118.
22. Anden NE, Stock G. Effect of clozapine on the turnover of dopamine in the corpus striatum and in the limbic system. J Pharm Pharmacol 1973; 25:346–348.
23. Michals MI, Crismon ML, Roberts S, Childs A. Clozapine response and adverse effects in nine brain-injured patients. J Clin Psychopharmacol 1993;13:198–203.
24. Schou M. Lithium treatment of manic-depressive illness. JAMA 1988;259:1834–1836.

25. Erwin CW, Gerber J, Morrison SD, James JF. Lithium carbonate and convulsive disorders. Arch Gen Psychiatry 1973;28:646–648.

26. Ballenger JC, Post RM. Carbamazepine in manic-depressive illness: a new treatment. Am J Psychiatry 1980;137:782–790.

27. Shukla S, Cook BL, Mukherjee S, et al. Mania following head trauma. Am J Psychiatry 1987;144:93–96.

28. Folks DG, King LD, Dowdy SB, et al. Carbamazepine treatment of selected affectively disordered inpatients. Am J Psychiatry 1982; 139:115–117.

29. Rall TW, Schleifer LS. Drugs effective in the therapy of the epilepsies. In: Gilman AG, Goodman LS, Rall TW, et al., eds. The pharmacological basis of therapeutics. 7th ed. New York: Macmillan, 1985:446–472.

30. McElroy SL, Pope HG, Keck PE. Sodium valproate: its use in primary psychiatric disorders. J Clin Psychopharmacol 1987;7:16–24.

31. McElroy SL, Pope HG. Use of anticonvulsants in psychiatry: recent advances. Clifton, NJ: Oxford Health Care, 1988.

32. Pope HG, McElroy SL, Satlin A, et al. Head injury, bipolar disorder, and response to valproate. Compr Psychiatry 1988;29:34–38.

33. Freeman TW, Clothier JL, Pazzaglia P, et al. A double-blind study of valproate and lithium in the treatment of acute mania. Am J Psychiatry 1992;149:108–111.

34. McElroy SL, Keck PE, Pope HG, Hudson JI. Valproate in psychiatric disorders: literature review and clinical guidelines. J Clin Psychiatry 1989;50:23–29.

35. Varney NR, Martzke JS, Roberts RJ. Major depression in patients with closed head injury. Neuropsychology 1987;1:7–9.

36. Cassidy JW. Fluoxetine: a new serotonergically-active antidepressant. J Head Trauma Rehabil 1989;4:67–69.

37. Spiker DG, Weiss JC, Dealy RS, et al. The pharmacological treatment of delusional depression. Am J Psychiatry 1985:142:430–436.

38. Eames P. Risk-benefit considerations in drug treatment. In: Wood RL, Eames P, eds. Models of brain injury rehabilitation. London: Chapman and Hall, 1989:164–182.

39. Humphries HR, Dixon PS. Hypomania following complex partial seizures. Br J Psychiatry 1988;152:571–572.

40. Silver JM, Yudofsky SC, Hales RE. Neuropsychiatric aspects of traumatic brain injury. In: Hales RE, Yudofsky SC, eds. Textbook of neuropsychiatry. Washington, DC: American Psychiatric Press, 1987: 179–190.

41. Rao N, Jellinek M, Woolston DC. Agitation in closed head injury: haloperidol effects on rehabilitation outcome. Arch Phys Med Rehabil 1985;66:30–34.

42. Feeney D, Gonzalez A, Law W. Amphetamine, haloperidol, and experience interact to affect rate of recovery after motor cortex injury. Science 1982;217:855–857.

43. Jackson RD, Corrigan JD, Arnett JA. Amitriptyline for agitation in head injury. Arch Phys Med Rehabil 1985;66:180–181.

44. Mysiw WJ, Jackson RD, Corrigan JD. Amitriptyline for post-agitation. Am J Phys Med Rehabil 1988;67:29–33.

45. Riblet LA, Taylor DP, Eison MS, Stanton HC. Pharmacology and neurochemistry of buspirone. J Clin Psychiatry 1982;43:11–18.

46. Eison AS, Temple DL. Buspirone: review of its pharmacology and current perspectives on its mechanism of action. Am J Med 1986;80:1–9.

47. Levine AM. Buspirone and agitation in head injury. Brain Injury 1988;2:165–167.
48. Patterson JF. Akathisia associated with buspirone. J Clin Psychopharmacol 1988;8:296–297.
49. Haas JF, Cope N. Neuropharmacologic management of behavior sequelae in head injury: a case report. Arch Phys Med Rehabil 1985;66:472–474.
50. Chandler MC, Barnhill JL, Gualtieri CT. Amantadine for the agitated head-injury patient. Brain Injury 1988;2:309–311.
51. Elliott FA. Propranolol for control of belligerent behavior following acute brain damage. Ann Neurol 1987;1:489–491.
52. Volavka J. Can aggressive behavior in humans be modified by beta-blockers? Postgrad Med 1988:163–168.
53. Yudofsky S, Williams D, Gorman J. Propranolol in the treatment of rage and violent behavior in patients with chronic brain syndromes. Am J Psychiatry 1981;138:218–220.
54. Greendyke RM, Kanter DR, Schuster DB, et al. Propranolol treatment of assaultive patients with organic brain disease: double-blind, crossover placebo controlled study. J Nerv Ment Dis 1986;174:290–294.
55. Polakoff SA, Sorgi PJ, Ratey JJ. The treatment of impulsive and aggressive behavior with nandolol. J Clin Psychopharmacol 1986;6:125–126.
56. Greendyke RM, Kanter DR. Therapeutic effects of pindolol on disturbances associated with organic brain disease: double-blind study. J Clin Psychiatry 1986;47:423–426.
57. Rudd P, Blaschke TF. Antihypertensive agents and the drug therapy of hypertension. In: Gilman AG, Goodman LS, Rall TW, et al., eds. The pharmacological basis of therapeutics. New York: Macmillan, 1985:784–805.
58. Morrison SD, Erwin CW, Gianturco DT, Gerber CJ. Effect of lithium on combative behavior in humans. Dis Nerv Syst 1973;34:186–189.
59. Sheard MH. Lithium in the treatment of aggression. J Nerv Ment Dis 1975;160:108–118.
60. Hale MS, Donaldson JO. Lithium carbonate in the treatment of organic brain syndrome. J Nerv Ment Dis 1982;170:362–365.
61. Williams KH, Goldstein G. Cognitive and affective responses to lithium in patients with organic brain syndrome. Am J Psychiatry 1979;136:800–803.
62. Glenn MB, Wroblewski B, Parziale J, Levine L. Lithium carbonate for aggressive behavior or affective instability in ten brain-injured patients. Am J Phys Med Rehabil 1989;68:221–226.
63. Ratey JJ, Komry V, Gaffar K. Low-dose buspirone to treat agitation and maladaptive behavior in brain-injured patients: two case reports. J Clin Psychopharmacol 1992;12:363–364.
64. Gualtieri CT, Evans RW. Stimulant treatment for the neurobehavioral sequelae of traumatic brain injury. Brain Injury 1988;2:273–290.
65. Lipper S, Tuchman MM. Treatment of chronic post-traumatic organic brain syndrome with dextroamphetamine: first reported case. J Nerv Ment Dis 1976;162:366–371.
66. Evans RW, Gualtieri CT, Patterson D. Treatment of chronic closed head injury with psychostimulant drugs: a controlled case study and an appropriate evaluation procedure. J Nerv Ment Dis 1987;175:106–110.
67. Mooney GF, Haas LJ. Effect of methylphenidate on brain injury-related anger. Arch Phys Med Rehabil 1993;74:153–160.

68. Speech TJ, Rao SM, Osmon DC, Sperry LT. A double-blind controlled study of methylphenidate treatment in closed head injury. Brain Injury 1993;4:333–338.

69. Salzman C. Treatment of agitation in the elderly. In: Meltzer HY, ed. Psychopharmacology: the third generation of progress. New York: Raven Press, 1987.

70. Deberdt R, Bagley CR. Oxazepam in the treatment of anxiety in children and the elderly. Acta Psychiatr Scand 1978;274(s):104–110.

71. Colenda CC. Buspirone in treatment of agitated dementia patients. Lancet 1988;1:1169.

72. Eames P, Haffey WJ, Cope DN. Treatment of behavioral disorders. In: Rosenthal M, Griffith ER, Bond MR, Miller JD, eds. Rehabilitation of the adult and child with traumatic brain injury. Philadelphia: F.A. Davis, 1990:410–432.

73. Wood RL, Eames P, eds. Models of brain injury rehabilitation. London: Chapman and Hall, 1989.

74. Diagnostic and statistical manual of mental disorders. 4th ed. Washington, DC: American Psychiatric Press, 1994.

Index

Abducens nerve, anatomic relationships of, 4, 5–6
Abscess, cerebral, 162
Acceleration/deceleration injuries, traumatic brain injuries as, 106, 127, 308
Acetylcholine, as memory deficit treatment, 90, 91
Acquired immunodeficiency syndrome (AIDS) dementia complex, 164
Activities Assessment Algorithm, 222–235
  action plan organization assessment, 229–230
  attention assessment, 222–224
  complex mental action plans assessment, 231–233
  language deficits assessment, 225–226
  memory assessment, 233–234
  organizing complex instrumental action plans assessment, 230–231
  perceptual function assessment, 226–227
  praxis assessment, 227–229
  spatial attention assessment, 226–227
Activities of daily living (ADLs) impairments
  Activities Assessment Algorithm for, 222–235
    action plan organization assessment, 229–230
    attention assessment, 222–224
    complex mental action plans assessment, 231–232
    language deficits assessment, 225–226
    memory assessment, 233–234
    organizing complex instrumental action plans assessment, 230–231
    perceptual function assessment, 226–227
    praxis assessment, 227–229
    spatial attention assessment, 226–227
  embolic stroke–related, 216
  left parietal stroke–related, 216–217
  multiple sclerosis–related, 196, 197
Acupuncture, as multiple sclerosis therapy, 196
Adult respiratory distress syndrome, 131, 309

Affective disorders, traumatic brain injury–related, 311
Age, effect on course of recovery, 25, 26
Aggression
  amygdala in, 9
  anoxic-hypotensive brain injury–related, 154, 158, 167
  persistent, in outlier patients, 312
  traumatic brain injury–related, 124, 312, 320–324
Agitation
  anoxic-hypotensive brain injury–related, 150
  buspirone treatment of, 323
  propranolol treatment of, 321
  traumatic brain injury–related, 133–137
  Wernicke's aphasia–related, 68
Agnosia
  stroke-related, 221
  visual, 139–140, 226–227
Agraphia, 39
Alpha-blockers, as personality disorder treatment, 322
Alternative therapies, for multiple sclerosis, 196
Alzheimer's disease
  acetylcholine treatment for, 90
  dementia of, 41, 49–50, 55
  memory deficit treatment in, 90
Amantadine
  as aggressive disorder treatment, 321
  in multiple sclerosis, 200
Ambulation
  balance training for, 263
  evaluation of, 259, 277–278
  by multiple sclerosis patients, 195
  in neurologic syndromes, 44
  by stroke survivors, 33–34
γ-Aminobutyric acid, role in memory function, 91
Amitriptyline, as aggressive disorder treatment, 320
Amnesia, 60
  anoxic-hypotensive brain injury–related, 151, 152, 157–158, 167–168
  anterior communicating artery syndrome-related, 85–89

339